The Benzodiazepines Crisis

THE BENZODIAZEPINES CRISIS

The Ramifications of an Over-Used Drug Class

Edited by
Senior Editor
John F. Peppin, DO, FACP
Clinical Adjunct Professor
Marian University College of Osteopathic Medicine
Indianapolis, IN, USA

Editors
Joseph V. Pergolizzi Jr., MD
Chief Operating Officer
NEMA Research
Naples, FL, USA

Robert B. Raffa, PhD
Professor Emeritus and Past Chair
Temple University School of Pharmacy
Philadelphia, PA, USA
Adjunct Professor
University of Arizona College of Pharmacy
Tucson, AZ, USA
Chief Scientific Officer
Neumentum
Palo Alto, CA, USA

Steven L. Wright, MD, FAAFP, FASAM
Physician Consultant
Alliance for Benzodiazepine Best Practices
Littleton, CO, USA

OXFORD
UNIVERSITY PRESS

OXFORD
UNIVERSITY PRESS

Oxford University Press is a department of the University of Oxford. It furthers
the University's objective of excellence in research, scholarship, and education
by publishing worldwide. Oxford is a registered trade mark of Oxford University
Press in the UK and certain other countries.

Published in the United States of America by Oxford University Press
198 Madison Avenue, New York, NY 10016, United States of America.

Library of Congress Cataloging-in-Publication Data
Names: Peppin, John F., editor. | Pergolizzi, Joseph V., Jr., editor. |
Raffa, Robert B., editor. | Wright, Steven L., editor.
Title: The benzodiazepines crisis : the ramifications of an over-used drug class/
senior editor, John F. Peppin ; editors, Joseph V. Pergolizzi Jr.,
Robert B. Raffa, Steven L. Wright.
Description: New York, NY : Oxford University Press, [2021] |
Includes bibliographical references and index.
Identifiers: LCCN 2020025885 (print) | LCCN 2020025886 (ebook) |
ISBN 9780197517277 (paperback) | ISBN 9780197517291 (epub) |
ISBN 9780197517307 (online)
Subjects: MESH: Anti-Anxiety Agents | Benzodiazepines—adverse effects |
Substance Withdrawal Syndrome
Classification: LCC RM666.B42 (print) | LCC RM666.B42 (ebook) |
NLM QV 77.9 | DDC 615.7/882—dc23
LC record available at https://lccn.loc.gov/2020025885
LC ebook record available at https://lccn.loc.gov/2020025886

9 8 7 6 5 4 3 2 1

Printed by Marquis, Canada

To Professor C. Heather Ashton, DM FRCP (1929–2019)

It was all very well to say "Drink me," but the wise little Alice was not going to do that in a hurry. "No, I'll look first," she said, "and see whether it's marked 'poison' or not."

—Lewis Carroll, *Alice in Wonderland*

CONTENTS

OVERVIEW

- Benzodiazepines were developed to treat legitimate medical needs. However, unbridled success and prescribing beyond their intended duration of use and the available data have led to excessive prescribing, extended utilization beyond good therapeutic practice, and unintended adverse effects and substance use disorder.
- This book is the first to bring to light and discuss the largely unrecognized and enigmatic problem of an exceedingly prolonged withdrawal syndrome from benzodiazepines that can persist for months or years in susceptible patients, the medical need for better evidence-based prescribing of benzodiazepines, and a call for the recognition and better treatment of the prolonged withdrawal syndrome.
- Unfortunately, many of the negative aspects of benzodiazepines and their ineffective or unsafe use (e.g., to treat pain or concomitant use with opioids) are not widely known, but the potential extreme duration of the withdrawal syndrome is virtually unknown to most healthcare providers and to regulatory agencies.
- Most healthcare prescribers believe that benzodiazepines produce one and only one pharmacologic effect: positive allosteric modulation of $GABA_A$ receptors located in the brain. Unfortunately, the simplicity of this belief has distracted researchers, clinicians, and regulators from studying and appreciating the negative consequences of the prolonged use of these drugs—and even other aspects of their pharmacology. A glaring example is an almost universal lack of awareness of peripheral benzodiazepine receptors. The peripheral benzodiazepine receptors affect mitochondrial function (energy supply), cholesterol transport, and immune function.
- Therefore, there exists a significant and pressing medical and societal need for an updated overview of benzodiazepine physiology, pharmacology, side effects, and abuse potential, as well as clinical efficacy and application.
- All stakeholders involved in the use of benzodiazepines (e.g., psychiatrists, primary care physicians, pain physicians, substance use disorder health care practitioners, regulatory, legislative, hospice and palliative care healthcare providers, and patients) should benefit from the information contained in this book.

FOREWORD: ADDICTION

A. J. REID FINLAYSON, MD
Vanderbilt University Medical Center, Nashville, TN, USA

This book is a much-needed compilation and examination of the risks and benefits of the long-term use of benzodiazepine drugs. Named to elicit thoughts of equilibrium, peaceful valleys, rest, relaxation and halcyon days, benzodiazepine minor tranquilizers provide safer sedation than the barbiturates that were in general use 60 years ago. Although these drugs are approved for use in seizure disorders, generalized anxiety, and panic disorders, benzodiazepines are no longer considered first-line treatment. The benzodiazepine class of sedating drugs carries significant risks that involve depression, dependence, addiction, amnesia, and overdose death, especially when combined with other agents that affect the central nervous system. Benzodiazepines are useful in emergency settings and operating theaters and to avert the consequences of withdrawal from alcohol and sedating drugs.

The illicit use of benzodiazepines is quite common because the medications have been generally believed to be safe. Minor tranquilizers have also become popularized as a safe solution to many varieties of the unpleasant feelings of distress that often accompany growth-promoting change in life circumstance. Increasingly, chronic benzodiazepine use appears to be detrimental to patients with chronic psychiatric illnesses and substance use disorders. Once thought to be protective against suicidal impulses, benzodiazepines are more often associated with suicide and overdose deaths. Benzodiazepine abuse is common among persons who abuse other substances, particularly opioids. Also, reports of forged benzodiazepine tablets containing fentanyl confirm the strength of the illicit demand for these still widely prescribed and available controlled substances.

The debate about the advantages of prescribing benzodiazepines over psychologic treatment modalities (e.g., cognitive-behavioral therapy, acceptance commitment therapy, various psychotherapies) is ending for common emotional symptoms like insomnia and anxiety disorders. Additionally, there may be perverse logic in reserving chronic benzodiazepine prescribing for the severely mentally ill. Disagreement persists about the advantages of chronic benzodiazepine prescription for schizophrenia, bipolar illness, and complex posttraumatic stress disorder. These are populations in which relevant randomized controlled trials are rare and disagreement about benzodiazepine efficacy abounds. Allowing that debate to remain unresolved rationalizes support for chronic prescribing at the expense of extremely vulnerable patient populations.

There are similarities to consider and lessons to learn from the role of pharmaceutical industry promotion in the current opioid crisis. In America, managed care facilitates benzodiazepine prescribing by providing increased reimbursement of physicians for prescribing medication that exceeds psychotherapy reimbursement. Since attending a Swiss Upjohn conference on alprazolam (Xanax) in the early 1990s, I have witnessed first-hand how market forces actively influence medical practice by obfuscating negative results.

This book assembles the best evidence-based information to guide caring and support for patients who are continuing long-term benzodiazepine use and may wish to stop. Physicians should learn to apply this knowledge to avoid unintended consequences of legislative prescribing regulations similar to those that have occurred in the management of chronic pain.

FOREWORD: PAIN

LYNN WEBSTER, MD
Vice President Scientific Affairs, Neurosciences
PRA Health Sciences, Salt Lake City, UT, USA

How can it be that a book like this has not been previously published? It is surprising, considering the length of time benzodiazepines have been around and the problems associated with them.

Over the past 50 years, more than 2,000 different benzodiazepines have been developed, but only about 15 are currently approved by the Food and Drug Administration in the United States.

The current opioid crisis has overshadowed the contribution of benzodiazepines to our larger drug crisis. The title of a 2018 *New England Journal of Medicine* commentary by Lembke et al., "Our Other Prescription Drug Problem," shines a light on the benzodiazepine stealth crisis of the last half century—and the problem is not unique to America.

A study of six European countries (Belgium, France, Italy, Germany, the Netherlands, and Spain) found that anxiolytics, including benzodiazepines, were the most commonly used psychotropic drugs in these countries, with an overall prevalence of 9.8%.[1] In fact, a 2006 study showed that 12.5% of people 18 and older in France were prescribed benzodiazepines.[2] The common use of benzodiazepines has also been reported in Canada,[3] Australia,[3] Finland,[3] Thailand,[4] and Brazil.[4] Surprisingly to many, Japan has been reported to have the highest consumption rate of benzodiazepines in the world.[5]

Between 1996 and 2013, the quantity of benzodiazepines prescriptions filled by adults in the United States increased by 67%, from 8.1 million to 13.5 million.[6] A 2008 study showed that benzodiazepines were prescribed twice as often for women as for men.[7] This may be due to attitudes toward women in society more than an absolute increase in anxiety with females.

Benzodiazepines have been extraordinarily beneficial for millions of people with anxiety disorders. However, clinical problems occur wherever benzodiazepines have been prescribed, although they are less widely acknowledged than those caused by other drugs. The lack of attention paid to the risks of benzodiazepines increases their danger. That is why this book is so desperately needed, and so timely.

I cannot think of editors who are more highly qualified to tell the story we need to hear. They have assembled authors who cogently explain the reality of the use and abuse of benzodiazepines. The information provided in this book is obviously important for all clinicians, but it is also very instructive for a public that increasingly demands more facts about the medications prescribed to them.

This is not the first avant-garde academic publication by senior editor John F. Peppin. I first learned of his academic prowess through his international expertise in medical ethics. That is not the subject of this book, but it certainly contributes to the reason he has championed a book on this topic. He is an authority in many areas, with deep roots in clinical medicine and research. A palliative care physician and scholar, Peppin is a prolific author who has penned or edited some of the most-cited publications in the field of pain medicine on topical analgesics, opioid-induced constipation, urine drug testing, and opioid abuse.

Co-editors Joseph Pergolizzi and Robert Raffa are equally well known and prolific. Between them, they have written more than 500 peer-reviewed publications including books, chapters, and manuscripts. This diverse group of editors produces informative, science-based, and clinically meaningful content.

THE ROOT OF THE PROBLEM

It may be useful to briefly examine why benzodiazepines have been so commonly prescribed and abused. For better or worse, benzodiazepines have been the gold standard for pharmacologic treatment of anxiety, despite the growing problem of their abuse and misuse—and people appear to have more anxiety and stress now than at any time in our history.

At the turn of the twentieth century, approximately 60% of the American population lived in rural areas.[8] By 2018, only 18% of the population remained on farms.[9] Most people who lived in rural areas early in the twentieth century channeled their anxiety into physically demanding jobs, which mitigated their stress. Urban and suburban dwellers can go to the gym and eat the right foods, but that isn't enough. Sedentary lifestyles and crowded conditions in less rural communities have been associated with an increase in stress.[10]

There are numerous other factors that contribute to an individual's ability to cope with stress; for example, approximately 20% of veterans of recent wars experience posttraumatic stress disorder.[11] These factors and many more help to explain why benzodiazepines have become so widely prescribed.

THE CONSEQUENCES OF BENZODIAZEPINES

According to the National Institute on Drug Abuse, overdose deaths involving benzodiazepines rose between 1999 and 2017, from 1,135 to 11,537.[12] Despite this trend, the adverse effects of benzodiazepine overuse, misuse, and addiction continue to go largely unacknowledged. Three-quarters of deaths involving benzodiazepines also involve an opioid,[13] which may explain why, in the context of a widely recognized opioid problem, the dangers associated with benzodiazepines have been overlooked.

We only have to scan news stories about many high-profile deaths in recent years to see that benzodiazepines were often a major contributor. The presence of benzodiazepines apparently played a role in the deaths of Anna Nicole Smith, Heath Ledger, Amy Winehouse, Whitney Houston, and many others, despite uncertainty about the exact causes of their demise.

Death is only one potential consequence of benzodiazepine misuse; unfortunately, there are others. For example, benzodiazepines have also been used as "date rape" drugs. Bill Cosby was convicted of using Quaaludes, which are similar to benzodiazepines, to incapacitate his victims.

And not least on our list of concerns is the fact that benzodiazepines amplify the effects of opioids on respiratory depression. It wasn't until about 2004 when I (and I believe most other physicians) became aware that benzodiazepines could render lethal what would otherwise be a safe dose of an opioid.

A sleep specialist made me aware that chronic opioid therapy could cause an abnormal breathing pattern, which he described as "biots breathing,"[14] during sleep. This is an irregular (similar to the rhythm of atrial fibrillation) breathing pattern and a form of sleep-disordered breathing.

I was puzzled and didn't know what to believe, because the American Pain Society and the American Academy of Pain Medicine had published a statement in 1996 that stated, "Respiratory depression induced by opioids tends to be a short-lived phenomenon, generally occurs only in the opioid-naive patient, and is antagonized by pain. Therefore, withholding the appropriate use of opioids from a patient who is experiencing pain on the basis of respiratory concerns is unwarranted."[15]

This seemingly conflicting information led me to do a study. What I discovered was new to most of us in the field and very disturbing. Although the focus of the study was on opioids, the more profound observation was the contribution benzodiazepines had on creating life-threatening sleep-disordered breathing.[16]

In this study, combining a benzodiazepine with an opioid dramatically increased the risk of central sleep apnea. Usually, central sleep apnea is limited to people with neurologic disorders or advanced cardiac disease. These conditions were not generally present among my pain patients. Furthermore, there were no clinical signs to warn me that patients could have a life-threatening condition due to co-prescribing opioids with benzodiazepines.

It took a few years, but eventually, other scientific literature began to report similar findings. As a result, some professionals now suggest that benzodiazepines are contraindicated when opioids are prescribed. I believe that may be an overreach, for reasons Gary Reisfield explained in the 2013 publication, "Benzodiazepines in Long-Term Opioid Therapy."[17] However, in recent years, benzodiazepines have deservedly been prescribed with more caution to patients using opioids.

Today, more than ever, providers are expected to understand the risks of drugs that can be abused—while formal medical education has failed to provide that understanding. Patients, too, are asking for a more thorough understanding of the trade-offs and possible consequences involved in the use of these drugs.

In the quest to help ensure these valuable drugs are used as safely as possible, benzodiazepine prescribers and users alike will be well directed by this book.

REFERENCES

1. Ohayon, M. M., Lader, M. H. (2002). Use of psychotropic medication in the general population of France, Germany, Italy, and the United Kingdom. *Journal of Clinical Psychiatry, 63*, 817–825.
2. Rosman, S., Marc, L. V., Nathalie, P. -F. (2011). Gaining insight into benzodiazepine prescribing in general practice in France: A data-based study. *BMC Family Practice, 12*, 28. Retrieved from http://doi.org/10.1186/1471-2296-12-28.
3. Hartikainen, S., Rahkonen, T., Kautiainen, H., Sulkava, R. (2003). Kuopio 75+ study: Does advanced age predict more common use of psychotropics among the elderly? *International Clinical Psychopharmacology, 18*, 163–167.
4. Horta, B. L., de Lima, M. S., Faleiros, J. J., Weiderpass, E., Horta, R. L. (1994). Benzodiazepines: prescription study in a primary health care unit. *Revista da Associação Medica Brasileira, 40*, 262–264.
5. Uchida, H., Suzuki, T., Mamo, D. C., Mulsant, B. H., Kikuchi, T., Takeuchi, H., Tomita, M., Watanabe, K., Yagi, G. (2009). Benzodiazepine and antidepressant use in elderly patients with anxiety disorders: a survey of 796 outpatients in Japan. *Journal of Anxiety Disorders, 23*, 477–481.
6. Bachhuber, M. A., Hennessy, S., Cunningham, C. O., Starrels, J. L. (2016). Increasing benzodiazepine prescriptions and overdose mortality in the United States, 1996–2013. *American Journal of Public Health, 106*(4), 686–688. doi:10.2105/AJPH.2016.303061
7. Olfson, M., King, M., Schoenbaum, M. (2015). Benzodiazepine use in the United States. *JAMA Psychiatry, 72*(2), 136–142. doi:10.1001/jamapsychiatry.2014.1763
8. Hoyt,J.(2019,April29).1800–1990:Changesinurban/ruralU.S.population.*SeniorLiving.* Retrieved from https://www.seniorliving.org/history/1800-1990-changes-urbanrural-us-population/
9. World Bank. (n.d.). Rural population (% of total population). Retrieved from https://data.worldbank.org/indicator/sp.rur.totl.zs
10. Teychenne, M., Costigan, S. A., Parker, K. (2015). The association between sedentary behaviour and risk of anxiety: a systematic review. *BMC Public Health, 15*, 513. doi:10.1186/s12889-015-1843-x
11. Gradus, J. L. (2019). U.S. epidemiology of PTSD. *U.S. Department of Veteran Affairs.* Retrieved from https://www.ptsd.va.gov/professional/treat/essentials/epidemiology.asp
12. National Institute on Drug Abuse. (2019). Overdose death rates. Retrieved from https://www.drugabuse.gov/related-topics/trends-statistics/overdose-death-rates
13. Bachhuber, M. A. Hennessy, S., Cunningham, C. O., Starrels, J. L. (2016). Increasing benzodiazepine prescriptions and overdose mortality in the United States, 1996–2013. *American Journal of Public Health, 106*, 686–688.
14. Walker, J., Farney, R. J., Rhondeau, S. M., Boyle, K. M., Valentine, K., Cloward, T. V., Shilling, K. C. (2007). Chronic opioid use is a risk factor for the development of central sleep apnea and ataxic breathing. *Journal of Clinical Sleep Medicine, 3*(5), 455–461.
15. Approved by the American Academy of Pain Medicine Board of Directors on June 29, 1996. Approved by the American Pain Society Executive Committee on August 20, 1996.
16. Webster, L. R., Choi, Y., Desai, H., Webster, L., Grant, B. J. B. (2008). Sleep-disordered breathing and chronic opioid therapy. *Pain Medicine, 9*(4), 425–432. doi:10.1111/j.1526-4637.2007.00343.x
17. Reisfield, G. M., Webster, L. R. (2013). Benzodiazepines in long-term opioid therapy. *Pain Medicine, 14*(10), 1441–1446. doi:10.1111/pme.12236

FOREWORD: PATIENT ADVOCACY

BERNIE SILVERNAIL
President, Alliance for Benzodiazepine Best Practices
www.benzoreform.org

Our journey into the "dark side" of benzodiazepines began about nine years ago. After intermittent use of alprazolam for anxiety and misdiagnosed atrial fibrillation, my wife Carrie, an RN, through her own research discovered that the strange and confusing symptoms she was experiencing were actually due to benzodiazepine withdrawal syndrome (BZWS). Our subsequent journey through the medical system left us frustrated and confused. We consulted over a dozen prescribers, and none of them had heard of BZWS. But all were willing help with what they knew: prescribing other medications, often other benzodiazepines, to help with symptom management. We eventually located a benzo-wise naturopath, but by then Carrie was well into a self-administered plan for tapering off of her benzodiazepine prescriptions. We discovered that there are thousands of BZWS sufferers who have had similar experiences, who have found their way out of the dark via the twisty unreliable path of website-based support groups.

We were looking for a way to prevent this from happening to others when we attended the International Benzodiazepine Symposium in 2017 and met its founder Marjorie Merit-Carmen, who is also a BZWS sufferer. In addition, we met authors Steven L. Wright, MD, and Robert Raffa, PhD, and several other "benzo-wise" medical professionals and BZWS sufferers. This was the genesis of the Alliance for Benzodiazepine Best Practices, a nonprofit organization that is dedicated to providing evidence-based benzodiazepine and Z-drug (collectively benzodiazepine receptor agonists [BzRAs]) information to prescribers and patients. None of the funding for the Alliance comes from pharmaceutical companies, with the majority coming from "benzo survivors" and their loved ones. We have an admitted bias: the evidence shows that benzodiazepines and Z-drugs are usually harmful when used for more than two to four weeks, and we want this induced suffering to stop.

Why is a small nonprofit leading this charge toward evidence-based prescription? In the last 20 years the Food and Drug Administration and Drug Enforcement Administration have received over 300,000 BzRA complaints and noted over 65,000 deaths in the system they set up to protect the public (MedWatch), yet they have not investigated these drugs. There has been little grant money for academic research into these drugs for several years, and none of it focused on the withdrawal and recovery problem. There are hundreds of scientific papers and books and thousands of personal stories and videos on the Internet, all connecting BzRAs to protracted withdrawal and suicide. Yet prescriptions of these drugs continue to increase, a trend that the makers of BzRAs are motivated to maintain.

This is a David-and-Goliath story with a couple of dozen grassroots organizations and the evidence of harm on one side and over $3 billion of annual benzodiazepine and Z-drug sales and more lobbyists than members of the US Congress on the other. When prescribed and used correctly, these drugs can be lifesavers. When not, they can be life-destroyers. This book presents the case for both sides, not just the arguments but the research basis, controversies, and gaps in knowledge. BzRAs have been in use for over 70 years, yet you will see how much and how surprisingly little is known about them. Even such basic questions as "What is the endogenous ligand of the benzodiazepine receptor?" have no accepted answer. Like the 1990s' "new generation" of opioids, BzRAs are generally considered "safe and effective," yet there is a trail of suicides and destroyed lives in the wake of their use. Even worse than the opioids, this book presents the evidence that shows that BzRAs can produce long-lasting neural damage.

Carrie has slowly healed since she finished her taper four years ago, but she is far from fully recovered. Thousands of others have, usually without help from their prescriber, determined the source of their persistent and ever-shifting symptoms. They suffer along with her. But they are almost certainly the lucky minority who had the tenacity and background to figure this out on their own. The vast majority still suffer in the dark. Our hope is that this book can bring the light of understanding to their prescribers and, through them, relief to current sufferers and avoidance of the creation of new sufferers.

FOREWORD: PATIENT

CARRIE SILVERNAIL

The story in this foreword describes in some detail the suffering of an individual patient in her goal of removing benzodiazepines from her life. It reflects in very personal terms the significant downside of an overused drug class. The editors would thank Carrie for her willingness to share her story and her agreement to have her name published in this volume.

Carrie Silvernail is a registered nurse by training and profession, living in Oregon, where she raised her children and now enjoys her grandchildren. Her story begins with some frightening runs of rapid heart rate without apparent reason a number of years ago. As a nurse, she knew the name of her condition (tachycardia) and understood that it can be dangerous, even life-threatening in some cases. She went to a doctor who diagnosed her with generalized anxiety disorder. The doctor prescribed 0.25 mg of alprazolam (Xanax®), which she was to take only as needed. Carrie was the perfect patient; she knew a lot about the drug and knew that benzodiazepines could cause dependence. She also knew she might develop tolerance to the drug if she took it too often. She was very careful to take only a little of the drug and only when necessary. She embarked on a stress-reduction regimen that included stress management techniques, more exercise, mindfulness meditation, yoga, and other natural ways to restore her emotional equilibrium.

"I used it theee for years," Carrie reported. "Sparingly. Less than directed." The benzodiazepines did nothing to help her tachycardia, and she was later diagnosed with atrial fibrillation. She eventually underwent an ablation that cured the arrhythmia. Unfortunately, at this point Carrie had a new problem. She had developed pelvic pain that waxed and waned, migrated around the body, and was sometimes diffuse and sometimes very localized. The pelvic pain was "weird" because the symptoms came from out of nowhere. Carrie eventually had a multidisciplinary team of clinicians look into these symptoms. Her clinical team included a neurologist and a gynecologist, and she underwent multiple diagnostic tests, including a lumbar magnetic resonance imaging scan, a pelvic ultrasound, and several other tests. Although the test results all came back normal, for Carrie, nothing was normal anymore.

Her physician suggested that she start taking the alprazolam every day to manage the increasing pain, and she increased her dose to a scheduled 1.5 mg/day. Additionally she was prescribed gabapentin (an anticonvulsant and pain reliever) as well as a diazepam vaginal suppository all to manage the pain. Desperate to relieve her overwhelming symptoms, Carrie precisely followed the doctor's instructions. But she had barely embarked on this regimen when she began experiencing extreme sedation. In response, she cut the doses of her medications by as much as half, and her function improved. For a very short span of time, she started to sleep well.

Then the unthinkable happened. For the first time in her life, Carrie experienced the dark despair of profound depression that was accompanied by suicidal thoughts. Her suicidality was so disabling that she had to quit her job. Her husband became her caretaker as she tried to navigate her way out of the darkness of depression. Whenever she had the energy and could manage it, she went online and started to research her symptoms. She had serious debilitating mental symptoms along with very painful physical symptoms. The pelvic pain that caused her to see a team of specialists had now spread to all parts of her body. There was not any part of her body or mind that did not seem to be caught up in her condition. "Then I found the Ashton Manual," Carrie reported as she started on her efforts to research the condition by herself. The Ashton Manual changed the trajectory of her disease. Written in 2002 by Professor Heather Ashton of the Institute of Neuroscience at Newcastle University in the United Kingdom, the little book explained how benzodiazepines worked and how to discontinue them and navigate withdrawal symptoms. The Ashton Manual also provided some very blunt information about just what benzodiazepines could do—the manual lists 90 symptoms or adverse effects of benzodiazepine use, which include everything from hallucinations to sensory hypersensitivity, memory deficits, and digestive disorders. The Ashton Manual told her that benzodiazepines can cause depression and suicidal thoughts. Carrie had a host of symptoms and had never categorized them as all being related to the benzodiazepines. Among her many symptoms related to benzodiazepines were myalgia; neuralgia; anorexia; problems with urination; hypersensitivity to sound, touch, and light; and visual disturbances, in addition to the other symptoms mentioned. "In 2012, I learned that I was benzodiazepine dependent," Carrie reported. "And I joined the ranks of the other 'accidental dependents.'" "Accidental dependent," the term she uses for her condition, is quite apt. Carrie had never had any intention of abusing benzodiazepines when she embarked on benzodiazepine use to treat a specific medical condition. She took the drugs carefully and only as prescribed by her physician. She tried hard to take as little as possible, but her physician told her, "I can't help you if you don't take all of the medications I prescribe for you." She thought she had understood the risks of tolerance and dependence, but it turned out she had underestimated the dependent nature of benzodiazepines and their multiple long-term effects. Carrie set up a new multidisciplinary team, this time with naturopaths, a massage therapist, a pharmacist, and an acupuncturist. She needed a primary care physician, and she visited a physician recommended to her by her growing new network of accidental dependent friends. The first time she told her story to the new doctor, he looked at her and replied, "I believe you. How can I support you on your journey?" His words encouraged Carrie more than what any other medical professional had before. "No one on my new team was an expert, but they were all curious and committed to helping me," Carrie related. In truth, there are few real experts in benzodiazepine tapering, withdrawal, dependency, and addiction. But Carrie had to work with the people who supported her, even if few of them were sure exactly what to do. Carrie and her team formulated a plan to slowly taper off benzodiazepines in a series of very tiny, gradual, decremental steps. She kept meticulous records of her symptoms and when symptoms increased, she slowed the taper. When symptoms stabilized, she decreased the dose a little more. The process was very slow, taking 38 months to discontinue benzodiazepines completely.

"During the taper, I never felt well," Carrie admitted, "but at times I felt less sick." When she was completely free of benzodiazepines, she found her symptoms persisted, but they were less severe and less frequent. Carrie spoke at a recent symposium about benzodiazepine use. "I've been off benzodiazepines for four years and two months," she said describing her current status, "and I'm not well, but I am better."

During Carrie's many years of suffering, even lapsing into disability, her husband cared for her, supported her, and encouraged her. Today, it is their work to promote projects like this book and other efforts to warn physicians, clinicians, and other prescribers and their patients about the risks of benzodiazepine therapy.

Carrie Silvernail's story is a patient voyage through the effects of benzodiazepines and their tapering. However, medical research needs to know the exact mechanisms of action of these side effects. More research is urgently needed, and we need to translate this research into clinical practice. We need practical, evidence-based answers to help us prevent patients like Carrie going through the difficult periods of benzodiazepine use and tapering she had to endure.

PREFACE

In September 2017, a remarkable symposium, The International Benzodiazepine Symposium, was held in Bend, Oregon and extended over three days. There were 19 invited speakers with an audience of 75. The conference was remarkable and, for many of us, life-changing. It was organized, financed, and run, not by physicians, researchers, or pharmaceutical companies, but by patients, their loved ones, and their supporters, which made it remarkable and would not have occurred without them. It was life-changing for us, each one a seasoned clinician, researcher, and educator of benzodiazepine/Z-drug receptor pharmacology and prescribing, because it revealed to us a little-known, neglected, and commonly discounted, disregarded, or even belittled aspect of either taking or discontinuing benzodiazepine medications. The scientific purpose of the symposium was achieved. Its intent was to elevate the concerns regarding the negative aspects of benzodiazepines, which have been known for many years, but have been largely ignored, perhaps forgotten. The speakers addressed a number of relevant issues, such as anxiety, anxiety disorders, posttraumatic stress disorder, benzodiazepine indications, contraindications, benzodiazepines and pain, nonpharmacologic approaches to anxiety states, benzodiazepine adverse outcomes, physical dependence, withdrawal, discontinuation, and much more. A much broader and perhaps more important purpose was to provide a safe environment in which to stimulate participation in cross-specialty and patient–provider interactions by being involved in ongoing discussions throughout the conference and to conclude with action steps so that what we learned did not stall as it has in the past.

At the outset, many of the professional medical speakers were, quite frankly, skeptical. Who were these individuals? What are these difficult-to-characterize (let alone explain) symptoms that seemed to have clear pharmacologic explanations. Maybe there were other, nonphysiologic explanations for their symptoms. But the more we listened, and the more we restudied the literature, we were shocked to learn that the data existed, and have been known for years. Further, there was now new basic science evidence supporting much of what the patients and attendees said they were experiencing.

Of the four editors of this volume, all have struggled with the issues surrounding benzodiazepine prescribing and use in internal medicine, family practice, pain medicine, addiction medicine, and psychiatry and in research. Benzodiazepine use is so prevalent, and the issues of tapering these medications from a patients' pharmacologic regimen present unique and serious challenges. So many of us had a long-standing foundation of distrust of this class of medications and a desire to remove them, especially from those patient on opioids and other central nervous system depressants. Anecdotally and early on, we found that removing these medications seemed to improve patients; however, the scientific basis for this improvement was not clear. This volume brings together years of research, investigation, clinical experience, and other information into one single volume. It describes our anecdotal and empirical experience and puts it into context with the scientific literature. Benzodiazepines have their place; however, they are clearly overused, and their side effects much more serious than previously perceived. This is the first time that many of our topics are discussed under one title, especially the issues of peripheral benzodiazepine receptors. Therefore we are proud to provide a new and unusual volume that discusses the downside of an overused drug class.

John F. Peppin, DO, FACP
Indianapolis, IN, USA

Joseph V. Pergolizzi Jr., MD
Naples, FL, USA

Robert B. Raffa, PhD
Tucson, AZ, USA

Steven L. Wright, MD, FAAFP, FASAM
Littleton, CO, USA

CONTRIBUTORS

Timothy J. Atkinson, PharmD, BCPS, CPE
Clinical Pharmacy Specialist, Pain
  Management
Veterans Affairs Tennessee Valley
  Healthcare System
Murfreesboro, TN, USA

John J. Coleman, PhD
Assistant Administrator for Operations
  (Ret.) at the U.S. Drug Enforcement
  Administration (DEA)
President, DrugWatch International, Inc.,
  a nonprofit drug-abuse prevention and
  education organization
Washington, DC, USA

Jeffrey Guina, MD, FAPA
Chief Medical Officer
Easterseals Michigan
Psychiatry Residency Program Director
Beaumont Health
Clinical Associate Professor
Wright State University and Michigan
  State University
Pontiac, MI, USA

Jamie L. Hansen, PhD
Clinical Associate Professor of Nursing
Carroll University
Waukesha, WI, USA

Jan M. Kitzen, BS, RPh, PhD
Pharmacist
Kitzen Pharmaceutical Consulting
Collegeville, PA, USA
Emeritus Adjunct Associate Professor of
  Pharmacology
Temple University School of Medicine
Philadelphia, PA, USA

George F. Koob, PhD
Director
National Institute of Alcohol Abuse and
  Alcoholism (NIAAA)
Professor on Leave
Scripps Research Institute
La Jolla, CA, USA

Jo Ann LeQuang, BA
President
LeQ Medical Communications
Angleton, TX, USA
Director of Scientific Communications
NEMA Research
Naples, FL, USA

Brian Merrill, MD, MBA
Assistant Professor
Director of Community Psychiatry
Department of Psychiatry
Wright State University
Dayton, OH, USA

Michael M. Miller, MD, FASAM, FAPA
Director
American Board of Addiction Medicine,
    and American College of Academic
    Addiction Medicine
Madison, WI, USA

Michael H. Ossipov, PhD
Research Professor Emeritus
University of Arizona College of
    Medicine
Tucson, AZ, USA

John F. Peppin, DO, FACP
Clinical Adjunct Professor
Marian University College of Osteopathic
    Medicine
Indianapolis, IN, USA

Joseph V. Pergolizzi Jr, MD
Chief Operating Officer
NEMA Research
Naples, FL, USA

Robert B. Raffa, PhD
Professor Emeritus and Past Chair
Temple University School of Pharmacy
Philadelphia, PA, USA
Adjunct Professor
University of Arizona College of
    Pharmacy
Tucson, AZ, USA
Chief Scientific Officer
Neumentum
Palo Alto, CA, USA

Steven L. Wright, MD, FAAFP, FASAM
Physician Consultant
Alliance for Benzodiazepine Best
    Practices
Littleton, CO, USA

BENZODIAZEPINES: A CHRONOLOGY

ca 460 BCE to ca 370 CE   Hippocrates
The Hippocratic Corpus (uncertain authorship) described "Nicanor's Affection" about a man in fear of the flute girl a drinking party.

106 BCE to 43 BCE   Cicero
Defined anxiety (*angor*) as a disorder (*aegritudo*) and a medical illness (*aegritudo*) in the Tusculan Disputations Book III, X.

1665–1750
The terms "vapors" and "melancholia" (*affection vaporeuse et mélancolique*) were used to describe nervous conditions.

1706–1767
Boissier de Sauvages published the first significant French medical nosology—the last major medical text written in Latin. He classified mental disorders (*vesaniae*) in four categories:
- Hallucinations, including hypochondriasis;
- Morositates, panophobia (terror at night without obvious cause), hydrophobia;
- Deliria; and
- Folies anomales, including agrypnia (i.e., insomnia).

1864
Barbituric acid first synthesized by Adolf von Baeyer; >2,500 structurally similar compounds have been synthesized.

1903
German scientists working at Bayer found that barbital put dogs to sleep; Marketed as Veronal.

1909
Emil Kraepelin described anxiety *(Angst)* as the most frequent abnormal affect.

1952
First edition of *Diagnostic and Statistical Manual of Mental Disorders* (DSM) published: psychoneurotic disorders—equivalent to anxiety.

1953
Miltown (meprobamate) first marketed as anxiolytic safer than the barbiturates.

1955 or 1957 (date uncertain)
Leo Sternbach discovered chlordiazepoxide (Ro 5-0690).

1958
Chlordiazepoxide patented; gamma-aminobutyric acid found to be inhibitory in mammalian central nervous system.

1960
Chlordiazepoxide (Librium) is introduced to the market.

1961
Major withdrawal reactions to chlordiazepoxide reported by Leo Holister.

1962
Rohypnol (flunitrazepam—"date-rape drug") was patented (available in 1974).

1968
Anxiety deemed the primary feature of the category "Neuroses."

1968–1981
Diazepam is the most widely prescribed drug of any kind in the Western market.

1975
Benzodiazepine class are placed in Schedule IV, where they remain.

1977
Peripheral binding of benzodiazepines is discovered.

1979
Kennedy hearings take place in the US Congress—no action was taken.

1980
Third edition of the DSM is published: Anxiety disorders categorized and criteria defined. Posttraumatic stress disorder and obsessive-compulsive disorder were included among the anxiety disorders.

1981
Alprazolam is introduced into the US market.

1983
Malcolm Lader published the first review on therapeutic uses and adverse reactions.

Late 1980s
First patient-support organizations established in the United Kingdom: Council for Involuntary Tranquilliser Addiction, Battle Against Tranquillisers, TRANX.

1991
Beers list first published indicating particular risk of benzodiazepines in elderly; Zolpidem introduced into the market.

1992

Peripheral benzodiazepine receptor (translocator protein) is isolated.

1999

Ashton Manual is published (revised in 2002; supplement in 2011); First online patient-support community was established: Benzodiazepine Withdrawal Support http://www.benzosupport.org/

2013

Fifth edition of the DSM regrouped disorders that included anxiety features into

Anxiety disorders

Trauma- and stressor-related disorders (e.g., posttraumatic stress disorder)

Obsessive-compulsive and related disorders (e.g., obsessive-compulsive disorder)

CHAPTER 1

Introduction

The Origins and Rise of Benzodiazepines

MICHAEL M. MILLER AND JOHN F. PEPPIN

The history of benzodiazepines begins with the preceding drug class, barbiturates.[1] Barbiturates first came to market for the pharmacological treatment of neuropsychiatric disorders that, at that time, had few treatment options. While they were effective for calming agitation in patients ranging from the mildly anxious to the seriously mentally ill, they were also associated with potentially fatal overdoses, respiratory depression, and impairments in cognition and motor skills, and their addiction potential was also recognized.[2] Pharmaceutical firms tried to discover newer molecules that would have the therapeutic benefits of barbiturates without some of the risks; this class of drugs were called nonbarbiturate sedative-hypnotics.

Meprobamate was the first nonbarbiturate sedative-hypnotic cleared for U.S. market release in 1955. Although it was originally developed as a muscle relaxant, the drug was found to have efficacy in other disease states, specifically anxiety.[3,4] Not having as narrow of a therapeutic window as the barbiturate class, it was widely prescribed. The brand name Miltown® became familiar and popular. However, the potential for addiction and the risk for oversedation and overdose were soon noticed.[5]

The medical community and many patients were hopeful that there would be newer medications available to treat anxiety and depression without the adverse effects and toxicities of barbiturates and the broad class of nonbarbiturate sedative-hypnotics. It was in this context that a new drug, and a new class of drugs, emerged: chlordiazepoxide, in the new drug class called benzodiazepines.[6] Since the introduction of chlordiazepoxide (brand name Librium®) in 1955 and diazepam (brand name Valium®) in 1963, benzodiazepines have been, and remain, among the most-prescribed drugs around the world.[7] These two new drugs were improvements over previously available therapeutic alternatives and achieved rapid utility in the medical community. Diazepam was actually developed from demoxepam, a metabolite of chlordiazepoxide; compared to the parent drug, it has higher potency and a shorter duration of action.[8] As these drugs were studied further and used more in naturalistic settings, it was discovered that they offered beneficial therapeutic effects as hypnotics, amnestics, and muscle relaxants. Purdue Pharma, known decades later as the manufacturer of another blockbuster drug, OxyContin®, was an early marketer of Valium, which quickly became the premiere drug in this emerging new class.[9] Lorazepam entered the U.S. market in 1977 under the brand name Ativan® with pharmacokinetic attributes which make is more advantageous to use in many populations than Valium® or Librium®; it is still listed on the World Health Organization's list of Essential Medicines.[10] With brisk sales of benzodiazepines in most Western nations, Upjohn Pharmaceuticals developed its entry, alprazolam (Xanax®), first sold in the United States in 1981.[11,12] For the next decade, benzodiazepines prescriptions were intensely marketed to the point they became among the most frequently prescribed drugs around the world, being consumed on a regular basis by 10% to 20% of adults in Western nations.[12,13] New benzodiazepines were being added to the marketplace at a brisk pace, offering less sedation and fewer adverse liver effects than barbiturates. In 2015, 35 benzodiazepines or benzodiazepine derivatives were commercially available for prescription in the United States, 21 of which were sold internationally.[14]

Benzodiazepines can lead to substance use disorder (SUD; as described in the fifth edition of the *Diagnostic and Statistical Manual of Mental Disorders*), particularly when prescribed to a person at elevated risk. SUD is evidenced by obsessive preoccupation with the drug, intense drug cravings, dosage escalation over time, impaired individual control over the dose taken, and a devotion of significant amounts of time to procuring the drug to the detriment of other more productive or socially beneficial activities.[15] (Note that not all of these features must be present in every individual for a diagnosis of SUD to be made, but these are among the diagnostic criteria for this disorder in the DSM-5, the most widely accepted diagnostic manual in the United States.) Regular use of benzodiazepines is associated with physiological dependence.[7] People taking benzodiazepines over the long term develop drug tolerance, a neuroadaptation that results in the need for increasing amounts of the drug to achieve the same result.[16] As with other substances that can result in physical dependence (yet another feature of SUD), the abrupt discontinuation or dose reduction of benzodiazepines can provoke withdrawal symptoms. In fact, it is tolerance (with escalating doses) and withdrawal symptoms that are frequently noticed by patients, more so that the cognitive behavioral components of SUD such as preoccupation and impairment of control over use. From a physiological and psychological viewpoint, sedative withdrawal symptoms are a powerful, albeit negative, reinforcement and create a vicious circle where users want to relieve their dysphoric state through the temporary relief gained by taking more of the very drug that is its cause.

In the United States, the Drug Enforcement Agency, through the statutory authority of the Controlled Substances Act, included benzodiazepines in its original list of controlled substances as Schedule IV substances, defined as follows: "abuse of the drug or other substance may lead to limited physical dependence or psychological dependence relative to the drugs or other substances in Schedule III."[17] The World Health

Organization stated that benzodiazepines were capable of creating dependence and benzodiazepines could cause depression of the central nervous system leading to disruption in motor function, behavior, and personality.[18] Although still prescribed in fairly high numbers in the United Kingdom, benzodiazepines are becoming less popular in that region.[19] Increasingly, in the United States, controls are being placed on the prescribing of benzodiazepines, such as through triplicate prescription laws[20] and the development of prescription drug monitoring programs; although these are state-by-state requirements, most states require monitoring of benzodiazepines.[21,22]

Benzodiazepines are effective at what they were designed to do: for reduction of anxiety in the short term, for sleep induction in the short term, and for helping patients better manage uncomfortable emotions and stress overall. Benzodiazepines have efficacy for certain nonpsychiatric conditions (e.g., acute treatment of seizure activity[23]) and in management of alcohol withdrawal.[24] However, benzodiazepines are double-edged swords, which offer benefits when used in carefully controlled circumstances but which are accompanied by risks when used inappropriately. Benzodiazepines reliably induce sleep but do so safely only for a couple of weeks. After about two weeks, they induce rebound insomnia, which traps the clinician and patient in an endless cycle.[25,26] A similar situation can occur with rebound anxiety.[27]

Rapid onset of action is one reason that benzodiazepines remain so popular. Patients suffering anxiety and depression often feel like they need help fast. However, benzodiazepines should only be used for a short time and in the carefully selected patient. They should not be taken continuously for more than two to four weeks, and for some patients, it is not unreasonable to prescribe them for only two or three days.[28,29] To treat long-term or chronic conditions, the prescriber should use other medication classes (e.g., SSRIs or SNRIs). While it may be possible that a patient may require prescribed benzodiazepines on a repeated basis—say, every several months—or in a future year, the role of a benzodiazepine should still be restricted to short-term therapy only whenever they are prescribed or represcribed to an individual, unless the reason for the prescription is a neurological or musculoskeletal condition rather than a psychiatric one.

The next set of novel agents introduced as sedative-hypnotics were the Z-drugs, with the first in this category, zolpidem (Ambien®) brought to market in 1992.[30] Zolpidem had many of the attributes of benzodiazepines but was technically not a benzodiazepine in its chemical structure. For prescribers eager to find a safer, better alternative to traditional benzodiazepines, the messaging surrounding this new product found resonance. Since zolpidem were considered "not a benzodiazepine," it was hoped that it might avoid the benzodiazepine risks of tolerance, physical dependence, addiction, and withdrawal. The problem with Z-drugs is that the receptors involved in their biological actions are the same receptors that benzodiazepines use.[31] As far as the brain is concerned, Z-drugs and benzodiazepines work the same way. Nowadays, knowledgeable clinicians and scientists recognize that Z-drugs are better described as benzodiazepine receptor agonists that activate benzodiazepine receptors exactly the same way that true benzodiazepines do. Thus, the risks associated with benzodiazepine use apply to the Z-drugs as well.

There is much that this book has to say about the risks of benzodiazepines and Z-drugs. But when are these drugs ever useful? Are they ever appropriate? The fact is that benzodiazepines and Z-drugs are effective and can be very helpful to patients when prescribed for short-term, carefully defined use under close clinical supervision. Benzodiazepines are also very important therapeutic options in the management of alcohol and other sedative withdrawal syndromes and in the management of some non-psychiatric conditions. Meanwhile, researchers may continue to search for the next-generation sedative-hypnotic agent or drug class, one that is not associated with risks of rebound insomnia, rebound anxiety, physiological dependence, withdrawal symptoms, misuse, and addiction. However, currently there are millions of people around the world who are struggling with benzodiazepine use because they find themselves stuck in a pattern of misuse, dependence and addiction. It is our sincere hope that this book presents the medical science as well as the personal encouragement for a better future for these and future individuals.

Not all physicians are fully appreciative of the dangers of benzodiazepines and even those who understand them may not be equipped to help navigate a patient through safe tapering and discontinuation. Unfortunately, physicians receive much more training on selection of agent and initiation of an agent than on safe dosage reduction and discontinuation of an agent with the potential for physical dependence, like sedative-hypnotics and opioids. It may be appropriate to refer long-term benzodiazepine-using patients to specialists in addiction medicine or addiction psychiatry for safe drug discontinuation or tapering. However, the number of general practice physicians prescribing these agents, even long term, far exceeds the other number of board certified addiction specialist physicians and psychiatrists. Thus, expecting others to manage this phase of a patient's care is unrealistic—the original prescribers need to develop the skills themselves in safe drug discontinuation and not think it is only within the scope of practice of a specialized consultant to do so. It should be encouraging that with our growing understanding of these drugs and our expanding knowledge of anxiety and sleep disorders, there is better understanding of how to avoid the long-term use of benzodiazepines for psychiatric conditions.

REFERENCES

1. Wick J. The history of benzodiazepines. Consult Pharm. 2013;28(9):538–548.
2. Norn S, Permin H, Kruse E, Kruse PR. [On the history of barbiturates]. Dan Medicinhist Arbog. 2015;43:133–151.
3. Harden RN, Argoff C. A review of three commonly prescribed skeletal muscle relaxants. J Back Musculoskeletal Rehabit. 2000;15(2–3):63–66.
4. Tone A. Listening to the past: history, psychiatry, and anxiety. Can J Psychiatry. 2005;50(7):373–380.
5. Mohr RC, Mead BT. Meprobamate addiction. N Engl J Med. 1958;259(18):865–868.
6. Lopez-Munoz F, Alamo C, Garcia-Garcia P. The discovery of chlordiazepoxide and the clinical introduction of benzodiazepines: half a century of anxiolytic drugs. J Anxiety Disord. 2011;25(4):554–562.
7. Agarwal SD, Landon BE. Patterns in outpatient benzodiazepine prescribing in the United States. JAMA Network Open. 2019;2(1):e187399.

8. Stronjny N, Bratin K, Brooks MA, de Silva JA. Determination of chlordiazepoxide, diaz-epam, and their major metabolites in blood or plasma by spectrophotodensitometry. J Chromatogr. 1977;143(4):363–374.

9. Cooper A. An anxious history of valium: what a drag it is getting old—or is it? Valium's heyday is long past, but it lives on as a cultural icon. WSJ. November 15, 2013.

10. World Health Organization. World Health Organization model list of essential medicines: 21st list 2019. Geneva: World Health Organization; 2019. hdl:10665/325771. WHO/MVP/EMP/IAU/2019.06. License: CC BY-NC-SA 3.0 IGO

11. Ait-Daoud N, Hamby AS, Sharma S, Blevins D. A review of alprazolam use, misuse, and withdrawal. J Addict Med. 2018;12(1):4–10. doi:10.1097/ADM.0000000000000350

12. Herper M. America's most popular mind medicines. Forbes. https://www.forbes.com/2010/09/16/prozac-xanax-valium-business-healthcare-psychiatric-drugs.html#4036a3782e05. Published September 7, 2010. Accessed October 13, 2019.

13. Ashton H. The diagnosis and management of benzodiazepine dependence. Curr Opin Psychiatry. 2005;18(3):249–255.

14. Soyka M. Medikamentenabhängigkeit. Stuttgart, Germany: Schattauer, 2015.

15. Hasin DS, O'Brien CP, Auriacombe M, et al. DSM-5 criteria for substance use disorders: recommendations and rationale. Am J Psychiatry. 2013;170(8):834–851.

16. Soyka M. Treatment of benzodiazepine dependence. NEJM. 2017;376(12):1147–1157.

17. Drug Enforcement Agency. Benzodizepines. https://www.deadiversion.usdoj.gov/drug_chem_info/benzo.pdf. Published 2019. Accessed September 30, 2019.

18. World Health Organization. Use and abuse of benzodiazepines. Bull World Health Org. 1983;61(4):551–562.

19. Mehdi T. Benzodiazepines revisited. BMJ. 2012;5(1):a501.

20. Miller MM, Brown RT. Prescription Drug Monitoring Programs. Am Fam Physician. 2007;75:810–811.

21. Worley J. Prescription drug monitoring programs, a response to doctor shopping: purpose, effectiveness, and directions for future research. Issues Ment Health N. 2012;33(5):319–328.

22. Bachhuber MA, Maughan BC, Mitra N, Feingold J, Starrels JL. Prescription monitoring programs and emergency department visits involving benzodiazepine misuse: early evidence from 11 United States metropolitan areas. Int J Drug Policy. 2016;28:120–123.

23. Betjemann JP, Lowenstein DH. Status epilepticus in adults. Lancet Neurol. 2015;14(6):615–624.

24. Wartenberg A. Management of Alcohol Intoxication and Withdrawal. In: Ries RK, Fiellin DA, Miller SC, Saitz R, eds. The ASAM Principles of Addiction Medicine (5th ed.). Lippincott Williams & Wilkins; 2014:635–651.

25. Kales A, Soldatos CR, Bixler EO, Kales JD. Rebound insomnia and rebound anxiety: a review. Pharmacology. 1983;26(3):121–137.

26. Sachdeva A, Choudhary M, Chandra M. Alcohol withdrawal syndrome: benzodiazepines and beyond. J Clin Diagn Res. 2015;9(9):VE01.

27. Kales A, Soldatos CR, Bixler EO, Kales JD. Rebound insomnia and rebound anxiety: a review. Pharmacology. 1983;26(3):121–137.

28. Bandelow B, Michaelis S, Wedekind D. Treatment of anxiety disorders. Dialogues Clin Neurosci. 2017;19(2):93–107.

29. Wilt TJ, MacDonald R, Brasure M, et al. Pharmacologic treatment of insomnia disorder: an evidence report for a clinical practice guideline by the American College of Physicians. Ann Intern Med. 2016;165(2):103–112.

30. Zolpidem tartrate. American Society of Health-System Pharmacists. https://www.drugs.com/monograph/zolpidem-tartrate.html. Accessed October 13, 2019.

31. Gunja N. The clinical and forensic toxicology of Z-drugs. J Med Toxicol. 2013;9(2):155–162. doi:10.1007/s13181-013-0292-0

CHAPTER 2

The Evolution of Benzodiazepine Receptor Agonists

Developments in Pharmacology and Toxicology

JAMIE L. HANSEN AND TIMOTHY J. ATKINSON

HIGHLIGHTS

- γ-aminobutyric acid (GABA) receptor variability is diverse yielding a wide array of clinical implications that are affected by a multitude of potential ligands including benzodiazepines.
- Benzodiazepine's primary effect is enhancement of the intrinsic response to endogenous GABA rather than increasing synthesis of GABA itself.
- Each benzodiazepine has a unique pharmacokinetic and pharmacodynamic profile, which contributes to variations in each individual agents' potency, half-life, and metabolism.
- Urine drug screens (UDS) are a valuable tool for monitoring potential misuse or diversion of benzodiazepines and require careful evaluation for proper interpretation.
- Z-drugs are a newer class of nonbenzodiazepine hypnotic agents that promote sleep by centrally enhancing GABA activity within the brain. Each possesses distinct differences in their mechanisms of action and receptor selectivity that appears to determine the differences in the agents' pharmacological profiles.

ORIGIN

Discovery of the benzodiazepine is credited to Austrian chemist Leo Sternbach.[1] While working for Hoffmann-La Roche labs in 1955, he identified the compound chlordiazepoxide which would go on to be marketed as Librium.[1] The benzheptoxdiazine derivative was a product of his earlier research as a student during which time he was attempting to discover new azo intermediates for the creation of usable dyes.[2] Sternbach's research was sparked by Roche's interest in developing a rival drug to meprobamate (Miltown), which had been introduced in 1953 and was marketed as being a safer anxiolytic option than barbiturates.[2] Prior to benzodiazepines, barbiturates were the primary anxiolytic drug class and their use can be traced back to as early as 1864 with the development of their parent drug of malonylurea by German chemist, Adolph von Baeyer.[3] Although barbiturates were rapidly viewed as miracle drugs for the treatment of neuroses, psychosis, insomnia, and epilepsy, shortly after their emergence in the clinical setting their potential to result in dependence was rapidly characterized in medical literature.[3] In addition to dependence, barbiturates have a narrow therapeutic index resulting in a significant convergence between the desired therapeutic and toxic dose-response curves.[4] At approximately three times the therapeutic dose, barbiturates virtually eliminate central nervous system (CNS)-mediated respiratory drive and at 10 times the therapeutic dose there is a potential for fatal overdose due to respiratory or cardiovascular depression.[4] The introduction of the benzodiazepine offered promises for improved safety due to fewer drug interactions, lower abuse potential, and decreased respiratory depression.

MECHANISM OF ACTION

While it is now widely recognized that GABA is the primary inhibitory neurotransmitter within the human CNS, this was not fully accepted until roughly 50 years ago, well after the development of benzodiazepines. In 1967, Krnjevic and Schwartz performed studies on cerebral cortical neurons that provided categorical evidence that solidified the role of GABA as an inhibitory transmitter.[5] GABA is found in high concentrations in the limbic system, particularly within the cerebral cortex where it's inhibitory action results in decreased neuron excitability, which produces a calming effect on the brain.[6] GABA is known to exert its effects on three receptors; $GABA_A$ and $GABA_C$, which are ionotropic in nature, and metabotropic $GABA_B$, which is a G protein-coupled receptor. The $GABA_A$ receptor has been the primary target for anxiolytics old and new including barbiturates, anticonvulsants, and the newer Z-drugs. The transmembrane $GABA_A$ receptor consists of five glycoprotein subunits that surround a centrally located chloride ion channel.[6] A common misconception is that benzodiazepines increase GABA synthesis when they actually work by enhancing your body's natural response to existing supplies of endogenous GABA.[7] Benzodiazepines bind at the juncture where the α and γ subunits meet, causing a conformational change in the GABA binding site on the central chloride channel causing an increase in the affinity for GABA. When GABA binds and activates the receptor, it causes an increase in the frequency of channel opening and chloride influx causing augmented hyperpolarization and a more profound decrease in cellular excitability.[8]

GABA$_A$ RECEPTOR DIVERSITY

Early hypotheses proposed the GABA$_A$ complex was composed of only α and β subunits, but evolving biochemical studies have postulated a more detailed chemical structure that yields a pentameric model containing two α subunits, two β subunits, and one γ subunit. Our current understanding is that multiple isoforms exist with identification of up to six α, four β, three γ, and one δ distinct subunit.[9,10] This heterogeneity among subunits yields hundreds of diverse receptor possibilities based on the multitude of genetic polymorphisms. The modern classification of GABA$_A$ receptors includes five predominant types based on the more commonly observed receptor compositions (Table 2.1).

Among the subunits, it is not surprising that the effects of α isomers are considered integral and are the best characterized among the subunits as they relate to the core benzodiazepine activity (Table 2.2). Notably, GABA$_A$ receptors containing α4 and α6 subunit isoforms are insensitive to benzodiazepines due to an arginine residue at this critical position.[11] Additionally, α6 is the most restricted and suspected to play a role in tolerance.[9] The problem with the oversimplification of effects based on solely the α subunit is that it cannot provide an explanation for the combined effects based on the presence of two α subunits that make up each receptor complex, nor does it address the multiple arrangements that can occur and likewise affect the resulting functional properties. It is because of these complexities, joined by genetic variations and uncharacterized effects of the other subunits and isoforms, that it becomes nearly impossible to fully pinpoint and describe how each component of the receptor complex exactly contributes to larger pharmacologic effects we see demonstrated by benzodiazepines.

Table 2.1 COMMON GABA$_A$ RECEPTOR COMBINATIONS

Type I: alpha1, beta2, gamma2
Type II: alpha2 or alpha3, beta2, gamma2
Type III: alpha5, beta3, gamma2
Type I: alpha6, beta2, gamma2
Type V: alpha1, beta1, gamma1

Source: Bourin.[9]

Table 2.2 α SUBUNIT PHARMACOLOGIC EFFECTS

Subunit	Effect
α1	Sedation, anticonvulsant, dependence, amnesia
α2	Anxiolysis, muscle relaxant
α3	Muscle relaxant
α5	Muscle relaxant, amnesia

There are currently 14 Food and Drug Administration–approved benzodiazepines that are commercially available within the United States; however, they are not used interchangeably and vary greatly by approved indications for use. Of the 14 approved agents, 9 benzodiazepines have a more established place in therapy; the remainder of this chapter will focus on describing the individual pharmacokinetic and pharmacodynamic characteristics to clarify key differences among the agents. The primary feature that determines the various agents' pharmacodynamics is their binding affinity while it is their differing half-lives $(t_{1/2})$ that defines their pharmacokinetics. One of the more common ways to classify benzodiazepines is by their half-life, which is the amount of time it takes for half of the drug to be eliminated from the body. By definition, the median elimination half-lives for short-acting agents is 1 to 12 hours versus 12 to 40 hours for intermediate-acting, and long-acting can extend up to 250 hours.[12] Preskorn developed a 2×2 model for conceptualizing benzodiazepines incorporating potency, as determined by binding affinity, and half-life providing a clearer relationship among the agents as it relates to the four primary chemical classes of benzodiazepines.[13] In general, 7-nitro-benzodiazepines (clonazepam) and 2-keto-benzodiazepines (diazepam, chlordiazepoxide, flurazepam) are considered to have long half-lives that exceed 24 hours. Conversely, triazolo-benzodiazepines (alprazolam, triazolam) and 3-OH-benzodiazepines (temazepam, lorazepam, oxazepam) are considered to have short half-lives of less than 12 hours. However, the same pairing cannot be used to apply relative potency, as 7-nitro-benzodiazepines and triazolo-benzodiazepines are classified as high potency agents versus 2-keto-benzodiazepines and 3-OH-benzodiazepines, which are low potency in comparison. (See Figure 2.1.)

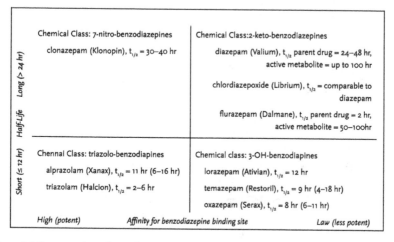

Figure 2.1 Conceptualizing benzodiazepines.
From Preskorn.[13]

PHARMACOKINETICS

The terms *pharmacokinetics* and *pharmacodynamics* are sometimes misused interchangeably but have very different definitions. Pharmacodynamics refers to the effect a drug has on the body while pharmacokinetics is the effect the body has on the drug. Specifically, pharmacokinetics is how the drug is absorbed, distributed, metabolized, and excreted by the body following administration. Two parameters that help describe a medication's properties for absorption are Tmax, or the time it takes for a medication to reach maximum serum concentration, and half-life, which was previously defined. In general, the time it takes to reach peak effect is similar among benzodiazepines and ranges from 0.5 to 2 hours, with some agents having an extended range of up to 4 hours for clonazepam or 6 hours for estazolam. As discussed earlier, half-life is a parameter that is frequently used to provide subclassifications for benzodiazepines. Clinically, half-life is a key factor to consider when determining the likelihood of an agent to precipitate dangerous withdrawals, as agents with shorter half-lives put patients at the highest risk. Chlordiazepoxide, diazepam, flurazepam, quazepam, and clorazepate are all long-acting agents with clonazepam, lorazepam, alprazolam, temazepam, estazolam, and oxazepam next in line as intermediate-acting. Midazolam and triazolam are the only short-acting agents that are available and used in clinical practice. Because each agent is metabolized differently within the body, you must consider the pharmacologic effect of both the parent drug and any active metabolites that are formed downstream (Table 2.3). For instance, 9 of the 14 benzodiazepines have active metabolites that have extended half-lives beyond that of the parent drug and can prolong the duration of activity with some active metabolites possessing a half-life that is nearly double that of the parent compound!

Following absorption, an agent's lipophilicity and protein binding affect distribution and the ability of the medication to diffuse from systemic circulation and penetrate the blood–brain barrier where it exerts its effects within the CNS. As a class, benzodiazepines are highly lipophilic and exhibit >85% protein binding, with most agents reaching >95% protein binding. Prior studies have revealed that there is no significant relationship between brain total serum concentration ratio and lipid solubility (measured by high performance liquid chromatography retention) or binding affinity (Ki). However, when brain uptake ratios are corrected to account for free benzodiazepine concentrations (as opposed to total serum concentration), there is a highly significant correlation with lipophilicity. This suggests that it is the benzodiazepine's physical property of lipophilicity that gives it the ability to first cross the blood–brain barrier and exert its effects within the CNS versus its binding affinity at the receptor.[14]

Although benzodiazepines have been touted as safer than barbiturates due to a decreased likelihood of serious drug–drug interactions, a large percentage of the agents within the class undergo phase I hepatic metabolism, primarily involving cytochrome 3A4 still making interactions a valid concern. Some agents act as substrates for additional cytochrome p450 enzymes such as 2C19 seen with clorazepate, diazepam,

Table 2.3 HEPATIC METABOLISM AND ACTIVE METABOLITES

Agent	Hepatic Metabolism	Active Metabolite
Phase I—CYP reactions (oxidation, reduction, hydrolysis)		
Alprazolam[15]	3A4	4-hydroxyalprazolam (weak)
		α-hydroxyalprazolam (weak)
Chlordiazepoxide[16]	3A4	Desmethylchlordiazepoxide
		Demoxepam
		Desmethyldiazepam
		Oxazepam
Clobazam[17]	3A4, 2C19 (minor), 2B6 (minor)	N-desmethylclobazam
Clonazepam[18]	3A4	
Clorazepate[19]	2C19, 3A4	Nordiazepam
Diazepam[20]	2C19, 3A4	Desmethyldiazepam (major)
		Temazepam (minor)
		Oxazepam (minor)
Estazolam[21]	3A4	
Flurazepam[22]	3A4	N-desalkylflurazepam
Midazolam[23]	3A4	1-hydroxy-midazolam
Quazepam[24]	3A4, 2C9, 2C19	2-oxoquazepam
		N-desalkyl-2-oxoquazepam
Triazolam[25]	3A4	
Phase II—Conjugation reactions (acetylation, glucuronidation, sulfation)		
Lorazepam[26]	Glucuronidation	Lorazepam glucuronide
Oxazepam[27]	Glucuronidation	
Phase I and II		
Temazepam[28]	Glucuronidation	
	2C19, 3A4	Oxazepam

quazepam, temazepam, and clobazam. Quazepam and clobazam also have ternary activity as a substrate for 2C9 and -2B6, respectively. For the previously discussed agents that act as substrates for either 3A4, 2B6, 2C9, or 2C19, concomitant use of strong inhibitors for the corresponding CYP isozyme pose an increased risk for adverse effects and benzodiazepine toxicity. Specifically, potential fatal respiratory depression is of concern and use of CYP3A4 inhibitors are contraindicated with the use of alprazolam and triazolam. A few notable exceptions are the handful of benzodiazepines that undergo phase II hepatic metabolism involving conjugation reactions, such as glucuronidation or acetylation, and have a lower propensity for drug–drug interactions including lorazepam, temazepam, and oxazepam. Following metabolism, the benzodiazepines are excreted primarily in the urine with clorazepate, clobazam, and quazepam exhibiting minor excretion in the feces.

THERAPEUTIC USE

All benzodiazepines have varying degrees of hypnotic, anxiolytic, antiepileptic, muscle relaxant, and amnestic properties with their primary effect varying among the individual agents and determining their indications for use. Most benzodiazepines are used as anxiolytics, sleep aids, or in the setting of alcohol withdrawal syndrome with some individual agents carrying additional indications for use including panic disorder, preoperative anxiety, and treatment of seizure disorders. There is no widely recognized singular source for definitive guidance on benzodiazepine dose equivalencies. Based on known differences that occur for any given individuals' metabolism and subsequent pharmacokinetics, it seems more appropriate to list as a range versus a hard-set value in most cases. Figure 2.1 shows the more commonly accepted dose equivalences with the figures in bold representing the dose established by the extensive studies performed by Ashton's research team.[7]

TERATOGENICITY

As recently as the mid-1990s benzodiazepines were among the most widely prescribed medications during pregnancy, with approximately 30% to 40% of pregnant women being prescribed a benzo at some stage of their pregnancy.[29] Although they were widely prescribed, there was little emphasis placed on establishing their safety in pregnancy. It is no surprise that diazepam, being the most frequently prescribed benzodiazepine, had the most data available to extrapolate to other agents within its class. However, despite growing research for other agents in the class the data regarding teratogenicity remains inconsistent. There greatest concerns for fetal defects arose from studies performed in the 1970s that implicated first trimester exposure to benzodiazepines in utero resulted in facial clefts, cardiac abnormalities, and other malformations in infants.[29] It is important to note that these studies were primarily studied in pregnant women taking diazepam or chlordiazepoxide and may not accurately represent the risk posed by other agents in the class. An additional confounder to consider is that many of the women included in the studies had risk factors for complicated pregnancies including psychiatric illnesses, epilepsy, diabetes, or were on multidrug therapy, which makes it difficult to establish a direct correlation between the use of benzodiazepines and the observed malformation. Data from later studies did not provide evidence of a significant increase in either the overall incidence of malformations or of any defect. More reliable evidence indicates that use of benzodiazepines in the late third trimester and during the delivery period are associated with a more significant risk to the fetus and neonate.[29] Infants who are exposed to benzodiazepines at this stage can develop floppy infant syndrome, which is marked by hypotonia and may result in difficulty feeding as decreased tone in their mouth muscles cannot properly establish a good breast-feeding latch or maintain an adequate suck–swallow pattern.[30] Other symptoms related to benzodiazepine exposure include mild sedation apneic spells, cyanosis, and impaired metabolic responses to cold stress, and neonatal withdrawal symptoms.[29] Due to the previously discussed evidence, the majority of benzodiazepines carry a former pregnancy class rating of D, except for clobazam, which carries a C rating. However, some agents bear a higher level of precaution with an X rating and are considered contraindicated during pregnancy including estazolam, flurazepam, triazolam, temazepam, and quazepam.

URINE TOXICOLOGY

Urine drug screens are an essential component of medication monitoring for controlled substances and have become a standard part of practice when prescribing opioids and benzodiazepines. Although UDS are a valuable tool to assess medication compliance, they can often be difficult to interpret, and the results may appear misleading to the untrained practitioner. As discussed previously in the pharmacokinetics section of this chapter, the majority of agents yield one or more active metabolites and developing an understanding of the which metabolites are detected in a urine drug screen will allow the practitioner the clinical judgement needed to properly assess the patient's use. There are inconsistencies that influence what a standard UDS is able to detect based on the performing lab's techniques and detection limits. Most UDS's utilize a traditional immunoassay that will commonly detect agents that yield the metabolites nordiazepam, oxazepam, and a-hydroxyalprazolam. Thus, parent drugs of diazepam, chlordiazepoxide, temazepam, and chlorazepate could result in a positive UDS result based on the presence of these metabolites. Likewise, alprazolam would result in a positive UDS result based on the presence of a-hydroxyalprazolam. (See Figure 2.2.) Unfortunately, due to their chemical structures clonazepam and lorazepam are not likely to be detected by the standard UDS and often require a specialized benzodiazepine immunoassay or a confirmatory test that utilizes mass spectrometry to detect their respective metabolites of 7-aminoclonazepam and lorazepam glucuronide. Additionally, because of the likelihood of cross-reactivity a confirmatory test should also be ordered following a positive UDS if the practitioner suspects the use of an alternative agent than what is prescribed. For example, both temazepam and diazepam could result in a positive UDS based on the presence of oxazepam. If a patient is only prescribed temazepam, ordering a confirmatory test will often allow specific detection of both individual agents versus the resulting metabolite only. Due to the high cross-reactivity of most UDS, it is also possible to get a false positive for a nonbenzodiazepine medication. Common agents that may result in false positives include nonsteroidal anti-inflammatory drugs and selective serotonin reuptake inhibitors, with oxaprozin and sertraline being the most likely agents from each class, respectively.

Z-DRUGS

Similarly to how the search for an improved anxiolytic resulted in the discovery and development of benzodiazepines, in the 1980s and 1990s the focus turned to finding an agent with more targeted sedative activity. The goal was to develop a sleep aid that

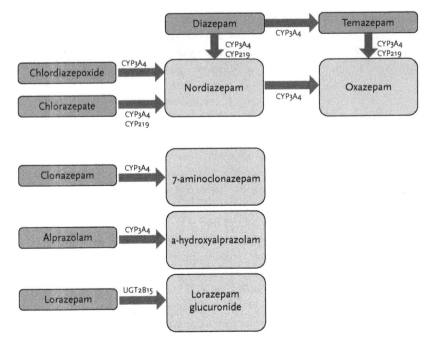

Figure 2.2 Detection of benzodiazepines by metabolites.
Figure adapted from Craven et al.[31]

lacked the undesirable qualities of benzos with an improved safety profile and ergo a new class of nonbenzodiazepine hypnotic agents, or Z-drugs, were born. There are currently three Z-drugs available within the United States, with zolpidem being first to market in 1992, followed by zaleplon in 1994, and finally eszopiclone in 2004. Z-drugs share the common characteristic of being short-acting in nature and are proposed to cause less disruption in the normal sleep cycle than benzodiazepines. Additional advantages advertised by manufacturers include decreased psychomotor and memory impairment, respiratory depression, rebound insomnia, abuse potential, and withdrawal symptoms when compared to longer-acting benzodiazepines. Each of these agents promote sleep by centrally enhancing GABA activity within the brain, but in vitro and animal studies have demonstrated distinct differences in in their receptor selectivity and mechanisms of action.[32] All three agents act as agonists at the ω-1 benzodiazepine receptor, which is also referred to as the benzodiazepine or omega receptor, which is associated with the GABA$_A$ receptor.[32] However, it is the differing selectivity between benzodiazepine 1 (BZ1) and benzodiazepine 2 (BZ2) receptors that appears to determine the differences in the agents' pharmacological profiles. To obtain a better grasp of how each agent's selectivity impacts its primary effect as well as observed adverse effects, we must first understand the functionality and distribution of the individual receptor subtypes. The BZ1 receptor contains the α1 isoform, which is responsible for sedative, antiepileptic, and amnestic qualities as seen with benzodiazepines. The BZ1 receptor is primarily distributed within the brain and is highly concentrated in the cortex, thalamus, and cerebellum.[6]

In contrast, BZ2 receptors contain the α2 isoform, which is responsible for anxiolytic and muscle relaxant effects observed with benzodiazepines. The BZ2 receptor is also heavily distributed within the CNS, particularly the dorsal horn of the spinal cord and the limbic system but is also highly concentrated within motor neurons of the peripheral nervous system.[6] Among the Z-drugs, zolpidem demonstrates the greatest selectivity for α1-containing BZ1 receptors with lesser agonist activity at α2 and α3 subunits and very little at the α5 subunit on BZ2 receptors. The roughly ninefold greater affinity for BZ1 renders it a potent sedative and hypnotic with minimal anxiolytic efficacy. While zaleplon also exhibits a slightly greater affinity for α1-containing BZ1 receptors, it also possesses low affinity and potency at α2 and α3 subunits of BZ2 receptors. The development of eszopiclone (the S-enantiomer of zopiclone; not available in the United States) still possesses activity at α1-containing BZ1 receptors, but without the R-enantiomer, it appears to have less selectivity due to increased efficacy at the α2 and α3 subunits when compared to its racemic counterpart. Zolpidem and eszopiclone have each shown efficacy in sleep induction and maintenance, but due to zaleplon's incredibly short half-life it is only recommended for sleep induction.[33]

In summation, benzodiazepines and Z-drugs, although widely prescribed, remain controversial agents in mainstream medicine. And while it would be hard to argue that they do not have a valuable place in therapy, it is equally important to understand their key differences and limitations to ensure appropriate prescribing. Taking into consideration pharmacokinetics, approved indications, and drug interactions are imperative in the proper selection of an agent.

REFERENCES

1. Wick JY. The history of benzodiazepines. *The Consultant Pharmacist.* 2013;28(9):538–548. doi:10.4140/tcp.n.2013.538.
2. Oransky I. Leo H. Sternbach. *The Lancet.* 2005;366(9495):1430. doi:10.1016/s0140-6736(05)67588-5.
3. López-Muñoz F, Ucha-Udabe R, Alamo C. The history of barbiturates a century after their clinical introduction. *Neuropsychiatric Disease and Treatment.* 2005;1(4):329–343.
4. Harrison N, Mendelson WB, de Wit H. Barbiturates. *American College of Neuropsychopharmacology.* www.acnp.org/g4/GN401000173/CH169.html. Published 2000.
5. Bowery NG, Smart TG. GABA and glycine as neurotransmitters: a brief history. *British Journal of Pharmacology.* 2009;147(Suppl 1):S109–S119. doi:10.1038/sj.bjp.0706443.
6. Griffin CE, Kaye AM, Bueno FR, Kaye AD. Benzodiazepine pharmacology and central nervous system-mediated effects. *Ochsner Journal.* 2013;13(2):214–223.
7. Ashton H. Benzodiazepine dependence and withdrawal: an update. *Northern Regional Health Authority Drug Newsletter, 31.* www.benzo.org.uk/drcha.htm. Published April 1985.
8. Booth, R. Psychotherapeutic drugs: antipsychotic and anxiolytic agents. In: Lemke TL, Williams DA, eds., *Foye's Principles of Medicinal Chemistry.* Philadelphia, PA: Williams & Wilkins; 2008:618–629.
9. Bourin M. The GABAA receptor and benzodiazepine acceptor site. *SOJ Pharmacy and Pharmaceutical Sciences.* 2018;5(2) 1–5. doi:10.15226/2374-6866/5/2/00176.

10. Sigel E, Steinmann ME. Structure, function, and modulation of GABAA receptors. *Journal of Biological Chemistry.* 2012;287(48):40224–40231. doi:10.1074/jbc.r112.386664.

11. Tan KR, Rudolph U, Lüscher C. Hooked on benzodiazepines: GABAA receptor subtypes and addiction. *Trends in Neurosciences.* 2011;34(4):188–197. doi:10.1016/j.tins.2011.01.004.

12. Fox C, Liu H, Kaye AD, et al., eds. Antianxiety agents. In: *Clinical Aspects of Pain Medicine and Interventional Pain Management: A Comprehensive Review.* Paducah, KY: ASIP Publishing; 2011:543–552.

13. Preskorn SH. A way of conceptualizing benzodiazepines to guide clinical use. *Journal of Psychiatric Practice.* 2015;21(6):436–441. doi:10.1097/pra.0000000000000114.

14. Arendt RM, et al. Determinants of benzodiazepine brain uptake: lipophilicity versus binding affinity. *Psychopharmacology.* 1987;93(1):72–76. doi:10.1007/bf02439589.

15. Xanax (alprazolam) [package insert]. New York, NY: Pfizer; 2011.

16. Librium (chlordiazepoxide) [package insert]. Bridgewater, NJ: Valeant Pharmaceuticals; 2005.

17. Onfi (clobazam) [package insert]. Deerfield, IL: Lundbeck; 2016.

18. Klonopin (clonazepam) [package insert]. San Francisco, CA: Genentech USA; 2013.

19. Tranxene (clorazepate) [package insert]. Deerfield, IL: Lundbeck; 2010.

20. Valium (diazepam) [package insert]. Nutley, NJ: Roche Pharmaceuticals; 2008.

21. Estazolam [package insert]. North Chicago, IL: Abbott Laboratories; 1996.

22. Dalmane (flurazepam) [package insert]. Aliso Viejo, CA: Valeant Pharmaceuticals; 2007.

23. Midazolam [package insert]. Kirkland, Quebec: Pfizer Canada; 2017.

24. Doral (quazepam) [package insert]. Marietta, GA: Cutis Health; 2016.

25. Halcion (triazolam) [package insert]. NY, NY: Pfizer; 2016.

26. Ativan (lorazepam) [package insert]. Bridgewater, NJ: Biovail Pharmaceuticals; 2007.

27. Oxazepam [package insert]. Princeton, NJ: Sandoz; 2016.

28. Restoril (temazepam) [package insert]. Hazelwood, MO: Mallinckrodt Inc; 2008.

29. Mcelhatton PR. The effects of benzodiazepine use during pregnancy and lactation. *Reproductive Toxicology.* 1994;8(6):461–475. doi:10.1016/0890-6238(94)90029-9.

30. Carney PR. The floppy infant syndrome. In: Carney PR, Geyer JD, eds., *Pediatric Practice: Neurology.* New York, NY: McGraw Hill; 2010:401–408.

31. Craven C, Fileger M, Woster P. Demystifying benzodiazepine urine drug screen results. *Practical Pain Management.* https://www.practicalpainmanagement.com/treatments/addiction-medicine/drug-monitoring-screening/demystifying-benzodiazepine-urine-drug. Published February 2014. Updated March 1, 2019.

32. Sanger DJ. The pharmacology and mechanisms of action of new generation, non-benzodiazepine hypnotic agents. *CNS Drugs.* 2004;18(Suppl 1):9–15. doi:10.2165/00023210-200418001-00004.

33. Gunja N. The clinical and forensic toxicology of Z-drugs. *Journal of Medical Toxicology.* 2013;9(2):155–162.

CHAPTER 3

Benzodiazepine Therapy

The Good, the Bad, and the Ugly

JEFFREY GUINA, BRIAN MERRILL, AND JO ANN LEQUANG

HIGHLIGHTS

- Historically, benzodiazepines (BZDs) were considered an advance in pharmaco-therapy over older sedatives like barbiturates.
- Although BZDs are some of the most widely prescribed medications, commonly their use is not evidence-based, particularly when used for longer than two to four weeks.
- The evidence for and against the use of BZDs needs to take into account many factors, such as real vs perceived efficacy, adverse effects, significant lack of evidence-based support for use beyond 2 to 4 weeks, development of physical dependence and withdrawal phenomena, and the availability of more effective and safer alternatives.

INTRODUCTION

Since their introduction in the 1960s, BZDs have been and remain among the most frequently prescribed medications worldwide and while they provide treatment for certain indicated conditions, they are often used off-label with little to no evidence for safety and efficacy.[1,2] BZDs are considered to be sedative-hypnotic agents, much like alcohol. Alcohol has a similar mechanism of action as BZDs, it has a synergistic effect when used together with BZDs, and it can produce symptoms of intoxication and withdrawal similar to BZDs. However, owing to cultural and medical perceptions, alcohol is not generally perceived as a sedative-hypnotic drug, including in the fifth edition of the *Diagnostic and Statistical Manual of Mental Disorders* (DSM).[3]

As early as the 19th century, other specific sedative-hypnotic agents were developed including chloral hydrate, paraldehyde, meprobamate, and a broad class of drugs known as barbiturates. By the mid-20th century, barbiturates became hugely popular as tranquilizers even though—or possibly because—their considerable abuse potential was already starting to emerge. The true ramifications of addiction were not well understood at the time: people who misused barbiturates were "pill poppers," and the drugs were benignly described as "habit forming." In addition, barbiturates were associated with adverse effects, could be toxic, could cause fatal overdose, and had an association with suicide. Even in the 1950s and 1960s, barbiturates were being taken intravenously by some users to enhance their psychoactive effects and often at high doses, multiples of the therapeutic dose level.[4] It was into this arena that BZDs appeared as a new and safer alternative. Ironically, BZDs were marketed to prescribers as having little to no risk for dependence or adverse effects.[1,4] The story of BZDs is an account of the good, the bad, and the ugly, as very little of it is really good.

THE GOOD: BENEFITS OF BENZODIAZEPINE THERAPY

At first, BZDs found great resonance among physicians and their patients. BZDs were soon prescribed for a laundry list of conditions including anxiety, seizures, muscle tension, psychosis, depression, and insomnia. They helped people cope with stress and psychological problems. They soothed nerves and calmed spirits. They were used for anesthesia and a variety of diffuse psychosomatic problems. The Rolling Stones' song, "Mother's Little Helper," from 1966 described the widespread prescribing of BZDs to housewives ("and though she's not really ill, there's this little yellow pill"). BZDs were also sometimes used to pharmacologically treat a condition then known as "combat neurosis," which today is called posttraumatic stress disorder (PTSD).[5]

Both the sedative and hypnotic effects of BZDs are produced because these agents potentiate the effects of gamma-aminobutyric acid (GABA), the most widely distributed inhibitory neurotransmitter in the central nervous system (CNS). BZDs have an allosteric effect on the $GABA_A$ receptors by binding to the BZD receptor complex.[6] This interaction allows for more frequent opening of ion channels which increases the influx of chloride ions, thus increasing membrane polarization and reducing the firing of neurons. In this way, BZDs depress the CNS.[4,7] All BZDs rely on this basic mechanism of action, and all of them produce both sedative and hypnotic effects even though individual BZDs have specific indications. Prescribing choices of a BZD for a specific patient are often made based on pharmacokinetic (e.g., half-life) rather than pharmacodynamic characteristics, as the pharmacodynamics of all BZDs are very similar.[8]

The GABA receptors are being explored as potential bases for a variety of anxiety disorders. Stressors and traumatic events may downregulate or modulate certain GABA receptors in some individuals.[9] GABA receptor dysfunction in different regions of the brain have been implicated in common anxiety symptoms. For examples, GABA dysfunction in the amygdala has been related to impaired emotional regulation and fear conditioning. GABA dysfunction in the prefrontal cortex has been linked to attention deficits and problems with working memory. In the hippocampus, GABA dysfunction may be associated with impaired memory formation while in the striatum, salience reactivity and misinterpretation of negative stimuli have been suggested.[9,10] Although GABA receptors are distributed throughout the CNS, it appears that BZD activity in specific brain regions is associated with specific effects; for example, when BZDs can normalize a hyperactive amygdala, they reduce anxiety and enhance sleep.[11]

BZDs are approved by the U.S. Food and Drug Administration (FDA) for treatment of acute anxiety, acute insomnia, anesthesia, and for short-term use in the treatment of alcohol/BZD withdrawal symptoms (Table 3.1).[12,13] Because the DSM did not set forth specific diagnostic criteria for specific conditions until 1980, pre-existing BZDs were approved for diffuse "anxiety states" and "anxiety disorders" that were not defined by scientific criteria. As a result, BZDs were used to treat a range of conditions, many of which would be considered off-label, that is, use without an FDA disease-specific approval. A good case-in-point is PTSD, which was first recognized as a disorder with the third edition of the DSM (published in 1980) but grouped with anxiety disorders. In the fifth edition of the DSM (published in 2013), PTSD was moved to the new trauma- and stressor-related disorder category and separated out from the anxiety disorders. The only FDA-approved medications to treat PTSD are the selective serotonin reuptake inhibitors (SSRIs) sertraline and paroxetine. Yet it has been reported that 37% to 74% of patients with PTSD are still prescribed sedative-hypnotics, which is an off-label use and is not supported by evidence-based clinical guidelines.[14–16]

Table 3.1 U.S. FOOD AND DRUG ADMINISTRATION–APPROVED INDICATIONS FOR BENZODIAZEPINES

Drug	FDA-Approved Indications
Alprazolam	Anxiety, panic disorder
Chlordiazepoxide	Anxiety, alcohol withdrawal, preoperative anxiety
Clorazepate	Anxiety, alcohol withdrawal, seizure
Clobazam	Lennox-Gastaut syndrome (adjunctive use)
Clonazepam	Anxiety, panic disorder, periodic limb movement disorder, neuralgia, seizure
Diazepam	Anxiety, alcohol withdrawal, seizure, muscle spasms, preoperative anxiety
Estazolam	Insomnia, short-term use only
Flurazepam	Insomnia, short-term use only
Lorazepam	Anxiety, chemotherapy-induced nausea/vomiting, insomnia short-term use only, preoperative sedation, seizure
Midazolam	Procedural sedation
Oxazepam	Anxiety, alcohol withdrawal
Temazepam	Insomnia, short-term use only
Triazolam	Insomnia, short-term use only

It has been argued to "limit benzodiazepine prescriptions to emergency situations where a rapid symptomatic amelioration is required."[17] Such situations include significant lack of sleep associated with mania or severe panic attacks.

There are only a few mental health disorders for which there is any evidence in support of the use of BZDs: panic disorder, generalized anxiety disorder, social anxiety disorder, and insomnia.[17-24] In these four conditions, BZDs are not recommended as first-line therapy but rather only in the event that first-line and even in some cases second-line drugs have failed. For treatment-resistant cases of those four disorders, BZDs have shown some evidence of being effective, but only short-term use is recommended, defined as two to four weeks of treatment at most. A particular danger in using BZDs for anxiety, insomnia, and similar mental health conditions is that those conditions are often persistent, prolonged, and even chronic, and BZD therapy is recommended for short duration only. While BZDs may be effective in relieving the acute symptoms of anxiety and insomnia, there are other, better treatment options that should be used first for chronic anxiety. According to clinical practice guidelines, serotonergic agents such as SSRIs are first-line treatments for anxiety disorders[21,25-33] along with psychotherapy, such as cognitive behavioral therapy (CBT) or other approaches. Anxiety can be challenging to treat. Not all patients respond to pharmacological therapy or respond only partially. The role of BZDs is as a short-term treatment option for patients who have failed psychotherapeutic interventions and multiple antidepressant therapy regimens and other adjunctive agents.

One way to approach the treatment of any anxiety disorder is to determine whether the anxiety disorder would respond better to short-term versus long-term treatment. There are cases of occasional acute anxiety provoked by circumstances that might respond well to short-term treatment, such as fear of flying or undergoing a serious medical procedure. While a BZD might work well in such a situation, they are not the only option, and non-BZD agents should be considered as well, such as propranolol, a beta-blocker that is sometimes used to treat performance anxiety. When a patient is dealing with anxiety that is persistent, prolonged, or diffuse, which is typical in generalized anxiety disorder, BZDs are not usually appropriate drugs, and other pharmacological options would be safer and more effective.

BZDs clearly have a role to play in our pharmacological armamentarium. They can be safe and effective for short-term use to control acute anxiety or acute insomnia. They are helpful in anesthesia and perioperatively. They are also effective in helping people manage symptoms of alcohol or BZD withdrawal. But these "wonder drugs" have very limited, very specific uses.[13]

THE BAD: HOW BENZODIAZEPINES BECAME PRESCRIBED WHERE THEY WERE CONTRAINDICATED

BZDs are far from the ideal tranquilizer they once seemed to be. By 1975, BZD abuse potential caused these drugs to be restricted by the FDA.[34] Tolerance to BZDs, that is, the need to take higher doses of the agent to obtain the same level of therapeutic benefit, had been observed anecdotally but was not confirmed in controlled clinical trials until the 1980s.[1] In the early years of BZD therapy, it was not unusual for patients to take BZDs long term, and it was also observed by clinicians that patients who tried to discontinue BZDs after extended exposure to the drugs exhibited withdrawal symptoms. By 1990, the American Psychiatric Association described BZD dependence as a risk associated with the drug class.[4,35] Concerns about the safety of BZDs along with the emergence of new anti-anxiety drugs such as SSRIs and others, along with the growing popularity of CBT in the 1980s, provided safe and effective alternatives to BZDs.[7] The Department of Veterans Affairs reduced its use of BZDs for PTSD from 1999 to 2009 mainly by opting for evidence-based treatments, including CBT.[36,37]

However, BZDs remain among the most frequently prescribed drugs in the world, even today. They are indicated only for short-term use of no longer than two to four weeks, yet healthcare providers often prescribe BZDs for long-term use in patients, even over the course of many years.[1] One way in which BZDs are inappropriately prescribed occurs when they are administered to a patient in an open-ended or long-term use for any condition. Even in the cases where there is evidence of the short-term efficacy of a BZD, long-term use of these drugs is problematic. Although BZDs are indicated for short-term use, many patients are started off with a 90-day supply.[36,38] Some patients seem to get open-ended BZD prescriptions; that is, they start BZDs and continue them indefinitely. The risks of BZDs were not—and even today are not—as well known as they should be, and many people who take them may view them as more or less harmless. While concerns were being raised about BZD safety, their consumption actually increased from 1999 to 2014, mainly due to the fact that so many people were taking them long term.[39] They still remain widely prescribed and often are recommended to patients who are not counseled about their risks. In any given year, about 15% of the U.S. population has taken a BZD, and about 6% of the U.S. population has abused sedative-hypnotic agents in that same time period.[7]

Among healthcare professionals, there had long been the notion that primary-care physicians were prescribing BZDs liberally only for their long-term BZD patients to enter the care of psychiatrists and other mental health specialists who had to deal with the aftermath of BZD dependence. But a large study ($N = 356,958$) dispelled that notion when it was found mental health providers prescribed more BZDs than other physicians—at a rate of more than two to one.[15] This is not to say that BZD prescribing rates are uniform or follow much of a pattern. BZD prescribing varies vastly among facilities and among prescribers. There are reasons for this: organizational culture can shape prescribing practices at a given healthcare facility, and many clinicians do not adhere to clinical practice guidelines in making prescribing choices for individual patients.[38] Furthermore, many people struggling with BZDs are legacy patients, meaning they were started on BZDs before guidelines were published or while in the case of another clinical team or even in different medical circumstances and are now being treated by other clinicians.[15,40]

Tolerance is the expected result of exposure to certain drugs, which in the case of BZDs means that over time, patients need higher and higher doses of the BZD to achieve the same level of therapeutic effect. Physiologically, tolerance develops when long-term exposure to BZDs causes intraneural gene expression and GABA receptor functionality to change. Although this mechanism has not entirely been elucidated, it likely involves the downregulation of the binding sites on the $GABA_A$ receptors where BZDs attach, resulting in the uncoupling of the allosteric link of BZD to GABA receptor complex and may involve alterations in the receptor subunit. This would be similar to what happens when people who drink alcohol over time become increasingly tolerant of its effects. It is also possible that persistent enhancement of the GABA system by BZDs results in some compensatory mechanisms over time.[1,4,18,41,42] With some drugs, tolerance builds up slowly, but with BZDs tolerance may develop much more swiftly, even within days.[1,18,41] While tolerance to therapeutic effects often parallels the development of tolerance to adverse effects with many drugs, this is not the case with BZDs.[18] Patients build up tolerance to the therapeutic effects of the BZDs but still experience side effects, which may worsen as doses increase. The bottom line in clinical practice is that patients who build up BZD tolerance must periodically increase their BZD dose to maintain the same effectiveness; in some cases, patients take more than one type of BZD.[1,3,4,43] BZDs have multiple effects, and it appears that tolerance to various effects develops at different rates. For instance, tolerance to the sedative effects of BZDs often builds up much more rapidly than tolerance to its depressant effects on the brain stem, with the result that patients may take higher doses or more BZDs to have the desired anxiolytic or hypnotic effect and experience hypotension and potentially life-threatening respiratory depression.[3] For those individuals who abuse BZDs by taking them recreationally, tolerance can pose a serious problem as the dose of BZD must escalate over time to maintain the same level of euphoria or psychoactive effects.[3]

Despite the fact that BZDs may be effective in certain treatment-resistant cases of panic disorder, generalized anxiety disorder, and insomnia, they must be considered with caution and used only when first-line treatments have failed and the clinician has a clear exit strategy to discontinue BZD use after two to four weeks. BZDs are frequently prescribed too liberally for these disorders, are often prescribed for conditions for which there is no evidence of efficacy, and even prescribed for patients with comorbidities that contraindicate their use.

While some prescribers start BZDs at the same time as serotonergic agents to give the latter time to start working, there is no evidence in support of this approach, which actually adds new risks.[2,25,44] Increasingly, first-line serotonergic agents such as SSRIs and other newer agents are used for anxiety and PTSD, but there can be challenges with these drugs since the onset of action with serotonergic agents can take four to six weeks,[45] and even after that initial period, they still may need to be adjusted to provide the patient with real relief. During this time period, BZDs are sometimes prescribed to help the patient manage acute symptoms. The thinking behind this not-all-that-uncommon prescribing regimen is that the BZDs would be used only for a few weeks and would be discontinued as soon as the right dose of serotonergic agent can be achieved.[19-21,46] There is no evidence to support the idea that SSRIs or similar agents are made more effective by co-prescribing them with BZDs or that anxiety outcomes are improved beyond using SSRIs alone.[2,22] Adding BZDs to a new prescription for SSRIs may actually increase the risk of adverse events. Perhaps the worst and most dangerous aspect of all is the fact that once BZDs are initiated in such a situation, it is not unusual for BZD therapy to continue indefinitely. About 12% of patients who start an SSRI with BZDs wind up taking BZDs for six months or more.[2] A subset of these patients wind up taking BZDs even after they have discontinued the SSRI, which only demonstrates how difficult it can be for patients to discontinue BZD therapy. Despite these risks, physicians prescribing BZDs as a stop-gap while waiting to achieve therapeutic efficacy with an SSRI or similar agent have almost doubled from 2001 to 2014.[2]

While BZDs may be indicated for short-term use for insomnia, insomnia tends to be a chronic condition. BZDs have been "weakly" recommended by guidelines for the short-term treatment of insomnia, defined as fewer than four weeks.[47] Sleep disorders are complex, and insomnia is not a homogeneous condition. Some patients experience insomnia as a primary sleep disorder, but for others, it is secondary to illness, stress, or may be a side effect of medications.[48] The sedative effects of BZDs may cause patients to mistakenly think they are sleeping better when, in reality, the sedation encourages the early phases of sleep while preventing deep sleep and its more restorative benefits.

Studies have found that BZD prescribing is significantly higher for individuals with anxiety disorders, PTSD, borderline personality disorder,[14,16,38,49-51] substance use disorders,[14,16,49,52] inpatient psychiatric care,[14,50] prolonged duration of one of these disorders,[36,38] a higher degree of disability in the Veteran's Administration system,[14,38] having a current prescription for opioid analgesics,[49,52] having a prescription for other BZDs,[52] and having a higher number of traumatic events.[51] In studying the pattern of BZD prescribing, a BZD prescription can be associated with a number of things, many of which are not evidence-based (e.g., personality disorders) or are even contraindications (e.g., PTSD, substance use, concurrent opioid prescriptions).

There is no evidence that either short-term or long-term BZD therapy is effective in the treatment of many well-known mental health conditions including PTSD[19,23,33,53] and phobias.[54] As a matter of fact, BZDs can actually be harmful for such patients. BZD can induce anxiety when it is discontinued (withdrawal symptoms) or exacerbate underlying pathologies such as the hypothalamic–pituitary–adrenal axis stress response.[54] Patients suffering from anxiety must rely in part on the fear extinction response to overcome their anxiety,[55] but BZDs can interfere with and even prevent fear extinction.[56] In other words, BZDs may treat anxiety well for a few days, but they paradoxically make it worse over the long term.

Exposure therapy has been used to help patients work through anxiety by exposing them to anxiety-producing stimuli in a controlled therapeutic setting with the goal that repeated exposures would gradually alleviate the anxiety response. Back in the 1960s, it was assumed that low anxiety levels caused by BZDs would facilitate exposure therapy and drive quicker results, but in the 1980s the opposite was found to be the case in that patients came to believe that their reduced levels of fear and anxiety were the result of the drug rather than exposure therapy.[53] In such cases, patients experienced an eroded sense of self-efficacy and were reticent to give up the drug; it became clear that BZDs can both directly and indirectly worsen anxiety. Once a patient becomes dependent on BZDs, those affective states that had been most numbed by sedation become the most intense (and most uncomfortable) during withdrawal. In dealing with withdrawal, patients sometimes assume that the withdrawal symptoms are not withdrawal at all, but rather their normal baseline unmedicated state. This causes the patient to urgently seek BZD therapy again to "manage" those symptoms. Overall, anxiety is a typical symptom of BZD withdrawal but based on subjective reports from patients giving up BZDs, anxiety decreases markedly after about five weeks, often to the point that it is less than the anxiety level experienced during BZD therapy. Other symptoms, such as avoidance and social functioning can take much longer to improve.[1,18]

BZDs are contraindicated for a number of mental health conditions as well as for long-term use, which is a defining characteristic of many psychiatric disorders. The problem is that many of these mental health conditions are comorbid with anxiety disorders and insomnia. When such patients seek out clinical care, they often present as highly distressed individuals in great suffering and despair; many feel misunderstood and neglected by the healthcare profession, who may prescribe BZD in an effort to provide some degree of rapid relief. A patient may present with the more obvious symptoms of anxiety or insomnia, and the true underlying pathology may only emerge over weeks or months of care. Treating the immediate symptoms of anxiety and/or insomnia sets in motion a very vicious circle: the intended short-term use of BZDs with its brief period of relief becomes prolonged and then starts to contribute to the patient's symptoms.

There are a number of other prominent contraindications for BZD therapy. These include hypersensitivity to BZDs, pulmonary disease (such as sleep apnea and chronic obstructive pulmonary disease), Parkinson's disease, hepatic disease, closed-angle glaucoma, and others.[57] Pediatric patients under the age of 18 are contraindicated for BZD use as are pregnant and nursing mothers.[57] Prescribing physicians should take care in not prescribing BZD to patients with sleep apnea, whose symptoms of fatigue, poor-quality sleep, and irritability may be misdiagnosed as insomnia or anxiety. People with Parkinson's disease often develop comorbid anxiety disorders but should not be prescribed BZDs even when anxiety symptoms are prominent. While obesity is not a contraindication for BZDs, caution should be exercised in prescribed BZDs in this population. The literature suggests that lorazepam-associated carcinogenesis may occur in obese and overweight individuals.[58] Obesity may also cause the BZD to accumulate in the system.[57]

THE UGLY: BENZODIAZEPINE-ASSOCIATED ADVERSE EVENTS

An ideal anxiolytic agent might selectively inhibit the GABA receptors in the hyperactive amygdala, which has been implicated in anxiety. In reality, GABA receptors are widely distributed throughout the brain and CNS with the result that BZDs nonselectively target all areas of the brain. The wide range of adverse effects of BZDs are summarized in Table 3.2. In many cases, the adverse effects of BZDs are similar to the signs and symptoms of anxiety disorder or other conditions, making it difficult to ascertain if a certain symptom is caused by the drug or the underlying disorder. Since most mental health conditions, including depression and PTSD, are associated with a hypoactive

Table 3.2 A PARTIAL SUMMATION OF POSSIBLE ADVERSE EFFECTS
ASSOCIATED WITH BZDS, MANY OF WHICH OCCUR IN ANXIETY OR OTHER
MENTAL DISORDERS

BZD Adverse Effect	May Also Occur With These Disorders
Behavioral symptoms	
Changes in appetite, overeating, anorexia, weight gain/loss	Anxiety, depressive disorder, substance use disorder, eating disorder
Insomnia	Anxiety, generalized anxiety disorder, depressive disorder, substance use disorder, posttraumatic stress disorder
Avoidance disorder, agoraphobia	Anxiety, posttraumatic stress disorder
Impulsivity, disinhibition	Posttraumatic stress disorder, substance use disorder, personality disorder, bipolar disorder
Agitation, restlessness	Anxiety, generalized anxiety disorder, mood disorders, somatic disorders
Cardiovascular symptoms	
Bradycardia, tachycardia	Anxiety, panic disorder, posttraumatic stress disorder, somatic disorders
Hypotension, hypertension	Anxiety, panic disorder, posttraumatic stress disorder, somatic disorders
Central nervous system symptoms	
Dizziness, vertigo, syncope, light-headedness	Anxiety, panic disorder, somatic disorders, dissociative disorders
Slurred speech	Substance use disorder, inebriation
Lack of coordination, poor reaction time, impaired motor skills, weakness	Anxiety, panic disorder, somatic disorder
Seizures	Anxiety disorder, somatic disorder
Cognitive symptoms	
Sedation, fatigue, drowsiness, somnolence	Anxiety, generalized anxiety disorder, depressive disorder, substance use disorder
Inattention, inability to concentrate	Anxiety, generalized anxiety disorder, depressive disorder, substance use disorder
Nightmares	Anxiety, posttraumatic stress disorder
Intrusive thoughts	Anxiety, posttraumatic stress disorder
Memory problems, amnesia	Anxiety, posttraumatic stress disorder, substance use disorder
Impaired judgment	Substance use disorder, psychotic disorder, bipolar disorder
Illusions, hallucinations	Posttraumatic stress disorder, psychotic disorder, dissociative disorder, substance use disorder
Dissociation, perceptual deficits	Posttraumatic stress disorder, psychotic disorder, dissociative disorder, substance use disorder

(*continued*)

Table 3.2 CONTINUED

BZD Adverse Effect	May Also Occur With These Disorders
Suicidality	Anxiety, posttraumatic stress disorder, depressive disorder, substance use disorder, personality disorder
Homicidal ideations	Substance use disorder, personality disorder
Paranoia, hypervigilance	Substance use disorder, psychotic disorder
Delirium, coma, stupor	Substance use disorder
Rash	Anxiety, somatic disorder
Drug dependency symptoms	
Drug dependence	Substance use disorder
Tolerance	Substance use disorder
Withdrawal symptoms	Substance use disorder
Drug misuse, drug abuse	Posttraumatic stress disorder, personality disorder, substance use disorder
Dysphoria, depression	Anxiety, posttraumatic stress disorder, depressive disorder substance use disorder
Emotional symptoms	
Emotional numbness, disengagement	Anxiety, posttraumatic stress disorder, depressive disorder substance use disorder, dissociative disorder
Anger, rage, irritability, mood swings, hostility, violence	Anxiety, generalized anxiety disorder, substance use disorder, personality disorder, bipolar disorder
Anxiety, phobias, panic	Anxiety, posttraumatic stress disorder substance use disorder
Euphoria, excessive excitement, histrionics	Anxiety, substance use disorder, bipolar disorder, personality disorder
Mania	Substance use disorder, bipolar disorder
Gastrointestinal symptoms	
Nausea, vomiting	Anxiety, panic disorder, somatic disorder, dissociative disorder
Hematologic and circulatory symptoms	
Blood disorders	Somatic disorders
Neuropathic symptoms	
Paresthesia, neuropathic pain	Anxiety, panic disorder, somatic disorder
Physical symptoms	
Muscle pain, muscle spasms, tense muscles	Anxiety, generalized anxiety disorder, posttraumatic stress disorder, somatic disorders
Nasal congestion	
Fever	Anxiety, panic disorder, posttraumatic stress disorder, somatic disorder
Respiratory symptoms	
Respiratory depression	Anxiety, panic disorder, posttraumatic stress disorder, somatic disorder
Hyperventilation	Anxiety, panic disorder, posttraumatic stress disorder, somatic disorder
Visual impairment, photophobia, tinnitus, strange tastes	Anxiety, panic disorder, somatic disorder
Sexual symptoms	
Sexual dysfunction	Anxiety, somatic disorders, depressive disorders, substance use disorder
Menstrual irregularities	Anxiety, somatic disorders, depressive disorders, substance use disorder

Note: Some of these signs and symptoms may occur with other conditions such as drug interactions, stress, and other conditions.

prefrontal cortex, this global inhibition of CNS by BZDs may lead to an exacerbation of many mental health conditions.

As is the case with many other drugs, adverse effects are more likely to occur in vulnerable patients, such as the elderly, the frail, those with renal or hepatic dysfunction, and other conditions. Further, BZD adverse effects may be exacerbated in patients using other CNS depressants such as alcohol, opioids, antihistamines, anticonvulsants, neuroleptic drugs, and sedating antidepressants.[59-61] It remains controversial as to whether or not BZD use increases the risk of death, but a study of two databases found that the use of BZDs was associated with a small but statistically significant increase in all-cause mortality.[62]

BZD use must be judiciously considered in patients at risk for other conditions. For instance, in patients with asthma, the use of BZDs may exacerbate asthma and increase their risk of mortality.[63] Patients at risk for falls, such as the elderly, or respiratory depression, such as those taking CNS depressants and/or with pulmonary conditions, may experience symptomatic exacerbation. The elderly should be mentioned specifically because of changes in distribution, metabolism, and elimination of pharmaceutical agents, which means that drugs can accumulate in the system, potentiating their effects including their adverse events. Drug dosing modifications are often recommended for older patients. In addition, with old age can come hepatic dysfunction, renal impairment, and brain deficits that can further complicate BZD use.[18,64,65] Of all the BZD drugs, diazepam's long half-life makes it least appropriate for use in geriatric patients, which is why clinicians may talk about "L.O.T" drugs for seniors, meaning lorazepam, oxazepam, and temazepam, because they have no active metabolites and do not require oxidative hepatic metabolism. The issue of BZD in geriatric patients with dementia is particularly challenging, because agitation and anxiety are all prevalent in this population. In some cases, the use of BZD to mitigate symptoms of agitation short term may be appropriate, but the recommendation is to use the lowest effective dose of BZD for the shortest duration of time. However, even at therapeutic doses for short courses, BZD toxicity may still occur and can be associated with cognitive impairment.[35] Many older patients are prescribed BZD therapy for extended periods of time; BZD dependence is an important problem in the elderly population, particularly those in long-term care facilities.[64]

BZDs are considered class D teratogens, meaning these drugs have shown positive evidence of risk to the human fetus although potential drug benefits may warrant its use in certain specific situations.[66] This means BZDs should not be used without very careful deliberation for women who are or who may become pregnant, and they are contraindicated in nursing mothers.[67] There is a paucity of evidence about BZDs in pregnant women, and the early evidence suggesting BZDs cause facial malformations remains controversial.[68] However, there is evidence that taking BZDs during pregnancy can be associated with preterm birth, difficult or prolonged childbirth, low birth weight and symptoms in the neonate including withdrawal, respiratory depression, temperature dysregulation, apnea, sedation, hypotonia, lethargy, and others. Congenital cardiac abnormalities, neural tube defects, limb deficiencies, "floppy baby" syndrome, lower Apgar scores, and feeding problems have also been reported.[59,69-73] BZDs are secreted in breast milk,[74] and taking these drugs while nursing has not been well studied but may be appropriate in some instances.[75]

It is clinically troubling that many of the more frequently reported adverse effects associated with BZDs are similar to those that occur in mental health disorders, which can make it difficult to ascertain if these effects are due to the patient's underlying anxiety, other mental health disorders, or are the result of BZD use. It may be that BZDs synergistically exacerbate the natural symptoms of underlying anxiety, which can be clinically misinterpreted as a primary exacerbation of the patient's anxiety, which may result in inappropriate treatment. There have been studies that support the idea that BZDs synergistically worsen the patient's underlying anxiety, because psychiatric symptoms, cognitive performance, and general physical well-being improve when BZD use is stopped.[1]

The cognitive side effects of BZDs are so well known they merit their own name: BZD-induced neurocognitive disorder. People with anxiety, generalized anxiety disorder, and other mental health conditions typically have challenges when it comes to focus, attention, and memory, which can be exacerbated with BZD use. BZD-induced neurocognitive disorder may occur during BZD toxicity, BZD withdrawal, or BZD-related delirium, or it may occur as a side effect of normal and therapeutic BZD therapy.[3] While BZD-induced neurocognitive disorder is more common among those taking high doses of BZDs or those on long-term BZD therapy, such side effects may arise even from a single dose and can occur in patients taking low doses.[3,64] The elderly are particularly vulnerable to such BZD-induced neurocognitive disorder, and in some cases, it is misdiagnosed as progressive dementia. In fact, about 10% of older individuals referred to memory clinics turn out to have medication-induced cognitive dysfunction, sometimes involving BZDs.[64] Other cognitive side effects of BZDs are drowsiness, fatigue, and sedation. While such symptoms sometimes improve over time, there are numerous problems with cognition possible with BZDs that do not get better with continued use. These include troubles with concentration, learning skills, working memory, verbal and nonverbal memory, problem-solving, sensory processing, motor performance, and others.[1,7,18,59,76,77] It appears that some people are at higher risk than others for BZD-induced neurocognitive disorder. Risk factors include age over 50 years,[3,7,49,76] use of some other substance including alcohol, those with traumatic brain injury, those with neurocognitive deficits, those with primary psychiatric disorders, and those using BZDs for long periods of time.[3] These risks are so pronounced that BZDs are contraindicated for patients with a history of substance use disorder, traumatic brain injury, depression, and neurocognitive deficits. For example, an older patient with Alzheimer's disease would be contraindicated for long-term BZD therapy even if the patient periodically experiences spells of being anxious or agitated. Sometimes people who enter psychotherapy are taking BZDs, and it is generally recommended that BZD therapy stop before commencing psychotherapy because the cognitive effects of BZDs can reduce the effectiveness of psychotherapy.[78,79] BZDs can make it difficult for such psychotherapy patients to understand, process, and remember the materials they work on with their therapists. It has been reported from research that many mental functions including attention, reaction time, and information processing improve when BZDs are discontinued.[64] However, this effect is not immediate, and many cognitive symptoms caused by BZDs may persist even after cessation of the BZDs. This condition is also so prevalent it also has its own name: BZD-induced persisting amnestic disorder.[1,3,7,76]

It can be counterproductive to give BZDs to patients actively struggling with symptoms such as depression, agitation, phobias, and social avoidance, because those are among the very side effects associated with BZD use. Of particular concern is the fact that while BZDs can alleviate anxiety at first, over the course of time, BZDs paradoxically worsen the anxiety. Nicotine has a similar effect; it tends to decrease anxiety at first, only to worsen anxiety over the long term.[80] Opioids likewise have a paradoxical effect in that they tend to relieve pain effectively at first, only to cause increased pain with long-term use.[81,82]

BZDs are not indicated for depression, may exacerbate the depressive symptoms, promote dysphoria, and have been associated with suicidality.[18,27,43,54,83–85] BZD intoxication as a one-time occurrence or as an ongoing condition has been linked to suicidality as have high doses of prescribed BZDs and underlying depression.[3,49,86] When a clinician treats a patient with comorbid anxiety and depression, there is a risk that the anxiety will mask the depression. Treating the anxiety with BZD may exacerbate the depression. The symptoms of anxiety and depression tend to overlap. For example, here are some symptoms that commonly occur in people with anxiety, depression, or both: negative thought patterns, insomnia, irritability, fatigue, and suicidal thoughts.[17,25,26,87,88] BZDs may reduce anxiety over the short term, but the anxiolytic effects of BZDs decrease as tolerance to the drug builds up, and depressive symptoms may develop or worsen.[18] While use of an SSRI can result in improved depression over time, with BZDs used in patients with depressive symptoms, the opposite is more likely: the longer a BZD is used, the worse the depression gets. This may partially explain why BZDs may be used for generalized anxiety disorder but not PTSD, since generalized anxiety disorder involves only anxiety while PTSD likely involves a depressive component.

The use of BZDs in the treatment of PTSD is particularly disturbing, as BZDs are actually contraindicated for this condition.[89] Impaired sleep is a frequently reported comorbidity with PTSD, and BZDs are considered contraindicated for such long-term treatments as well.[90] This is evidenced in that most clinical practice guidelines do not support the use of BZDs in PTSD.[33,87,91–93] Despite this knowledge, BZDs were prescribed to active-duty service members with a diagnosis of PTSD at rates of 20.9% in 2007, increasing to 22.3% in 2010, and 24.7% in 2013.[94] Among the general population, prescribing rates were similar with 24.4% of patients with primary PTSD prescribed a BZD.[95] The ongoing use of BZD therapy for PTSD may be the result of the erroneous clinical assumption that because BZDs can temporarily reduce anxiety, they are helping the patient with PTSD when, in fact, they are not addressing the underlying pathology (e.g., hypoactivity in the prefrontal cortex and hippocampus) and will eventually exacerbate the anxiety.[27] Indeed, for combat veterans, the use of BZDs is associated with an increased risk of hospitalization and other morbidity.[96] Veterans with PTSD who were prescribed BZD therapy have higher rates of healthcare utilization and are more likely to attempt and commit suicide than similar patients not prescribed BZDs.[97]

Patients may continue to take BZDs even when they cause side effects for several reasons. First, people may be unsure how to assess their symptoms and assume that side effects are just part of their underlying condition. In other words, not all people who take BZDs fully recognize their side effects or even know that BZDs have side effects. Finally, patients may experience withdrawal symptoms when they try to taper or quit BZDs and erroneously assume that withdrawal symptoms are due to their underlying condition and demonstrate that they need the BZDs to feel better. While people often perceive the immediate effect of BZDs on anxiety, they can be much less aware of the slow, progressive decline these drugs can produce in mood, well-being, and anxiousness. BZDs may actually induce anxiety by withdrawal symptoms, causing rebound anxiety, and enhancing the natural fear response.[98–100] In some cases, BZDs can erode the patient's self-confidence and sense of self-efficacy, making patients feel as if they cannot cope with their stress without the aid of BZDs.[101] BZDs in some cases can promote active avoidance of social situations, can thwart normal fear extinction processes, inhibit the healthy cognitive processing of past adversities and trauma, and block the normal desensitization to anxiety that can and should occur in healthy individuals who experience anxiety in their environment or in controlled therapeutic settings.[27,36,44,49,51,53,54] In other words, BZDs can undermine the patient's normal responses and abilities that might otherwise promote mental health and wellness.

The ugly issues of drug misuse, abuse, dependence, and addiction have been somewhat clouded by shifts in terminology. Aberrant drug-taking behaviors include *misuse*, in which drugs are taken in ways other than as prescribed, such as seeking multiple sources of BZDs (e.g., other prescribers), obtaining them illegally (e.g., through theft or the black market), taking prescribed BZDs in higher doses or more frequently than prescribed, or combining BZDs with other substances (including prescribed or illicit drugs, or alcohol) in potentially dangerous ways. *Abuse* refers to continued use despite evidence of harm (e.g., physical or mental adverse effects; legal or social problems; occupational or academic impairment). *Dependence* is the expected effect of prolonged exposure to certain drugs, such as BZDs, that involves tolerance and/or withdrawal symptoms if the drug is discontinued abruptly. This condition is sometimes called physical or physiological dependence. *Addiction* (which is considered a stigmatizing term by some who prefer other terms such as *use disorder*, but is also used by many advocacy groups and treatment modalities) refers to the biopsychosocial phenomenon around compulsive drug use and is characterized by intense cravings for the drug. Individuals who take BZDs over a protracted period of time can become dependent on them.[3]

People with a history of substance use disorder are at higher risk for aberrant drug-taking behaviors and are thus contraindicated for BZD therapy.[14,16] Moreover patients with substance use disorders present with concomitant anxiety rates as high as 33% to 50%.[54,102] These patients may be prescribed BZD to help manage symptoms that may in fact be caused to their substance use, which may delay effective treatment.[14,16,37,49,103] More concerning yet, taking BZDs along with other substances can be dangerous and potentially fatal. People with an active substance use disorder are at elevated risk to misuse BZDs and develop BZD use disorder (BUD). In fact, about half of all patients with an active substance use disorder or a history of substance use disorder will develop BUD if exposed to BZDs.[1] The exception to this is the use of BZDs for managing withdrawal in patients suffering from acute alcohol withdrawal or acute withdrawal from sedative hypnotics, but in those cases, the use of BZDs is not long term but rather is bracketed around the time period of the withdrawal.

Distinguishing BUD from iatrogenic physical dependence without aberrant drug-taking behaviors can lead to confusion. Table 3.3 helps to better define the various BZD-related disorders. Tolerance and withdrawal symptoms are not sufficient by themselves to diagnose BUD.[3] A very large proportion of people prescribed long-term BZD therapy, ranging from 58% to 100%, become physically dependent on the BZDs.[1,7] Other aberrant drug-taking behaviors may occur in individuals with chronic pain or in the elderly who find that tolerance develops over time, requiring them to increase the dose or find a new prescriber to achieve the same results. The latter case can be particularly challenging to diagnose as it may occur without true intention to abuse BZDs and develop slowly, over time, and in a way that may be difficult to distinguish from appropriate use as prescribed.[1] BZD dependence can occur with any BZD description and may occur faster in some patients than others, although it appears to be more likely to occur with higher doses of BZDs and short-acting formulations of BZDs.[1,19,37] Many people taking BZDs long term come to recognize that they cause side effects and worsen anxiety but may continue to take the drugs to prevent unpleasant withdrawal symptoms or because they do not know what else to do.[1] This begins a vicious circle as continuing use of the BZD increases tolerance and may cause the patient to need higher and higher doses of BZDs which then worsen withdrawal symptoms if the BZDs are tapered or even discontinued. In medical terms, BZD tolerance and withdrawal are caused by a chronic long-term desensitization of the GABA receptors and the concomitant hypersensitization of the glutamate receptors. Apart from BZDs, the natural situation in which GABA receptors are hypoactive and glutamate receptors are hyperactive describes physiological anxiety.[1,42] Thus, chronic BZD use enhances the pathophysiology of anxiety rather than relieves it. This also explains why prolonged exposure to BZDs results in paradoxical anxiety, which, unfortunately, is sometimes misinterpreted as a worsening of the underlying anxiety disorder, which, in turn, can cause the patient and prescriber to increase the BZD dose.

In general, one could sketch out four thumbnail portraits of typical chronic BZD patients:

- Older patients with (multiple) diagnosed medical illnesses, who are taking many medications, including BZDs. Among these patients, BZDs are rarely prescribed by psychiatrists.
- Patients of all ages who are diagnosed with panic disorder or agoraphobia.
- Patients of all ages with chronic symptoms of dysphoria and vague symptoms of malaise and depression.
- Patients with chronic insomnia.

With these four thumbnail sketches of BZD patients, it can be said that the latter two groups are more likely to misuse BZDs, such as taking them with alcohol or taking them in ways other than prescribed, compared to the first two groups.[38] A wide range of risk factors have been defined that can make a person vulnerable to BUD. (See Table 3.4.)

Table 3.3 BZD DISORDERS AS DEFINED MEDICALLY

	BZD Use Disorder	BZD Intoxication	BZD Withdrawal
Onset/duration	At least 2 of the signs or symptoms below within a 12-month period	Onset during or shortly after taking BZD	Onset following taper or discontinuation of BZD after a prolonged period of use
Definition	At least 2 of the following items	Clinically significant maladaptive behaviors, impaired judgment, inappropriate behaviors and at least one of the items below	Clinically significant impairment or distress in function in the social, occupational settings or in other areas important to the patient and at least one of the items below
Signs/Symptoms	Use of higher doses or over a longer time than originally intended Desire to reduce use Spending a lot of time obtaining BZDs Cravings for BZDs Failure to fulfill important obligations or social roles Continuing use despite interpersonal problems and social problems caused by BZD use Giving up or cutting back on activities once important to the patient Use of BZDs even in physically hazardous situations Use of BZDs in spite of physical and/or psychological problems Tolerance Withdrawal symptoms	Slurred speech Lack of coordination Unsteady gait Nystagmus Cognitive deficits, such as attention problems or memory loss Stupor or coma	Autonomic hyperactivity, such as profuse sweating or tachycardia Hand tremors Insomnia Nausea and/or vomiting Transient visual, tactile, or auditory hallucinations or illusions Psychomotor agitation Anxiety Grand mal seizures

Note: These categories may overlap somewhat.[3] BZDs = benzodiazepines.

Table 3.4 SOME OF THE RISK FACTORS FOR BENZODIAZEPINE USE DISORDER

Risk Factor	Considerations	Is BZD Use Appropriate?	Comments
Active or recent substance use disorder	Particularly other central nervous system depressants such as opioids, alcohol, marijuana	BZDs may be indicated short term to help with alcohol or opioid withdrawal	Polydrug abuse is very common among those with substance use disorder
Family history of substance use disorder	This describes substance use disorder in a parent or sibling	No	This is also a risk factor for other drugs and alcohol use disorder
Chronic pain and/or chronic medical conditions	These are persistent conditions for which the patient may have little relief	No but people with chronic conditions may have anxiety or insomnia	BZDs do not treat pain or chronic conditions but mental health disorders are often comorbid with chronic pain
Chronic insomnia	Insomnia is often persistent and BZDs are useful only for short-term treatment of acute insomnia	Insomnia is an indication for BZDs or the so-called Z-drugs	Insomnia is often comorbid with mental health disorders
Chronic dysphoria	An inability to feel pleasure or take ordinary enjoyment out of life	No, but such patients may express anxiety or have insomnia	
Impulsivity	This condition is associated with many types of risk-taking behaviors, including substance use	No	Impulsivity may be comorbid with mental health disorders
Personality disorders	Borderline personality disorder and dependent personality disorders are particularly associated with BZD use	No, although sometimes prescribed off-label	Personality disorders may have a component of anxiety or insomnia

Notes: BZD = benzodiazepine.
Sources: Ashton,[1] American Psychiatric Association,[3] Pary and Lewis,[7] Mohamed and Rosenheck,[14] Harpaz-Rotem,[16] Michelini,[18] Salzman et al.,[35] Kaufmann et al.,[38] and Hawkins et al.[49]

Note that risk factors do not automatically mean a person will develop BUD, even if prescribed a BZD. Conversely, people with none of these risk factors can develop BUD.

Street or illicit BZDs are available and are typically sold to individuals who seek the drugs for recreational purposes because BZDs possess both psychoactive effects and may enhance or potentiate the effects of other drugs.[1,3] In fact, about 80% of the people who buy illicit BZDs use them with other substances.[1] BZDs are thought to enhance or boost intoxication of CNS depressants such as opioids, marijuana, and alcohol.[4] Combining CNS depressants elevates the risk of a potentially life-threatening respiratory depression.[3] Alcohol may be of particular risk to BZD users as its dangers when used concomitantly with BZDs are not well recognized, even by providers, and may be trivialized by recreational users.[3,4] Illicit BZDs are also sometimes used by substance users trying to self-medicate opioid withdrawal or alcohol withdrawal, and they are also sometimes used by people who abuse stimulants to help ease transitions from highs to lows.[1,3] The combination of stimulants such as amphetamines or cocaine to induce wakeful activity followed by BZDs to bring on sleep can cause unpredictable alterations in behavior, cognitive deficits, and memory loss.[4] It should be noted that purely recreational users of BZDs often prefer to insufflate or "snort" BZDs or inject it intravenously.[1,3] Intravenous drug use is associated with its own risks, such as infections, which exceed the scope of this chapter. It should be noted that polydrug abuse, that is, combining BZDs with other drugs or alcohol, non-oral use of BZDs, and taking BZDs in ways other than as prescribed all increase the risk of toxicity.

Unlike with many other drugs, there are no clandestine labs that manufacture illicit or street BZDs. When BZDs are obtained from street dealers or when they are described as illicit, it is because prescription products were diverted to street trade. Because BZDs are only manufactured by pharmaceutical companies and prescribed to patients, BUD is commonly iatrogenic and the result of overprescribing.[1] In most communities, the prevalence of BUD will correlate with its medical availability.[4] Sources for BZDs include legitimate prescriptions, inappropriate or stolen prescriptions, friends, theft, online sources, and street dealers.

CONCLUSION

For most psychiatric disorders, there is little or no hard evidence to support the effectiveness of BZDs. For evidence-based indications such as panic disorder, generalized anxiety disorder, and insomnia, BZDs can offer rapid anxiolysis and rapid sedation but they should be reserved for treatment-resistant cases and limited to short-term use. Indeed, these drugs are being used chronically with very little supporting evidence for their long-term efficacy and disturbing observations about their long-term safety. BZDs should only be prescribed when the patient is fully informed that these drugs are habit forming and that they are associated with numerous risks and side effects, including suicidality and dementia. Patients should also be informed not only that long-term use of BZDs can result in dependence and withdrawal symptoms but also that BZDs over a prolonged exposure may actually worsen symptoms like anxiety and sleeplessness. BZDs should only be prescribed with a clear and defined exit plan so that the patient never expects their chronic use. That being said, there may be times when BZDs are appropriate, but they should be administered only at the lowest effective dose for the shortest period of time possible. The longer the course of BZD treatment, the greater the risks to the patient. The addictive potential of BZDs must be better appreciated by providers and patients. There are alternative drugs to BZDs with higher therapeutic efficacy and substantially lower risk. Indeed, BZDs are not first-line therapy for any condition—except for alcohol or BZD withdrawal—and are best used in specific settings requiring acute remedy for a specific and well-defined short duration of time.

REFERENCES

1. Ashton H. The diagnosis and management of benzodiazepine dependence. *Curr Opin Psychiatry.* 2005;18(3):249–255.
2. Bushnell GA, Sturmer T, Gaynes BN, Pate V, Miller M. Simultaneous antidepressant and benzodiazepine new use and subsequent long-term benzodiazepine use in adults with depression, United States, 2001–2014. *JAMA Psychiatry.* 2017;74(7):747–755.
3. American Psychiatric Association. *Diagnostic and Statistical Manual of Mental Disorders.* 5th ed. Arlington, VA: American Psychiatric Association; 2013.
4. Wesson D, Smith D, Ling W, Sabnani S. Substance abuse: sedative, hypnotic, or anxiolytic use disorders. In: Tasman A, Kay J, Liberman J, eds. *Psychiatry.* Vol 1. Chichester, England: Wiley; 2008:1186–1200.
5. Friedman MJ. Biological approaches to the diagnosis and treatment of Post-Traumatic Stress Disorder. *J Trauma Stress.* 1991;4(1):67–91.
6. Maramai S, Benchekroun M, Ward SE, Atack JR. Subtype selective gamma-aminobutyric acid type a receptor (GABAAR) modulators acting at the benzodiazepine binding site: an update. *J Med Chem.* 2020;63(7):3425–3446.
7. Pary R, Lewis S. Prescribing benzodiazepines in clinical practice. *Resident Staff Physician.* 2008;54(1):8–17.
8. Geuze E, van Berckel BN, Lammertsma AA, et al. Reduced GABAA benzodiazepine receptor binding in veterans with post-traumatic stress disorder. *Mol Psychiatry.* 2008;13(1):74–83.
9. Bremner JD, Innis RB, Southwick SM, Staib L, Zoghbi S, Charney DS. Decreased benzodiazepine receptor binding in prefrontal cortex in combat-related posttraumatic stress disorder. *Am J Psychiatry.* 2000;157(7):1120–1126.
10. Fujita M, Southwick SM, Denucci CC, et al. Central type benzodiazepine receptors in Gulf War veterans with posttraumatic stress disorder. *Biol Psychiatry.* 2004;56(2):95–100.
11. Song Y, Liu J, Ma F, Mao L. Diazepam reduces excitability of amygdala and further influences auditory cortex following sodium salicylate treatment in rats. *Acta Otolaryngol.* 2016;136(12):1220–1224.
12. Olfson M, King M, Schoenbaum M. Benzodiazepine use in the United States. *JAMA Psychiatry.* 2015;72(2):136–142.
13. Guina J, Merrill B. Benzodiazepines I: upping the care on downers: the evidence of risks, benefits and alternatives. *J Clin Med.* 2018;7(2):17.
14. Mohamed S, Rosenheck RA. Pharmacotherapy of PTSD in the U.S. Department of Veterans Affairs: diagnostic- and symptom-guided drug selection. *J Clin Psychiatry.* 2008;69(6):959–965.

15. Abrams TE, Lund BC, Bernardy NC, Friedman MJ. Aligning clinical practice to PTSD treatment guidelines: medication prescribing by provider type. *Psychiatr Serv.* 2013;64(2):142–148.

16. Harpaz-Rotem I, Rosenheck RA, Mohamed S, Desai RA. Pharmacologic treatment of posttraumatic stress disorder among privately insured Americans. *Psychiatr Serv.* 2008;59(10):1184–1190.

17. Bourin M, Lambert O. Pharmacotherapy of anxious disorders. *Hum Psychopharmacology.* 2002;17(8):383–400.

18. Michelini S, Cassano GB, Frare F, Perugi G. Long-term use of benzodiazepines: tolerance, dependence and clinical problems in anxiety and mood disorders. *Pharmacopsychiatry.* 1996;29(4):127–134.

19. Bastien DL. Pharmacological treatment of combat-induced PTSD: a literature review. *Br J Nurs.* 2010;19(5):318–321.

20. Hoffman EJ, Mathew SJ. Anxiety disorders: a comprehensive review of pharmacotherapies. *Mt Sinai J Med.* 2008;75(3):248–262.

21. van Dijk KN, de Vries CS, ter Huurne K, van den Berg PB, Brouwers JR, de Jong-van den Berg LT. Concomitant prescribing of benzodiazepines during antidepressant therapy in the elderly. *J Clin Epidemiol.* 2002;55(10):1049–1053.

22. Bourin M, Lambert O. Pharmacotherapy of anxious disorders. *Hum Psychopharmacology.* 2002;17(8):383–400.

23. Sateia MJ, Buysse DJ, Krystal AD, Neubauer DN, Heald JL. Clinical practice guideline for the pharmacologic treatment of chronic insomnia in adults: an American Academy of Sleep Medicine clinical practice guideline. *J Clin Sleep Med.* 2017;13(2):307–349.

24. Spaulding AM. A pharmacotherapeutic approach to the management of chronic posttraumatic stress disorder. *J Pharm Pract.* 2012;25(5):541–551.

25. Ravindran LN, Stein MB. Pharmacotherapy of PTSD: premises, principles, and priorities. *Brain Res.* 2009;1293:24–39.

26. Jeffreys M, Capehart B, Friedman MJ. Pharmacotherapy for posttraumatic stress disorder: review with clinical applications. *J Rehabil Res Dev.* 2012;49(5):703–715.

27. National Institute for Health and Care Excellence. Generalised anxiety disorder and panic disorder in adults: management. https://www.nice.org.uk/guidance/cg113/chapter/1-Guidance#principles-of-care-for-people-with-generalised-anxiety-disorder-gad. Published 2011. Updated July 2019. Accessed July 30, 2019.

28. Asnis GM, Kohn SR, Henderson M, Brown NL. SSRIs versus non-SSRIs in post-traumatic stress disorder: an update with recommendations. *Drugs.* 2004;64(4):383–404.

29. Berger W, Mendlowicz MV, Marques-Portella C, et al. Pharmacologic alternatives to antidepressants in posttraumatic stress disorder: a systematic review. *Prog Neuropsychopharmacol Biol Psychiatry.* 2009;33(2):169–180.

30. Tasman A, Kay J, Lieberman J. *Psychiatry.* Vol 1. 3rd ed. Chichester, England: Wiley; 2008.

31. American Psychological Association. Clinical practice guideline for the treatment of posttraumatic stress disorder (PTSD). *American Psychological Association.* https://www.apa.org/ptsd-guideline/ptsd.pdf. Published 2017. Accessed November 20, 2019.

32. American Psychological Association. Practice guideline for the treatment of patients with acute stress disorder and posttraumatic stress disorder. https://psychiatryonline.org/pb/assets/raw/sitewide/practice_guidelines/guidelines/acutestressdisorderptsd.pdf. Published 2004. Updated March 2009. Accessed November 20, 2019.

33. Department of Veterans Affairs. VA/DOD clinical practice guideline for the management of posttraumatic stress disorder and acute stress disorder. https://www.healthquality.va.gov/guidelines/MH/ptsd/VADoDPTSDCPGFinal012418.pdf. Published 2017. Accessed November 20, 2019.

34. Rickels K. Use of antianxiety agents in anxious outpatients. *Psychopharmacology.* 1978;*58*(1):1–17.
35. Salzman C. The APA Task Force report on benzodiazepine dependence, toxicity, and abuse. *Am J Psychiatry.* 1991;*148*(2):151–152.
36. Lund BC, Bernardy NC, Alexander B, Friedman MJ. Declining benzodiazepine use in veterans with posttraumatic stress disorder. *J Clin Psychiatry.* 2012;*73*(3):292–296.
37. Bernardy NC, Lund BC, Alexander B, Friedman MJ. Prescribing trends in veterans with posttraumatic stress disorder. *J Clin Psychiatry.* 2012;*73*(3):297–303.
38. Lund BC, Bernardy NC, Vaughan-Sarrazin M, Alexander B, Friedman MJ. Patient and facility characteristics associated with benzodiazepine prescribing for veterans with PTSD. *Psychiatr Serv.* 2013;*64*(2):149–155.
39. Kaufmann CN, Spira AP, Depp CA, Mojtabai R. Long-term use of benzodiazepines and nonbenzodiazepine hypnotics, 1999–2014. *Psychiatr Serv.* 2018;*69*(2):235–238.
40. Guina J, Merrill B. Benzodiazepines II: waking up on sedatives: providing optimal care when inheriting benzodiazepine prescriptions in transfer patients. *J Clin Med.* 2018;*7*(2):E20.
41. Allison C, Pratt JA. Neuroadaptive processes in GABAergic and glutamatergic systems in benzodiazepine dependence. *Pharmacol Ther.* 2003;*98*(2):171–195.
42. Morissette SB, Tull MT, Gulliver SB, Kamholz BW, Zimering RT. Anxiety, anxiety disorders, tobacco use, and nicotine: a critical review of interrelationships. *Psychol Bull.* 2007;*133*(2):245–272.
43. Lydiard RB, Brawman-Mintzer O, Ballenger JC. Recent developments in the psychopharmacology of anxiety disorders. *J Consult Clin Psychol.* 1996;*64*(4):660–668.
44. Dunlop BW, Davis PG. Combination treatment with benzodiazepines and SSRIs for comorbid anxiety and depression: a review. *Prim Care Companion J Clin Psychiatry.* 2008;*10*(3):222–228.
45. Fava M, Rush AJ, Alpert JE, et al. Difference in treatment outcome in outpatients with anxious versus nonanxious depression: a STAR*D report. *Am J Psychiatry.* 2008;*165*(3):342–351.
46. Bandelow B, Zohar J, Hollander E, et al. World Federation of Societies of Biological Psychiatry (WFSBP) guidelines for the pharmacological treatment of anxiety, obsessive-compulsive and post-traumatic stress disorders: first revision. *World J Bio Psychiatry.* 2008;*9*(4):248–312.
47. Riemann D, Baglioni C, Bassetti C, et al. European guideline for the diagnosis and treatment of insomnia. *J Sleep Res.* 2017;*26*(6):675–700.
48. Remi J, Pollmacher T, Spiegelhalder K, Trenkwalder C, Young P. Sleep-related disorders in neurology and psychiatry. *Dtsch Arztebl Int.* 2019;*116*(41):681–688.
49. Hawkins EJ, Malte CA, Imel ZE, Saxon AJ, Kivlahan DR. Prevalence and trends of benzodiazepine use among Veterans Affairs patients with posttraumatic stress disorder, 2003–2010. *Drug Alcohol Depend.* 2012;*124*(1-2):154–161.
50. Kosten TR, Fontana A, Sernyak MJ, Rosenheck R. Benzodiazepine use in posttraumatic stress disorder among veterans with substance abuse. *J Nerv Ment Dis.* 2000;*188*(7):454–459.
51. Sansone RA, Hruschka J, Vasudevan A, Miller SN. Benzodiazepine exposure and history of trauma. *Psychosomatics.* 2003;*44*(6):523–524.
52. Hermos JA, Young MM, Lawler EV, Rosenbloom D, Fiore LD. Long-term, high-dose benzodiazepine prescriptions in veteran patients with PTSD: influence of preexisting alcoholism and drug-abuse diagnoses. *J Trauma Stress.* 2007;*20*(5):909–914.
53. Matar MA, Zohar J, Kaplan Z, Cohen H. Alprazolam treatment immediately after stress exposure interferes with the normal HPA-stress response and increases vulnerability to subsequent stress in an animal model of PTSD. *Eur Neuropsychopharmacol.* 2009;*19*(4):283–295.

54. Wilhelm FH, Roth WT. Acute and delayed effects of alprazolam on flight phobics during exposure. *Behav Res Ther.* 1997;35(9):831–841.

55. King G, Scott E, Graham BM, Richardson R. Individual differences in fear extinction and anxiety-like behavior. *Learn Mem.* 2017;24(5):182–190.

56. Hart G, Holmes NM, Harris JA, Westbrook RF. Benzodiazepine administration prevents the use of error-correction mechanisms during fear extinction. *Learn Behav.* 2014;42(4):383–397.

57. Grant BF, Stinson FS, Dawson DA, et al. Prevalence and co-occurrence of substance use disorders and independent mood and anxiety disorders: results from the National Epidemiologic Survey on Alcohol and Related Conditions. *Arch Gen Psychiatry.* 2004;61(8):807–816.

58. Ku SC, Ho PS, Tseng YT, Yeh TC, Cheng SL, Liang CS. Benzodiazepine-associated carcinogenesis: focus on lorazepam-associated cancer biomarker changes in overweight individuals. *Psychiatry Investig.* 2018;15(9):900–906.

59. Lader MH. Limitations on the use of benzodiazepines in anxiety and insomnia: are they justified? *Eur Neuropsychopharmacol.* 1999;9(Suppl 6):S399–S405.

60. Brandt J, Leong C. Benzodiazepines and Z-drugs: an updated review of major adverse outcomes reported on in epidemiologic research. *Drugs R D.* 2017;17(4):493–507.

61. Benard-Laribiere A, Noize P, Pambrun E, et al. Comorbidities and concurrent medications increasing the risk of adverse drug reactions: prevalence in French benzodiazepine users. *Eur J Clin Pharmacol.* 2016;72(7):869–876.

62. Palmaro A, Dupouy J, Lapeyre-Mestre M. Benzodiazepines and risk of death: results from two large cohort studies in France and UK. *Eur Neuropsychopharmacol.* 2015;25(10):1566–1577.

63. Nakafero G, Sanders RD, Nguyen-Van-Tam JS, Myles PR. Association between benzodiazepine use and exacerbations and mortality in patients with asthma: a matched case-control and survival analysis using the United Kingdom Clinical Practice Research Datalink. *Pharmacoepidemiol Drug Saf.* 2015;24(8):793–802.

64. Curran HV, Collins R, Fletcher S, Kee SC, Woods B, Iliffe S. Older adults and withdrawal from benzodiazepine hypnotics in general practice: effects on cognitive function, sleep, mood and quality of life. *Psychol Med.* 2003;33(7):1223–1237.

65. Puustinen J, Lahteenmaki R, Polo-Kantola P, et al. Effect of withdrawal from long-term use of temazepam, zopiclone or zolpidem as hypnotic agents on cognition in older adults. *Eur J Clin Pharmacol.* 2014;70(3):319–329.

66. Andrade C. Gestational exposure to benzodiazepines, 3: clobazam and major congenital malformations. *J Clin Psychiatry.* 2019;80(6):19f13151.

67. Yonkers KA, Wisner KL, Stewart DE, et al. The management of depression during pregnancy: a report from the American Psychiatric Association and the American College of Obstetricians and Gynecologists. *Obstet Gynecol.* 2009;114(3):703–713.

68. Sundbakk LM, Wood M, Gran JM, Nordeng H. Impact of prenatal exposure to benzodiazepines and z-hypnotics on behavioral problems at 5 years of age: a study from the Norwegian Mother and Child Cohort Study. *PloS One.* 2019;14(6):e0217830–e0217830.

69. Wikner BN, Stiller CO, Bergman U, Asker C, Kallen B. Use of benzodiazepines and benzodiazepine receptor agonists during pregnancy: neonatal outcome and congenital malformations. *Pharmacoepidemiol Drug Saf.* 2007;16(11):1203–1210.

70. Wikner BN, Stiller CO, Kallen B, Asker C. Use of benzodiazepines and benzodiazepine receptor agonists during pregnancy: maternal characteristics. *Pharmacoepidemiol Drug Saf.* 2007;16(9):988–994.

71. Tinker SC, Reefhuis J, Bitsko RH, et al. Use of benzodiazepine medications during pregnancy and potential risk for birth defects, National Birth Defects Prevention Study, 1997–2011. *Birth Defects Res.* 2019;111(10):613–620.

72. Gonzalez de Dios J, Moya-Benavent M, Carratala-Marco F. ["Floppy infant" syndrome in twins secondary to the use of benzodiazepines during pregnancy]. *Rev Neurol.* 1999;29(2):121–123.

73. Wikner BN, Kallen B. Are hypnotic benzodiazepine receptor agonists teratogenic in humans? *J Clin Psychopharmacol.* 2011;31(3):356–359.

74. Beauchamp GA, Hendrickson RG, Horowitz BZ, Spyker DA. Exposures through breast milk: an analysis of exposure and information calls to U.S. Poison Centers, 2001–2017. *Breastfeed Med.* 2019;14(7):508–512.

75. Kelly LE, Poon S, Madadi P, Koren G. Neonatal benzodiazepines exposure during breastfeeding. *J Pediatr.* 2012;161(3):448–451.

76. Barker MJ, Greenwood KM, Jackson M, Crowe SF. Cognitive effects of long-term benzodiazepine use: a meta-analysis. *CNS Drugs.* 2004;18(1):37–48.

77. Poyares D, Guilleminault C, Ohayon MM, Tufik S. Chronic benzodiazepine usage and withdrawal in insomnia patients. *J Psychiatr Res.* 2004;38(3):327–334.

78. O'Connor K, Marchand A, Brousseau L, et al. Cognitive-behavioural, pharmacological and psychosocial predictors of outcome during tapered discontinuation of benzodiazepine. *Clin Psychol Psychother.* 2008;15(1):1–14.

79. Otto MW, Bruce SE, Deckersbach T. Benzodiazepine use, cognitive impairment, and cognitive-behavioral therapy for anxiety disorders: issues in the treatment of a patient in need. *J Clin Psychiatry.* 2005;66(Suppl 2):34–38.

80. West R, Hajek P. What happens to anxiety levels on giving up smoking? *Am J Psychiatry.* 1997;154(11):1589–1592.

81. Weber L, Yeomans DC, Tzabazis A. Opioid-induced hyperalgesia in clinical anesthesia practice: what has remained from theoretical concepts and experimental studies? *Curr Opin Anaesthesiol.* 2017;30(4):458–465.

82. Yi P, Pryzbylkowski P. Opioid Induced Hyperalgesia. *Pain Med (Malden, Mass).* 2015;16(Suppl 1):S32–S36.

83. Mellman TA, Byers PM, Augenstein JS. Pilot evaluation of hypnotic medication during acute traumatic stress response. *J Trauma Stress.* 1998;11(3):563–569.

84. Ader R. Psychoneuroimmunology. *Ilar J.* 1998;39(1):27–29.

85. Pfeiffer PN, Ganoczy D, Ilgen M, Zivin K, Valenstein M. Comorbid anxiety as a suicide risk factor among depressed veterans. *Depress Anxiety.* 2009;26(8):752–757.

86. Longo L, Johnson B. Addiction: Part I. Benzodiazepines—side effects, abuse risk, and alternatives. *Am Fam Physicians.* 2000;61(7):2121–2128.

87. Ballenger JC, Davidson JR, Lecrubier Y, et al. Consensus statement update on posttraumatic stress disorder from the international consensus group on depression and anxiety. *J Clin Psychiatry.* 2004;65(Suppl 1):55–62.

88. Jacobsen LK, Southwick SM, Kosten TR. Substance use disorders in patients with posttraumatic stress disorder: a review of the literature. *Am J Psychiatry.* 2001;158(8):1184–1190.

89. Guina J, Rossetter SR, De RB, Nahhas RW, Welton RS. Benzodiazepines for PTSD: a systematic review and meta-analysis. *J Psychiatr Pract.* 2015;21(4):281–303.

90. Lipinska G, Baldwin DS, Thomas KG. Pharmacology for sleep disturbance in PTSD. *Hum Psychopharmacology.* 2016;31(2):156–163.

91. Berger MJ, Ettinger DS, Aston J, et al. NCCN guidelines insights: antiemesis, version 2.2017. *JNCCN.* 2017;15(7):883–893.

92. Forbes D, Creamer M, Bisson JI, et al. A guide to guidelines for the treatment of PTSD and related conditions. *J Trauma Stress.* 2010;23(5):537–552.

93. Guina J, Nahhas RW, Welton RS. No role for benzodiazepines in posttraumatic stress disorder until supported by evidence. *Australas Psychiatry.* 2017;25(4):415–416.

94. Loeffler G, Coller R, Tracy L, Derderian BR. Prescribing trends in US active duty service members with posttraumatic stress disorder: a population-based study from 2007–2013. *J Clin Psychiatry.* 2018;79(4):17m11667.

95. Nobles CJ, Valentine SE, Zepeda ED, Ahles EM, Shtasel DL, Marques L. Usual course of treatment and predictors of treatment utilization for patients with posttraumatic stress disorder. *J Clin Psychiatry.* 2017;78(5):e559–e566.

96. Lee S, Heesch C, Allison K, Binns L, Straw-Wilson K, Wendel CS. Hospitalization risk with benzodiazepine and opioid use in veterans with posttraumatic stress disorder. *Fed Pract.* 2017;34(Suppl 2):S26–S33.

97. Deka R, Bryan CJ, LaFleur J, Oderda G, Atherton A, Stevens V. Benzodiazepines, health care utilization, and suicidal behavior in veterans with posttraumatic stress disorder. *J Clin Psychiatry.* 2018;79(6):17m12038.

98. Li S, Murakami Y, Wang M, Maeda K, Matsumoto K. The effects of chronic valproate and diazepam in a mouse model of posttraumatic stress disorder. *Pharmacol Biochem Behav.* 2006;85(2):324–331.

99. Gelpin E, Bonne O, Peri T, Brandes D, Shalev AY. Treatment of recent trauma survivors with benzodiazepines: a prospective study. *J Clin Psychiatry.* 1996;57(9):390–394.

100. van Minnen A, Arntz A, Keijsers GP. Prolonged exposure in patients with chronic PTSD: predictors of treatment outcome and dropout. *Behav Res Ther.* 2002;40(4):439–457.

101. Bandelow B, Reitt M, Rover C, Michaelis S, Gorlich Y, Wedekind D. Efficacy of treatments for anxiety disorders: a meta-analysis. *Int Clin Psychopharmacology.* 2015;30(4):183–192.

102. Cifu DX, Taylor BC, Carne WF, et al. Traumatic brain injury, posttraumatic stress disorder, and pain diagnoses in OIF/OEF/OND veterans. *J Rehabil Res Dev.* 2013;50(9):1169–1176.

103. Fossey MD, Hamner MB. Clonazepam-related sexual dysfunction in male veterans with PTSD. *Anxiety.* 1994;1(5):233–236.

CHAPTER 4

Use of Benzodiazepines and Z-Drugs in the Geriatric Population

JAN M. KITZEN

HIGHLIGHTS

- From 1999 to 2016, benzodiazepine-related overdose mortality increased from 0.6/100,000 adults to 4.4/100,000 adults.
- The long-term use of benzodiazepines increased steadily with age from a rate of 14.7% among young adults between the ages 18 to 35 to 31.4% in adults between the ages 65 and 80.
- Several physiological changes associated with the aging process such as decreases in renal and hepatic function, altered CNS function and changes in body composition can lead to impaired excretion of drug, higher plasma levels and accumulation of these drugs in the body. These age-related changes make the elderly population more sensitive to the effects of many drugs, especially anxiolytic and sedative-hypnotic drugs.
- The American Geriatrics Society has developed a set of guidelines known as the AGS Beers Criteria' for potentially inappropriate medication in the elderly. The use of all benzodiazepines and Z-drugs (zolpidem, zaleplon and eszopiclone) are not recommended for use in persons ≥ 65 years of age, except for a few specific conditions.
- Many studies have shown that when benzodiazepines or Z-drugs are used in elderly patients, side effects such as sedation, dizziness, cognitive impairment and diminished control of gait and balance functions place the elderly at greater risk for adverse events, especially falls and fractures that can lead to serious injury or death.
- For the management of anxiety and insomnia in the elderly, several nonpharmacological options are available including cognitive behavioral therapy, relaxation techniques and biofeedback. Alternative pharmacotherapies for insomnia

include low doses of doxepin, mirtazapine, melatonin extended release and the melatonin agonist ramelteon. Anxiety disorders can be managed with selective serotonin norepinephrine reuptake inhibitors such as venlafaxine and duloxetine or the atypical anxiolytic buspirone.

- Some studies have suggested that long-term use of benzodiazepines earlier in life may increase the risk of developing dementia later in life.

INTRODUCTION

There is little doubt that when the benzodiazepines (BZDs) were first introduced into clinical practice in the late 1950s and early 1960s, they represented a milestone breakthrough in the pharmacologic management of certain neuropsychiatric disorders that previously had limited treatment options for physicians. The earlier use of barbiturates as sedatives for management of anxiety disorders was associated with many undesirable effects such as respiratory depression and significant impairment of motor and intellectual skills. These negative actions, along with their abuse potential and potential for causing overdosing death, made them undesirable as their risks far outweighed their advantages.[1] The introduction of meprobamate, the first nonbarbiturate agent for treating anxiety, rapidly became the most popular psychotropic agent in the United States and was widely prescribed by psychiatrists and general practitioners. The overuse of meprobamate soon exposed the addiction potential, and clinicians found that the drug was similar in sedative and addiction potential as the barbiturates and nearly as dangerous in overdose. A few years after the introduction of meprobamate, chemists at Hoffman LaRoche laboratories in Switzerland synthesized two new compounds, chlordiazepoxide and then diazepam.[2] Ironically, early clinical trials with chlordiazepoxide were conducted in a small population of elderly patients at doses that were too high. Results of this trial led the patients to experience sedative effects along with severe ataxia and confused speech, leading the investigators to believe the molecule lacked significant clinical interest. Further clinical trials conducted at lower doses in a broader population of patients found more regularly in clinical psychiatric outpatient treatment showed that chlordiazepoxide was an effective anxiolytic drug with very few adverse effects and little effect on cognitive function. Expanded clinical trials in as many as 16,000 patients showed additional efficacy in the treatment of phobias and obsessive states, such that the Food and Drug administration (FDA) granted market approval in 1960 under the trade name Librium. The enthusiasm for this new class of drugs, the BZDs, was embraced by clinicians and led to further chemical modification by chemists in the pharmaceutical industry to identify more potent compounds with additional pharmacologic properties. The metabolite of chlordiazepoxide, demoxepam, later known as diazepam, was the next major pharmacologic advancement in the BZD family. Diazepam was commercialized in 1963 and given the trade name Valium. Diazepam was more potent than chlordiazepoxide, had a shorter duration of efficacy, and displayed dissociation between its anxiolytic and sedative effects.[2] As research expanded with clinical trials utilizing newly synthesized BZDs during the 1960s, it was soon discovered that they had additional pharmacologic actions including hypnotic, muscle relaxant, and amnesic properties.

The therapeutic impact of the BZDs from 1965 to 1975 was so profound that these drugs became the most widely prescribed in the world, and they had completely replaced the barbiturates and meprobamate in the treatment of anxiety. Between 1965 and 1970, BZD prescriptions increased by 110% versus just 9% for psychotropic drugs as a whole.[2] The use of this new class of psychotropic agents was such that they were consumed on a regular basis by 10% to 20% of adults in Western countries.[2] The medical establishment was so convinced of the safety, efficacy, and low addiction potential of these drugs that it was not until 1963, three years after the FDA approval of chlordiazepoxide, that the first case of BZD physiologic dependence was recognized.[2] In the following years, dependence to diazepam was identified, and by the 1970s their popularity began to decline in the United Kingdom and in the United States, the FDA included BZDs on its list of controlled substances (C-IV), and shortly thereafter the World Health Organization recognized that the BZDs were "clearly capable of creating a state of dependence and central nervous system (CNS) depression leading to disruptions in motor function, behavior and personality" (pp. 558–559).[2] Over the ensuing years, increased controls over these drugs made them subject to the same control measures as other drugs including opiates, barbiturates, and amphetamines. Today, many states have implemented prescription drug monitoring programs to track the use of these drugs by both patients and prescribers.[3] Currently, all 50 states, the District of Columbia, Guam, and Puerto Rico have prescription drug monitoring programs in place and collect data for drugs in schedules II to IV, while some also collect data for schedule V drugs.[4]

Patterns of Prescribing: Overall use of BZDs in the United States

Given that the development, the rise in popularity, and the ultimate recognition of the true hazards associated with the BZDs have been established, it is useful to discuss the prescribing patterns of BZD use as well as morbidity and mortality associated with their use today.

From 1999 through 2016, BZD-related overdose mortality had risen dramatically from 0.6/100,000 adults to 4.4/100,000.[5] Benzodiazepine use is also associated with emergency department visits and falls and fractures, as well as motor vehicle crashes and cognitive impairment.[5] In 2008, there were approximately 272,000 emergency department visits in the United States involving nonmedical use of BZDs, and 40% of this involved concomitant use of alcohol. This figure increased to 426,000 visits in 2011 with a somewhat lower (26.4%) association with the use of alcohol. Benzodiazepine use has also been found to affect other aspects of daily life such as mobility disability (defined as the inability to walk half a mile or climb stairs without assistance) and impairment in several activities of daily living including the inability to perform such activities as dressing, bathing, eating, toileting, and the ability to transfer from a bed to a chair.[6]

In a study conducted by Olfson et al. that utilized data from the IMS Health database (currently IQVIA), results showed a steady progressive increase in BZD use between

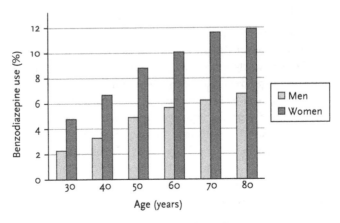

Figure 4.1 Percentage of 2008 US population using any benzodiazepine.
Adapted from Olfson et al.[7]

the ages of 18 and 80 in 2008.[7] The IMS study population received approximately 46.9 million prescriptions, which corresponded to about 75 million for the national population. For women, less than 2% of the population of 18-year-olds received BZDs, and, as shown in Figure 4.1, the percentage increased progressively in each age group with the highest usage rate at 11.9% in 80-year-old women. The usage rate was lower in men, beginning at <1% in 18-year-old males and peaked at approximately 6% to 7% in males between 60 and 80 years of age.

Other findings from this study showed that long-term use, defined as filling prescriptions for at least a 120 day supply, steadily increased with age from a rate of 14.7% among young adults between the ages of 18 and 35 to 31.4% in both men and women between the ages of 65 and 80. In all age and sex groups, fewer than 1 in 10 individuals using long-acting BZDs received a prescription from a psychiatrist. In an analysis that examined outpatient BZD prescribing patterns by medical specialty, Agarwal et al. utilized data obtained from the National Ambulatory Medical Care survey from January 1, 2003 through December 31, 2015.[5] Patient visits were divided into four categories of medical practice: (i) primary care physicians, consisting of those physicians involved in family medicine, internal medicine, geriatric medicine and obstetrics and gynecology; (ii) surgical specialties; (iii) psychiatry; and (iv) medical specialties. Results showed that nearly one-half of all visits to these four medical providers where a BZD was prescribed were by primary care providers: from 51.4% in 2003 to 47.7% in 2015. BZD-related visits by medical specialty are shown in Figure 4.2.

As shown in Figure 4.2, primary care providers were responsible for most of the prescriptions written for as many as 12 different BZDs.[5] The most common indication for these visits was anxiety and depression, which accounted for 26.6% of the total visits for 2003 and increased to 33.5% of visits in 2015. The other indications for BZD prescriptions included insomnia (26.9% and 25.5% for 2003 and 2015, respectively) and various neurologic reasons including headache, seizures, vertigo, and movement

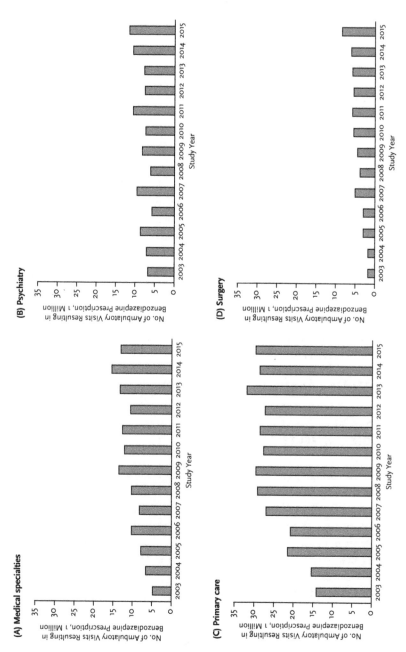

Figure 4.2 Benzodiazepine-related physician visits by medical discipline from 2003–2015. Note that primary care physicians prescribed BZDs far more frequently than physicians in other types of medical practices.
From Agarwal and Landon.[5]

disorders. The visit rate increases between 2003 and 2015 were statistically significant for all indications except for insomnia.

Although this study did not stratify BZD visits by age, the increases in prescribing over the time period of the study and the data provided by the Olfson study suggests that the trends observed here are likely applicable to the elderly, where BZD prescriptions showed an age-related increase in 2008, as shown in Figure 4.1.[7]

The increases in BZD prescribing are likely related to increases in adverse events and overdose mortality, since the increases in the number of BZD visits is indicative of an increasing total number of individuals receiving BZDs both for short-term and chronic use.

Overview of Statistics of Prescribing and Prevalence of Falls

Despite the extensive literature devoted to studying the role of BZDs and other psychotropic drugs and the risk of drug-related falls in the elderly that date back nearly three decades,[8,9] the rate of prescriptions filled for this segment of the population appears to continue at a high rate. In a study from 2015, Olfson et al. found that BZDs were prescribed at a rate of 8.7% to US adults aged 65 to 80 years over the course of one year (2008).[7] A more recent analysis of prescribing patterns conducted by Maust et al showed that during the period from 2007 to 2010 the rate of new BZD visits was relatively constant across age groups; however, the rate of continuation visits increased markedly with age from 61.7/1,000 persons in those aged 18 to 34 to 463.7/1,000 persons in those aged 80 years and older.[10] These prescribing rates all occurred prior to the first publication of the AGS Beers Criteria* in 2011 and the publication of the American Geriatrics Society and British Geriatrics Society recommendations, Clinical Guidelines for Prevention of Falls in Older Persons, in 2011.[11]

PHYSIOLOGICAL EFFECTS OF AGING

The aging process itself predisposes individuals to increased vulnerability to physical environmental challenges. Therefore, it is useful to consider the many biochemical and physiological changes related to the aging process, as many of these changes directly affect how elderly patients respond to drug therapy. Because the amount of information on geriatric physiology is beyond the scope of this chapter, only those systems that are related to drug metabolism or relevant to adverse events will be described. Some of the key age-related changes in physiologic function are summarized in Table 4.1, along with effects on drug action and expected possible adverse events.

Definition of Aging

The aging process can be defined in several ways; two of the more useful definitions that are relevant to drugs include incorporating the concepts of progressive functional

Table 4.1 AGE-RELATED CHANGES IN VARIOUS ORGAN SYSTEMS AND PHYSIOLOGICAL/PHARMACOLOGICAL CONSEQUENCES

Organ system	Change	Result	Effect of Drug	Possible Adverse Event
Kidney	↓ Renal mass, glomeruli ↓ GFR[16]	Prolonged half-life of drugs cleared by filtration	↓Drug excretion	↑ Risk of drug interaction; prolonged drug actions
Gastrointestinal	↓Esophageal and intestinal motility[16,19]	Difficulty swallowing solid dosage forms	Variable effects on drug absorption[19]	Constipation Abdominal pain[20,21]
Liver	↓ Hepatic blood flow[14,19] ↓ Hepatic clearance[16,19,22]	↑ In drug half-life ↓Phase I metabolism[14]	↑ Exposure to drugs	↑ Risk of drug interactions; accumulation of drug
Musculoskeletal	↓Lean muscle mass[16] ↓Bone density[16] ↑Adipose tissue[13,16,19]	↑ Volume of distribution ↑ Increased risk of fractures	Prolonged exposure to drugs	Delayed excretion of drug; accumulation in adipose tissue
Plasma	↓Plasma albumin synthesis[14,19]	↓ Decreased protein binding ↑ Free drug concentration	Enhanced response to higher levels of free drug	↑ Sedation ↑ Risk of drug interactions
CNS a) neurotransmitters and receptors b) visual & vestibular function	↓Ach, DA synthesis[27] ↑ Affinity for GABA$_A$ receptor[27,31] Impaired posture and gait[26] Visual impairment[26,27]	Impaired cognitive function Altered quality of sleep[27] ↑ Risk of falls ↓ Visuospatial perception	Enhanced response to BZDs[31,32] ↓ Mobility	Excessive drowsiness[32] Confusion Ataxia ↑ Risk of drug-related falls

Notes: Ach = acetylcholine. BZD = benzodiazepine. DA = dopamine. GABA = gamma amino butyric acid. GFR = glomerular filtration rate.

deterioration and inability to adapt to stress over time. Aging can be defined as the complex multifactorial processes that represent the gradual deterioration in function that occurs after maturity and ultimately leads to disability or death. Another definition of aging identifies it as the inability of the organism to respond to stress and maintain homeostasis when presented with a challenge, thereby decreasing the ability of the organism to survive detrimental changes occurring over time.[12]

The aging process affects many body organ systems and tissues in ways that can affect overall health and also alter responses to various drugs. In general, there is a decrease in lean muscle mass and an increase in adipose tissue. The elderly are generally less physically active than younger people and therefore have a lower energy expenditure that leads to an increase in body weight. There is an impaired ability to absorb micronutrients such as calcium and vitamin D and a decrease in secretion of intrinsic factor leads to impaired absorption of vitamin B_{12}.[13] The decrease in lean muscle mass can lead to increases in the volume of distribution of lipophilic BZDs, causing a prolonged elimination time[14] while decreases in vitamin D and calcium absorption may exacerbate the frail condition and possibly increase the postfall-related injury.

In a recent comprehensive analysis of 4,796 individuals (2,804 women and 1,992 men) obtained from the Osteoarthritis Initiative cohort, the authors assessed physiological aging by evaluating multiple key physiological components. Several hundred variables were used to evaluate physiologic aspects of aging by calculating a composite age using data associated with physical activity, mental health, nutrition, medications, body type, and heart health that were evaluated and used to correlate chronological aging versus physiological aging.[15] Results showed that the rate of physiological aging is not constant throughout chronological age. There is a period of slower aging before the age of 55 followed by more rapid aging between the ages of 55 and 60 years in both men and women. After the age of 60, there is a period of slower aging that increases again at about the age of 70. These findings of irregular rates of physiological aging throughout a person's chronological age may help explain the variability in individuals' response to drugs. Some of the more pertinent age-related physiological changes by specific organ systems are summarized in the following discussion.

Cardiovascular System

The cardiac output decreases linearly with age at about 1% per year after 30 years of age.[16] Cardiac muscle becomes less responsive to both endogenous and exogenous catecholamines.[16] There is a progressive stiffening of the arterial vasculature with age that imposes an increase in the cardiac afterload, making it more difficult for the heart to pump blood to the vasculature. In general, there is a progressive increase in blood pressure after the age of 10, and the elevation with age is more pronounced with systolic blood pressure than diastolic pressure due to the age-related loss in distensibility of the larger arteries, especially the aorta.[17] Although it is clearly important to lower blood pressure in these individuals, some antihypertensives such as the peripheral α1-adrenergic blocking drugs have been shown to increase the risk of falls in the elderly.[16-18]

There is also a progressive increase in atherosclerosis with age, and the incidence of myocardial infarction from coronary artery disease dramatically increases with age. Besides the well-known risk factors of high blood pressure, smoking, and plasma cholesterol, age is the next most important risk factor associated with myocardial infarction.[16]

Genitourinary System: Renal Function

There is a gradual decrease in the volume and weight of the kidneys with aging.[16] These decreases are associated with reduced blood flow to the kidneys at about 1% to 2% per year and a decline in the glomerular filtration rate.[14,16] There is also an age-related decline in the total number of glomeruli per kidney from about 1 million in persons less than 40 years of age to approximately 700,000 per kidney by the age of 65. This results in a decrease in creatinine clearance and can cause a prolongation in the half-life ($t_{1/2}$) of many drugs cleared by glomerular filtration such as aminoglycosides, digoxin, penicillin, and tetracycline.[16] There is also a decline in renal tubular function, which can lead to glucose thresholds ranging from 130 to 310 mg/dL in the elderly.[16] Dehydration and hyponatremia may result from the progressive deterioration of tubular concentrating and diluting abilities.[16] These changes in tubular function would not be expected to have any significant effects on the urinary excretion of BZDs. The decline in glomerular filtration rate would be expected to decrease the rate of renal clearance of BZDs.[14]

Gastrointestinal System

There are numerous age-related changes that take place in the various portions of the gastrointestinal system that can impact drug absorption.[16] In addition to an increase in the incidence of atrophic gastritis with age, there is also a decrease in esophageal and colonic motility. The former change can make it more difficult to swallow oral solid dosage forms while the latter leads to a decrease in transit time, leading to dehydration of the stool and constipation, a common finding in the elderly.[16] Other factors that can affect drug absorption include a decrease in gastric acid secretion and reduced splanchnic blood flow.[14,19] Overall, physiologic changes in the gastrointestinal tract may have little or variable effects on drug absorption.[19] Although not common, some gastrointestinal adverse effects including constipation and abdominal pain have been reported with BZDs,[20,21] and these could conceivably become enhanced in the elderly.

Hepatic Function and Drug Metabolism

Aging is associated with a reduction in both hepatic blood flow and in liver mass.[16,19] Although liver function tests show little change with age, there is a progressive decrease in the amount and distribution of the smooth endoplasmic reticulum.[16] Yet aging has not been associated with any change in hepatic microsomal protein content nor the activities of several enzymes including NADPH cytochrome P450 reductase and various cytochrome P450 enzymes.[19] Therefore, it has been postulated that the effects of aging on drug metabolism are secondary to a reduction in blood flow and liver size.[22] Any reduction in hepatic blood flow would only be expected to affect the concomitant decrease in the clearance of drugs with a high extraction fraction. Also, since protein binding of drugs can affect clearance, the age-related decrease in albumin synthesis would be expected to be associated with an increase in the fraction of unbound drug, offsetting any reduction in hepatic drug metabolism for those drugs where hepatic blood flow rate is an important factor in drug clearance.[19] Benzodiazepines in general are highly bound to plasma proteins with clonazepam being 85% and diazepam up to 98% protein bound.[20,21]

The effect of aging on Phase I drug metabolism (oxidation, reduction, hydrolysis, hydration) reactions does not appear to be directly affected by age, as shown in in vitro studies of CYP450 enzymes determined from microsomal preparations obtained from human liver resection specimens.[19] Yet Greenblatt et al. found that persons over the age of 60 years had a reduced capability to complete Phase I reactions involving N-demethylation and hydroxylation reactions for long acting BZDs resulting in prolonged half-lives and reduced total metabolic clearance.[23] There does not appear to be any significant reduction of Phase II drug metabolism (glucuronidation, sulfation, methylation, acetylation or amino acid conjugation) with age.[19] However, Phase I reactions are dependent on molecular oxygen as a substrate, which could be reduced under conditions of decreased hepatic blood flow. Unlike Phase I reactions, Phase II enzymes require oxygen indirectly for energy production in the form of NADPH or ATP. Therefore, Phase I reactions could be indirectly diminished with decreased hepatic blood flow while Phase II reactions are less likely to be affected.[19] Most of the BZDs are metabolized primarily by Phase I oxidation or reduction reactions primarily via CYP3A4. Others (oxazepam, lorazepam, and temazepam) are primarily metabolized by glucuronidation.[24]

Musculoskeletal

There is an age-dependent decline in lean body mass primarily due to the loss and atrophy of muscle cells.[16] Some muscles show a pronounced infiltration of collagen and fat.[16]

The decrease in lean muscle mass is a factor that contributes to increases in the volume of distribution of lipid soluble drugs, resulting in longer half-lives and drug accumulation with BZDs and other lipophilic psychotropic drugs.[25] Degenerative joint disease occurs in 85% of persons greater than 70 years of age and primarily occurs in weight-bearing joints.[16] The decrease in mobility in the elderly is largely due to affected joints. In addition, there is an age-related decrease in bone mass. Beginning in the fourth decade of life there is a linear decline in bone mass at a rate of approximately 10% per decade in women and 5% per decade in men.[16] This decrease is due to an increase in the rate of bone resorption over bone formation, and this age-related increase in fragility is a significant factor contributing to the increased susceptibility of the elderly to experience fractures associated with falls.[26] Hormonal factors play a role in the regulation of bone mass since women are more susceptible to develop osteoporosis than men, and the process accelerates in women after menopause.[16]

Central Nervous System

The age-related changes that occur in the CNS are multifactorial and certainly play a significant role in the response of the elderly to psychoactive medications. In general, homeostatic control mechanisms such as thermoregulation, baroreceptor control of orthostasis, postural control, and water and electrolyte balance are attenuated in the elderly relative to younger adults.[25] This factor may impair the elderly's physiological adaptation to pharmacological challenges.

Neuroanatomical Changes

There is an age-related decrease in the number and size of neurons, a loss of synapses and neuronal branching, and a reduced function in neurotransmitter systems.[27] Anatomically, there are structural changes in the hippocampal dentate gyrus and neocortex.[27] During the aging process, cortical neurons that furnish both long and short corticocortical projections undergo neurochemical changes, including a differential decrease in the cellular expression of the glutamate receptor subunit.[27]

Neurochemical and Biochemical Changes

Similar to the finding of regional differences in neuroanatomy, neurochemical data also show that there are regional differences in the distribution of various important substances such as serotonin (5-HT), which is increased in the frontoparietal cortex, hippocampus, hypothalamus, and raphe regions, while it is normal in the caudate-putamen regions.[27] Conversely, there is an age-related decline in dopamine levels in the striatum and some extrastriatal areas, and loss of dopamine synthesis is normal in the aging brain and begins at about the age of 60 and continues to decrease with advancing age.[27] There is also an age-related decline in the pineal gland's capacity to secrete melatonin during the night, and this decline occurs at an average rate of 10% to 15% per decade and may play a role in causing insomnia in the elderly.[27,28]

Neurotransmitters, Associated Enzymes, and Receptors

Age-related decreases in both biosynthetic and degradative enzymes associated with several neurotransmitter systems appear to decline at different rates in different regions of the brain.[27] Striatal dopamine synthesis is known to decrease with advancing age.[27] Choline acetyltransferase, the principal enzyme associated with the biosynthesis of acetylcholine, decreases with advancing age.[27] Dopamine β-hydroxylase, the enzyme that converts dopamine to norepinephrine, also shows an age-related decrease in concentration.[27] In addition to the various changes that take place with neurotransmitter-related enzymes of biosynthesis and biodegradation, it has been postulated that the aging process may lead to an increase in receptor sensitivity to BZDs. Animal studies have shown that there may be age-related changes in the molecular composition of the $GABA_A$ receptor complex that results in an increase in the binding affinity of BZDs for the GABA receptor.[29] This suggests that enhanced responsiveness to BZDs may be a pharmacodynamic effect as well as one related to changes in pharmacokinetics and may also account for the increased sedation, loss of gait, memory impairment, and disinhibition observed in response to BZD administration.[30] Direct pharmacological evidence for this enhanced pharmacodynamic responsiveness was obtained in the study by Bertz et al., who demonstrated that at similar plasma levels of alprazolam, elderly male subjects (mean age: 68.2 years; range: 65–75) had significant psychomotor impairment on multiple tests of cognitive function compared to younger subjects (mean age: 27.5 years; range: 22–35).[31] Possible explanations offered for these observations included a slower rate of tolerance development, blood–brain barrier alterations that may have led to increased concentrations of drug in brain tissue, and increases in BZD receptor binding and functionality.[31]

Vestibular System and Vision: Important Role in Maintenance of Balance and Equilibrium

Due to a loss of neural and sensory hair cells in the vestibular system with increasing age, vestibular dysfunction is common in older people.[26] This leads to impairment in posture and gait and is characterized by postural instability and a staggering gait with unsteadiness in making turns,[26] placing the older adult at increased risk of falls. The visual system plays an important role in the maintenance of body balance during motion. An intact vestibulo-ocular reflex is essential for maintaining stable vision during motion of the head. A decrease in visual acuity due to an impairment of the peripheral vestibular system may interfere with postural balance control, thereby placing an individual at increased risk of falling.[26]

Numerous types of age-related visual impairments such as macular degeneration, impaired depth perception, and decreased peripheral vision can affect the individual's ability to maintain balance and equilibrium.[26] These types of changes make it more difficult for an individual to judge distances and perceive spatial relationships, making it more difficult to make the fine-tuning of the muscular movements needed to move around safely in the environment, thereby also increasing the risk for falling.[26]

Many of the age-related changes in the various organ systems and tissues are summarized in Table 4.1 and indicate that the elderly are frail compared to younger adults and more susceptible to adverse events associated with BZD therapy as well as other drugs that interact with the GABA receptor such as the Z-drugs zolpidem, zaleplon, and eszopiclone.[32] Because of the effects of aging on the physiological processes associated with drug metabolism, excretion, and distribution and the effects of aging on psychomotor performance, it is reasonable to expect the elderly to experience exaggerated pharmacologic responsiveness to BZDs as shown by Bertz, et al.[31] and Greenblatt et al.[33]

For the Z-drugs, each of these is structurally different from the BZDs, yet they are capable of binding to the $\alpha 1$ subunit of the BZD_1 receptor.[32] These drugs have sedative-hypnotic activity and are used for the management of insomnia. As described in the next section, both the BZDs and the Z-drugs are not generally recommended for use in the elderly and must always be used with caution when they are administered.

THE AGS BEERS CRITERIA® FOR POTENTIALLY
INAPPROPRIATE MEDICATION IN THE ELDERLY

The American Geriatric Society Beers Criteria˙ is a list of potentially inappropriate medications that are best avoided in older adults under most circumstances.[18] The current criteria evolved from a 2008 publication "Health Outcomes Associated with Potentially Inappropriate Medication Use in Older Adults" by Fick et al.[34] The current criteria were developed by a panel of health care practitioners from a diverse range of medical specialties and various clinical practice settings including ambulatory care, acute hospital care, home care, skilled nursing facilities, and long-term care.[18] Additional input to the development of the criteria was provided by the Center for Medicare and Medicaid Services, the National Committee for Quality Assurance, and the Pharmacy Quality Alliance.[18] The members of this panel conducted extensive literature searches and reviewed hundreds of documents to determine which articles represented the best available evidence. Key criteria used in the literature review included methodologic quality, relevance to older adults, and concordance with desired evidence. The panel placed special emphasis on selecting meta-analysis articles and systematic reviews as these are considered to contain high-quality material since these are on the upper portion of the strength-of-evidence pyramid.[35,36] In addition, when other types of articles were reviewed, high-quality evidence consisted of "evidence obtained from one or more well designed and well-executed randomized controlled trials that yields consistent and directly applicable results" (Table 1 on p. 677).[18] "Evidence obtained from observational studies would typically be rated as low-quality evidence because of the risk for bias" and other compromising factors (Table 1 on p. 677).[18] The primary target audience for the AGS Beers Criteria˙ is practicing clinicians. The criteria are intended for use in adults aged 65 years and older in all ambulatory, acute, and institutional settings other than hospice or palliative care settings. The objective of the criteria is to improve medication selection, educate clinicians and patients, reduce the incidence of adverse events, and serve as a clinical tool for evaluating the quality of care, cost, and patterns of drug use in older adults. The criteria provide clinicians with the information they need to make important decisions about medication use in the elderly by avoiding potentially inappropriate medications that have an unfavorable benefit–harm ratio compared to alternative treatments.

The criteria are presented as a series of 10 tables with the drugs of interest arranged by pharmacologic category and recommendations to consider in healthy patients as well as those with concurrent medical conditions. Rationales for their criteria decisions are presented along with recommendations, the quality of evidence, and the strength of the recommendation. Usually when the quality of the evidence reviewed was considered either of moderate or high quality, the strength of the recommendations is strong. A strong recommendation was considered if the evidence suggested that use of a drug could lead to harm or adverse events and the risks clearly outweighed the benefits. A weak recommendation is one where drug use may cause harm or adverse events but the risks may not outweigh the benefits.[18]

Benzodiazepine and Z-Drug Use in Older Adults

The recommendation for all BZDs is to avoid using in this population based on the rationale that older adults have an increased sensitivity to BZDs and a decreased metabolism of long-acting agents. Other studies have shown that, in relation to younger adults, elderly patients also have an increased sensitivity to short acting BZDs such as alprazolam and triazolam, thus supporting the notion that all BZDs should be avoided in the elderly.[31,33] In general, all BZDs increase the risk of cognitive impairment, delirium, falls, fractures, and motor vehicle crashes in older adults.[18] The exception to this recommendation applies to those patients with seizure disorders, rapid eye movement sleep disorder, BZD or alcohol withdrawal, severe generalized anxiety disorder (GAD), and periprocedural anesthesia.[18] The quality of evidence for this rationale is considered moderate, and the strength of the recommendation is strong. This recommendation also applies to the Z-drugs with a similar quality of evidence and strength of recommendation.[18] The rationale for avoiding the Z-drugs is based on the findings that these drugs have a similar adverse event profile as those observed with the BZDs in older adults such as delirium, falls and fractures, and motor vehicle accidents, coupled with a minimal improvement in sleep latency and duration. In addition, the FDA recently required a boxed warning to be added to the labeling for zaleplon, zolpidem, and eszoplicone.[37] This decision was made following reports of injury (46 reports of nonfatal serious injury) and death (20 reports) resulting from sleepwalking, sleep driving, and engaging in other activities while not completely awake.[37]

Recommendations for Benzodiazepine and Z-Drug Use in Elderly Patients With a History of Falls and Fractures

The use of these drugs in this subpopulation of the elderly is also to be avoided unless safer alternatives are not available. The rationale, based on a high quality of evidence, is related to the facts that any of these drugs can cause ataxia, impaired psychomotor function, syncope, and additional falls.[18] Shorter acting BZDs are not safer than long-acting ones since studies have shown that at both long- and short-acting BZDs can increase the risk for falls[38] (see section on side effects/adverse events associated with BZDs and Z-drugs). Also, Greenblatt et al. showed that healthy elderly men and women (age range: 62–83 years) displayed enhanced sedative responsiveness and greater psychomotor impairment to equivalent doses of the short-acting BZD triazolam administered to young healthy adults (age range: 21–41 years).[33]

PREVALENCE OF ANXIETY DISORDERS AND INSOMNIA IN THE ELDERLY

Anxiety (phobias, GAD, and panic disorder) is the most prevalent type of psychiatric disorder and has lifetime prevalence in the overall population of approximately 29%, and the prevalence of persistent disorders ranges from 16% to 49% after one to six years of follow-up.[39,40] The incidence of newly diagnosed anxiety disorders later in life is low (1%–2% in persons older than 65), since they do not tend to newly emerge, and complaints of anxiety have usually already existed in 99% of individuals with anxiety disorder who are over the age of 65.[39] Systematic reviews and meta-regression analyses have led to the recent suggestion that the global prevalence of anxiety disorders is 7.3% (range: 4.8%–10.9%).[41] Anxiety disorders are frequently accompanied with comorbid conditions such as other anxiety disorders or depression.[39]

Insomnia, defined as difficulty in initiating or maintaining sleep, has a prevalence of 9% to 12% in the general population but is somewhat higher in individuals older than 65 with a prevalence of 25% to 40%.[42] In the United States and globally, pharmacotherapy with BZDs or Z-drugs is the most frequent treatment approach for insomnia, and it has been estimated that up to one-third of elderly people are prescribed either a BZD or a Z-drug for the management of sleep disturbances.[43]

PHARMACOTHERAPY OF INSOMNIA AND ANXIETY DISORDERS IN THE ELDERLY

Despite nearly three decades of awareness of the risks and harms associated with BZD use in the elderly, clinicians frequently fail to heed guideline recommendations: "Clinicians should endeavor to use the lowest BZD doses that are therapeutic and treat for the briefest period of time as indicated by the patient's own clinical condition. In addition, special caution should be taken when BZDs are prescribed to the elderly" (p. 792),[8,44] since prescribing patterns show that BZDs continue to be prescribed for use in the elderly as shown in Figure 4.1. A recent study by Maust et al. found that anxiety and insomnia were the most common diagnoses reported for a BZD visit, at 21.3% and 11.6%, respectively, of new BZD visits to primary care physicians.[10]

When these drugs are prescribed for treatment of GAD, the recommended duration of treatment is two to four weeks to prevent the development of tolerance and physiological dependence on therapeutic doses.[45] When patients are treated for four months or longer, approximately 40% to 80% experience withdrawal syndrome upon cessation of therapy, regardless of the half-life of the drug.[45]

If a patient has been receiving long-term BZD or Z-drug therapy for management of either insomnia or anxiety, it is recommended that the Z-drug or BZD should be gradually withdrawn to prevent withdrawal effects and an increase in anxiety. Tapering protocols are available in Markota et al.[46] and Tannenbaum et al.[47] and must be adjusted according BZD dose, frequency of dosing, and duration of therapy.[46,47] Tapering can take up to 22 weeks or longer, depending on the conditions encountered at the beginning of tapering. Once the tapering is initiated, the patient can be transferred to other more appropriate medication or suitable psychological therapies such as cognitive behavioral therapy (CBT) to manage these conditions.

Nonpharmacologic approaches to managing insomnia in patients previously treated with either a Z-drug or a BZD include several options: CBT for insomnia has been shown to be very effective as it combines different behavioral treatments such as sleep restriction/sleep compression and relaxation therapy.[48] Several studies have shown that CBT alone is less effective in restoring normal sleep than CBT plus pharmacological therapy, while long-term remission is more effective with CBT for insomnia alone.[49,50] Methods used in relaxation therapy include muscle relaxation, diaphragmatic breathing, meditation, and biofeedback. Further information on these approaches can be found in Markota et al. and Bloom et al.[46,48]

Pharmacologic approaches for management of insomnia that utilize lower doses of drugs listed in the AGS Beers Criteria[i] are shown in Table 4.2 and include doxepin (Silenor[i]) at doses ≤ 6 mg/day and mirtazapine. Both of these drugs can be used to manage insomnia, as they are antidepressants with sedative activity, due primarily to antihistamine activity. Of note, diphenhydramine and doxylamine, two very commonly used antihistamines, are both on the Beers list of drugs to be avoided in the elderly. Mirtazapine is only FDA-approved for the indication of major depressive disorder and therefore use for insomnia would be considered an off-label use of this drug.[51] Doxepin (Silenor[i]) at this low dose of 3 to 6 mg is FDA-approved for insomnia.[52] Other options include the use of melatonin and the melatonin agonist ramelteon. Clinical trials with melatonin at a dose of 2 mg found it to be ineffective in promoting sleep onset or maintenance.[53] However, when administered as a controlled release formulation, a dose of 2 mg was found to enable elderly patients (mean age: 68 years) to discontinue BZD use successfully while maintaining sleep quality.[54] Ramelteon has a longer half-life than melatonin and is a potent, selective agonist of melatonin receptors MT_1 and MT_2, thought to be involved in the regulation of circadian rhythms and synchronization of the sleep–wake cycle.[28] Agonist activation of MT_1 is thought to preferentially induce sleepiness, while MT_2 receptor activation preferentially influences regulation of circadian rhythms.[28] Clinical pharmacokinetic studies with ramelteon showed the drug has a higher area under the curve and C_{max} in elderly persons compared to younger adults (97% and 86% higher, respectively).[55] Despite this finding, a single nighttime dose of 8 mg did not impair middle-of-the-night balance, mobility, or memory functions relative

---

i. Silenor® is the only brand of doxepin available in 3 and 6 mg tablets for insomnia.

Table 4.2 NONBENZODIAZEPINE ALTERNATIVES FOR MANAGEMENT OF
INSOMNIA AND ANXIETY IN ELDERLY PATIENTS

Condition	Drug	Pharmacologic Category	Indications/Uses[a]	Recommended Oral Dose in Elderly
Insomnia	Doxepin/Silenor®	AD	MDD/insomnia	3-6 mg hs[b,46]
	Mirtazapine[c]	AD	MDD	7.5-15 mg hs[b,d, 51]
	Melatonin ER	MT$_1$, MT$_2$ agonist	Insomnia	2 mg hs[28]
	Ramelteon	MT$_1$, MT$_2$ agonist	Insomnia	8 mg hs[55]
Anxiety	Venlafaxine ER	SSNRI	MDD, GAD, PD	GAD: 75 mg/day[62]
			SAD	PD: 37.5 mg/day[62]
				SAD: 75 mg/day[62]
	Duloxetine[e]	SSNRI	MDD, GAD	GAD: 30 mg qd for 2 weeks, then 60 mg qd[63]
	Buspirone	Anxiolytic	GAD	7.5 mg bid, then ↑ by 5 mg/day over 2–3 day intervals; maximum dose: 60 mg/day[60]

Notes: AD = antidepressant, bid = twice daily, ER = extended release. GAD = generalized anxiety disorder. hs=at bedtime. MDD = major depressive disorder. MT = melatonin receptor. PD = panic disorder. SAD = social anxiety disorder. SSNRI=selective serotonin norepinephrine reuptake inhibitor.
[a]All approved indications as per FDA prescribing information
[b]Clearance is reduced 40% in elderly men and 10% in elderly women.[51]
[c]Subtherapeutic AD doses allow antihistamine (H$_1$) activity to cause sedation.[61]
[d]off label use
[e]Avoid in patients with creatinine clearance <30 ml/min.[46]

to placebo in this age group.[55] The efficacy and safety of ramelteon were evaluated in a double-blind randomized controlled clinical trial in men and nonpregnant women aged 18 to 64 years of age diagnosed with primary insomnia. The study duration was five weeks and was preceded by a two-night run-in phase with study subjects receiving placebo, and the latency to persistent sleep (LPS) was assessed using polysomnography. LPS, the primary measure of efficacy was defined as the "elapsed time from the beginning of the polysomnography recording to the onset of 10 minutes of continuous sleep" (p. 497).[56] Results showed that two doses of ramelteon, 8 and 16 mg, significantly decreased the LPS compared to placebo at weeks 1, 3, and 5. Change from baseline analyses showed that LPS was decreased by approximately 32 to 40 minutes with both doses of ramelteon compared to 17 to 23 minutes with placebo. This reduction in LPS was significant at the end of weeks 1, 3, and 5.[56] In a randomized double-blind placebo controlled study conducted in elderly patients (≥ 65 years) with chronic insomnia, ramelteon doses at 4 and 8 mg were found to reduce sleep latency significantly, but the effects were less pronounced compared to the effects in the younger adults studied.[57]

Nonpharmacologic approaches for management of anxiety include CBT, which has been shown to benefit older patients with GAD by diminishing worry and symptoms of depression.[39,58] Elderly persons who have fallen previously from a defective gait or some other age-related physiologic deficit develop a fear of falling again, and this can become worrisome and possibly develop into a phobia. The fear of falling itself may be a protective mechanism by limiting actions taken by an individual that may lead to a fall.[39,59]

One form of exercise, tai chi, has been suggested to be a useful approach to improving posture and balance by performing the various tai chi body posture movements.[39] These involve a wide range of changes in body posture and changing the base of support. This type of exercise develops flexibility and coordination and also promotes relaxation, awareness, and focus and can help individuals regain confidence in their ability to ambulate safely.[39]

Alternative pharmacotherapies for managing GAD are also summarized in Table 4.2 and include drugs such as the serotonin-norepinephrine reuptake inhibitors (SNRIs) venlafaxine and duloxetine (see next section). Each of these drugs are not only indicated for major depressive disorder, but are also approved for use in other anxiety-related conditions including GAD, panic disorder, and social anxiety disorder and may be used as these are not on the AGS Beers Criteria' list of drugs to be avoided except in those patients with a history of falls or fractures. Buspirone is a chemically unique nonsedating, non-BZD anxiolytic drug indicated for management of GAD.[45,60] Tricyclic antidepressants should be avoided due to their anticholinergic activity, which is problematic in the elderly due to sedative activity and the tendency to cause orthostatic hypotension.[18] When SNRIs or buspirone are used to manage anxiety, it is also recommended to minimize the use of other CNS active drugs that increase the risk of falls such as antiepileptics, opioid receptor agonists, and antipsychotics[18] and implement other strategies to reduce the risk of falls such as improved lighting, removal of trip hazards, and similar physical changes to an individual's home environment.[26]

SIDE EFFECTS/ADVERSE EVENTS ASSOCIATED WITH BENZODIAZEPINES AND Z-DRUGS

Common side effects among all BZDs include drowsiness, lethargy, and fatigue. Higher doses can cause impaired motor coordination, dizziness, vertigo, slurred speech, blurred vision, mood swings, and euphoria.[64]

The relatively slow elimination of most BZDs may lead to significant drug accumulation in fatty tissues with repeated dosing. Symptoms of overmedication include impaired thinking, confusion, disorientation, and slurred speech.[64] Long-term use can lead to tolerance, physiological dependence, and withdrawal and also increase the risk of cognitive decline.[64,65] The elderly are more sensitive to the cognitive impairing effects compared to younger adults. Characteristics of cognitive impairment include anterograde amnesia, inattentiveness, ataxia, increased forgetfulness, and a decrease in short-term recall.[30,64]

Side effects associated with the Z-drugs are relatively minor such as headache, gastrointestinal upset, and dizziness.[43] However, these drugs have a dangerous adverse event profile, which is why they are recommended to be avoided in the elderly according to the 2019 AGS Beers Criteria' (see section on Beers Criteria). The Z-drugs, especially zolpidem, have a peculiar adverse event of causing abnormal and complex sleep-related behaviors (parasomnias) such as sleep-driving, sleep-eating, sleep-talking, and sleep-sex. These behaviors are performed in a semi-awake state of consciousness after getting out of bed during sleep and are also associated with anterograde amnesia.[66] This type of adverse event endangers the safety of the individual and possibly others and is cause for concern.

Benzodiazepines, Z-drugs, and the Risks for Falls and Fractures

It has been estimated that exposure to BZDs increases the risk of falling by 50%, and BZDs are strongly associated with hip fractures, which is concerning since up to one-third of hip fracture patients die within a year.[46] Surveillance data from the Centers for Disease Control and Prevention show that almost 8 out of 10 traumatic brain injuries among older adults are caused by a fall.[67]

Deaths from unintentional injury are the seventh leading cause of death in adults aged 65 years or older with 55,951 injury related deaths occurring in 2017 and falls accounted for most of these deaths. In 2007, there were 18,334 deaths, and over the period 2007 to 2016 the rate of deaths from falls increased by 3% per year.[68,69] In many cases, these falls are preventable, and healthcare providers are encouraged to discuss falls and fall prevention during annual wellness visits when they should also assess fall risk, educate patients about falls, and make any necessary interventions. Results from more recent studies (2010 and beyond) of BZD-related falls in the elderly are summarized in the following discussion.

Benzodiazepines can increase the risk for falls by several mechanisms related to their pharmacologic properties such as causing an increase in reaction time, sedation, vertigo, impaired vision (diplopia), and disrupting gait and balance control.[46] As mentioned previously, older persons are already at risk of falls and fractures due to the age-related physiologic changes they have experienced. This makes it much more important to adopt safe medication practices when treating conditions that may require a BZD or a sedative-hypnotic.

Several studies have shown that when BZDs are prescribed to elderly persons, there is a clear increase in the risk for falls and fractures mostly attributable to BZDs with shorter elimination half-lives.[38,70,71] A retrospective cohort study ($N = 416$) of geriatric patients visiting a clinic to assess various parameters associated with cognitive function and mobility, who had a known fall within the past year ($n = 404$), found a strong association with frequent falls and the use of psychotropic medication. In this particular study, the total sample size for use of any psychotropic was 139, and the majority were females (76.3%). Only short-acting BZDs (oxazepam, temazepam, alprazolam, bromazepam, lorazepam, midazolam, and the Z-drugs) were significantly associated with more frequent falls (odds ratio [OR]: 1.94; 95% confidence interval [CI]: 1.10–3.42) while long-acting BZDs were not.

Interestingly, antidepressants, including duloxetine and venlafaxine (Table 4.2) were also associated with more frequent falls (OR: 3.35; 95% CI: 1.33–4.16).[71] These findings indicate that even when alternatives to BZDs for anxiety management are used, caution is required since there is still an increased risk for falls. These specific antidepressants are not included in the AGS Beers Criteria` as they do not increase the risk for falls in elderly patients who have not experienced a previous fall; however, the SSRIs and SNRIs, as a class are recommended to be avoided in patients with a history of falls or fractures.[18]

In a study that reviewed BZD use in an elderly population of patients on either Medicare or Medicaid, the effects of half-life, drug dose, and duration of therapy were examined as risk factors for hip fracture.[38] The study consisted of 1,222 patients with a history of hip fracture within the past year and compared them to a randomized sample of age- and gender-matched patients drawn from the larger study population with no history of hip fracture in a ratio of 1:4 ($n = 4,888$). The mean age of each group was 82, and both groups were mostly comprised of women. Both of the study groups had been exposed to BZDs and other psychoactive medications prior to the date of hospital admission for hip fracture surgery (index date) and the comparable date assigned to the nonhip fracture group. Benzodiazepine doses were converted to diazepam equivalent doses for comparison purposes. Hip fracture patients had a higher exposure to BZDs, antidepressants, antipsychotics, and other psychoactive medications compared to the nonhip fracture group. Hip fracture patients were found to have a greater exposure to more medications and have more comorbid illnesses relative to the comparison group. After adjusting for variables using logistic regression, it was possible to calculate the adjusted ORs for BZD use and relative risk for hip fracture. Results showed that for diazepam equivalent doses <3 mg/day, the risk for hip fracture was not significant. However, at diazepam equivalent doses ≥3 mg/day, the adjusted risk of hip fracture was increased by at least 50%. When duration of continuous use was less than 28 days, there was no increase in the risk for hip fracture. Continuous use beyond 28 days was associated with an 80% increase in risk of hip fracture. Results of this study also found no significant increase in risk of hip fracture with long-acting BZDs.[38]

Bakken et al. tracked over 900,000 individuals over the age of 65 for up to five years in a nationwide prospective cohort study.[72] Out of the initial study population, 204,532 people (69% women) received at least one prescription for an anxiolytic while 275,372 people (67% women) received a sedative-hypnotic agent, mostly a Z-drug. Altogether 39,938 individuals (72% women) experienced a hip fracture during the study period (mean age: 83 years). Risk of hip fracture was determined by calculating the standardized incidence ratio. Any number >1 indicates an increase in risk. Results of this study are summarized in Table 4.3.

Note the risk for long-acting BZDs was 1.2 while the standardized incidence ratio for short-acting BZDs was 1.5. The methods used in this study show that although the risk of fracture was higher for short-acting BZDs, there was no statistical method available to test for significant differences between these two groups. In general, it seems clear that the use of any BZD poses an increase of hip fracture and should be avoided.

Although the Z-drug hypnotics all have very short half-lives and were therefore initially considered to be safer than BZDs, more recent studies have shown that these drugs have the potential to cause residual postawakening effects related to cognition, memory, and parasomnia and, in addition, have a profound effect on nocturnal and next-day cognitive performance including body balance, multitasking ability, and reaction time.[43]

Table 4.3 EFFECTS OF EXPOSURE TO ANXIOLYTICS AND SEDATIVE
HYPNOTICS ON RISK OF HIP FRACTURE IN PERSONS >65 YEARS OLD

Drug	n	SIR	95% CI
Any anxiolytic[a]	2009	1.4	1.4–1.5
Short-acting BZD[b]	896	1.5	1.4–1.6
Long-acting BZD[c]	2141	1.2	1.2–1.3
Any hypnotic[d]	6583	1.2	1.1–1.2
Z-drug	5418	1.2	1.1–1.2

Notes: BZD = benzodiazepine. CI = confidence interval. SIR = standardized incidence ratio.
Source: Adapted from Table 2 in Bakken MS, Engeland A, Engesaeter LB, et. al. Risk of hip fracture among older people using anxiolytic and hypnotic drugs: a nationwide prospective cohort study. *Eur J Clin Pharmacol.* 2014;70(7):873–880.
[a]BZDs or hydroxyzine.
bOxazepam, alprazolam, or midazolam.
[c]Nitrazepam, flunitrazepam, or diazepam.
[d]BZDs, Z-drugs, or melatonin.

This poses a problem for those older individuals who may awaken and mobilize during the first few hours after ingestion of zolpidem, placing them at risk of imbalance and falls. The Z-drug zolpidem was found to increase the risk of hip fracture in persons >65 years of age by a factor of 2.55.[73] In another study that compared all three of the Z-drugs for risk of falls in a case-crossover study in elderly inpatients ($N = 37{,}833$, mean age = 83.4 years), results showed that zolpidem use 30 days prior to injury was significantly associated with an increase of hospitalizations due to traumatic brain injury (OR: 1.87, 95% CI: 1.56–2.25) and hip fracture (OR: 1.59, 95% CI: 1.41–1.79) but not eszopiclone (zaleplon was unable to be assessed due to insufficient statistical power).[42]

Comment: The Effect of Drug Half-Life and the Risk for Falls

In the preceding discussion, there was a great deal of emphasis placed on the role of a drug's pharmacokinetic half-life and the impact of this on the risk for causing falls. There is much confusion in the literature on this subject and for good reason. Many of the BZDs have half-lives with a wide range of durations, and they are generally recognized as either short- to intermediate-acting or long-acting, and various studies use a range of cut-off times. For example, the half-life of chlordiazepoxide ranges from 5 to 30 hours while the half-life for diazepam ranges from 20 to 80 hours.[64] In another reference, the half-lives for these drugs are given as 20 to 100 hours and 5 to 30 hours for diazepam and chlordiazepoxide, respectively.[23] In the study by Bakken et al., the authors defined a short-acting BZD as any BZD with a half-life <24 hours.[72] This would clearly include oxazepam (5–15 hours),[64] and midazolam (<5 hour) as well as many others.[23] However, alprazolam, with a half-life of 6.3 to 26.9 hours[64] can either be classified as a short-acting BZD, based on the lower range of the half-life, or as a long-acting BZD, based on the upper end of the value. Several authors cited here used a half-life cut-off time of 20 to

24 hours[71,72]; however, De Vries et al. used a cut-off time of 10 hours,[70] while Wang et al. did not specify a cut-off time but specified which were short-acting (alprazolam, temazepam, oxazepam, among others) and which were long-acting (diazepam, chlordiazepoxide, flurazepam, and clonazepam).[38] These various methods used to define a drug's half-life along with differences in study designs, dosage, duration of drug administration, sample sizes, and other confounding factors all contribute to the lack of clarity regarding the relationship between half-life and the risk for causing falls. Because of this, it is recommended that all BZDs, regardless of half-life, should be considered as high risk factors for causing falls.

Effect of Long-Term Benzodiazepine Therapy on Cognitive Function: Risk Factor for Dementia?

Because of the well-known effects of BZDs on memory and cognitive function, there has been significant interest in exploring the possibility that long-term use of BZDs may increase the risk for elderly individuals to develop dementia after several years of exposure. Several meta-analysis studies have pooled data from case control and prospective cohort studies with follow-up periods ranging from 4 to 25 years.[74,75] In the study by Zhong et al., nearly 1,600 studies were reviewed, and after selecting only those studies that met their inclusion criteria, the analysis was narrowed down to six studies with sample sizes ranging from 1,063 to 25,140 for a total of 45,391 participants across all six studies with a total of 11,891 cases of dementia.[75] Results of the meta-analysis showed ever-users of BZDs had a higher risk of developing dementia (risk ratio [RR] 2.03, 95% CI 1.56–2.63) compared to never-users, and recent-users had a higher risk of dementia compared to never-users (RR 1.93, 95% CI 1.33–2.79). The authors concluded that their analysis showed that long-term use of BZDs resulted in a 1.2 to 2-fold increase in the risk of developing dementia compared to patients who never used BZDs.

In a second meta-analysis that reviewed over 3,000 studies narrowed down to 10 studies (four cohort and six case-control studies) consisted of 171,939 subjects and 42,025 dementia cases in patients with a mean age of >70 years.[74] Results showed that patients who had ever used a BZD had an increased risk of dementia compared to never-users (rate ratio, RR 1.51, 95%CI 1.17–1.95, $P = 0.002$). Long-term use of any BZD was associated with an increased risk of dementia (RR 1.21) when compared to short-term use of any BZD. The definitions of short- and long-term use varied among the studies, but, in general, short-term use was considered to be use of any BZD for <120 days. Long-term use varied between ≥121 days to >180 days within a one-year period to use for as long as four years or longer.[74]

The use of long-acting BZDs, defined as any BZD with a half-life ≥20 hours, was not strongly related to risk of dementia (RR = 1.16) when compared to patients taking short-acting (half-life <12 hours) or medium-term acting BZDs (half-life =12–24 hours). This meta-analysis did not compare the risk of dementia associated with longer half-life BZDs versus never users. The results of this analysis did yield evidence that BZD use is associated with the development of dementia later in life, and the association was stronger in those patients using long-acting BZDs for longer durations.

Each of these studies was unable to distinguish between the role of BZDs and the two major subtypes of dementia (Alzheimer's and vascular) attributable to BZDs due to the limited number of studies included in these meta-analyses. It is noteworthy that each of these studies further supported the earlier findings of Gallacher et al. who showed in a prospective cohort study conducted in males ($N = 1,134$, 103 who had been using BZDs regularly) followed up for 22 years, showed a marked increase in the incidence of dementia (OR = 3.50, 95% CI 1.57–7.79, $P = 0.002$).[76]

CONCLUSIONS

The BZDs are clearly a valuable therapeutic class of drugs than can provide significant symptomatic improvement in many psychiatric and sleep-related disorders in the adult population. However, in the elderly population, there are numerous changes in many physiologic systems than can overtly affect how the elderly patient responds to challenge with any BZD. Since the aging process leads to a progression of gradual deterioration in many body tissues and systems over time, as humans age they become more susceptible to external environmental challenges, including the effects of drugs. Because of the changes that affect how the body handles drugs, specifically, metabolism, distribution, and excretion as well as enhanced pharmacologic responsiveness, it seems prudent to use only drugs that are the safest and possess the least amount of risk to endangering the well-being of the individual. The literature reviewed here strongly suggest that, as recommended in the AGS Beers Criteria', with few exceptions, the use of any BZD or Z-drug for the management of anxiety disorders or insomnia should not be used in elderly individuals because of the significant short-term and long-term risks they pose to a person's health. Short- and intermediate-acting BZDs may be appropriate to use in elderly patients with specific conditions such as seizure disorders, management of BZD or ethanol withdrawal, periprocedural anesthesia, severe GAD, and rapid eye movement sleep behavior disorder. The use of BZDs, whether short- or long-acting, and Z-drugs should be avoided for management of any other conditions in elderly patients due to the hazards and increased risks for falls and fractures that they pose to this special population.

REFERENCES

1. Anderson RJ. Sixty years of benzodiazepines. *Pharmacologist*. 2019;61(1):26–37.
2. Lopez-Munoz F, Alamo C, Garcia-Garcia P. The discovery of chlordiazepoxide and the clinical introduction of benzodiazepines: half a century of anxiolytic drugs. *J Anxiety Disord*. 2011;25(4):554–562.
3. Prescription Drug Monitoring Program Training and Technical Assistance Center. History of prescription drug monitoring programs. *Brandeis University*. http://www.pdmpassist.

org/pdf/PDMP_admin/TAG_History_PDMPs_final_20180314.pdf. Published 2018. Accessed September 26, 2019.

4. Prescription Drug Monitoring Program Training and Technical Assistance Center. Frequently asked questions. Published 2019. Updated September 20, 2019. Accessed September 26, 2019. https://www.pdmpassist.org/RxCheck/FAQ

5. Agarwal SD, Landon BE. Patterns in outpatient benzodiazepine prescribing in the United States. *JAMA Network Open.* 2019;2(1):e187399.

6. Gray SL, LaCroix AZ, Hanlon JT, et al. Benzodiazepine use and physical disability in community-dwelling older adults. *J Am Geriatr Soc.* 2006;54(2):224–230.

7. Olfson M, King M, Schoenbaum M. Benzodiazepine use in the United States. *JAMA Psychiatry.* 2015;72(2):136–142.

8. Thomson M, Smith WA. Prescribing benzodiazepines for noninstitutionalized elderly. *Can Fam Physician.* 1995;41:792–798.

9. Trewin VF, Lawrence CJ, Veitch GB. An investigation of the association of benzodiazepines and other hypnotics with the incidence of falls in the elderly. *J Clin Pharm Ther.* 1992;17(2):129–133.

10. Maust DT, Kales HC, Wiechers IR, Blow FC, Olfson M. No end in sight: benzodiazepine use in older adults in the United States. *J Am Geriatr Soc.* 2016;64(12):2546–2553.

11. Panel on Prevention of Falls in Older Persons, American Geriatrics Society, British Geriatrics Society. Summary of the updated American Geriatrics Society/British Geriatrics Society Clinical practice guideline for prevention of falls in older persons. *J Am Geriatr Soc.* 2011;59(1):148–157.

12. Gilca M, Stoian I, Atanasiu V, Virgolici B. The oxidative hypothesis of senescence. *J Postgrad Med.* 2007;53(3):207–213.

13. Elmadfa I, Meyer AL. Body composition, changing physiological functions and nutrient requirements of the elderly. *Ann Nutr Metab.* 2008;52(Suppl 1):2–5.

14. Schmucker DL. Aging and drug disposition: an update. *Pharmacol Rev.* 1985;37(2):133–148.

15. Lixie E, Edgeworth J, Shamir L. Comprehensive analysis of large sets of age-related physiological indicators reveals rapid aging around the age of 55 years. *Gerontology.* 2015;61(6):526–533.

16. Boss GR, Seegmiller JE. Age-related physiological changes and their clinical significance. *West J Med.* 1981;135(6):434–440.

17. Basile J. Hypertension in the elderly: a review of the importance of systolic blood pressure elevation. *J Clin Hypertens (Greenwich).* 2002;4(2):108–112, 119.

18. American Geriatrics Society. 2019 updated AGS Beers Criteria(R) for potentially inappropriate medication use in older adults. *J Am Geriatr Soc.* 2019;67(4):674–694.

19. McLean AJ, Le Couteur DG. Aging biology and geriatric clinical pharmacology. *Pharmacol Rev.* 2004;56(2):163–184.

20. Genentech. Klonopin tablets prescribing information. South San Francisco, CA, Genentech USA; 2016.

21. Genentech. Valium tablets prescribing information. South San Francisco, CA, Genentech USA; 2016.

22. Woodhouse K. Drugs and the liver. Part III: Ageing of the liver and the metabolism of drugs. *Biopharm Drug Dispos.* 1992;13(5):311–320.

23. Greenblatt DJ, Shader RI, Divoll M, Harmatz JS. Benzodiazepines: a summary of pharmacokinetic properties. *Br J Clin Pharmacol.* 1981;11(Suppl 1):S11–S16.

24. Raj A, Sheehan D. Benzodiazepines. In: Schatzberg AF, Nemeroff CB, eds. *Textbook of Psychopharmacology.* 3rd ed. Washington, DC: American Psychiatric Publishing; 2004:371–389.

25. Roose SP, Pollack BG, Devanand DP. Treatment during late life. In: Schatzberg AF, Nemeroff CB, eds. *Textbook of Psychopharmacology*. 3rd ed. Washington, DC: American Psychiatric Publishing; 2004:1083–1108.

26. Ambrose AF, Paul G, Hausdorff JM. Risk factors for falls among older adults: a review of the literature. *Maturitas*. 2013;75(1):51–61.

27. Anyanwu EC. Neurochemical changes in the aging process: implications in medication in the elderly. *Scientific World Journal*. 2007;7:1603–1610.

28. Turek FW, Gillette MU. Melatonin, sleep, and circadian rhythms: rationale for development of specific melatonin agonists. *Sleep Med*. 2004;5(6):523–532.

29. Rissman RA, De Blas AL, Armstrong DM. GABA(A) receptors in aging and Alzheimer's disease. *J Neurochem*. 2007;103(4):1285–1292.

30. Madhusoodanan S, Bogunovic OJ. Safety of benzodiazepines in the geriatric population. *Expert Opin Drug Saf*. 2004;3(5):485–493.

31. Bertz RJ, Kroboth PD, Kroboth FJ, et al. Alprazolam in young and elderly men: sensitivity and tolerance to psychomotor, sedative and memory effects. *J Pharmacol Exp Ther*. 1997;281(3):1317–1329.

32. Greenblatt DJ, Harmatz JS, Shapiro L, Engelhardt N, Gouthro TA, Shader RI. Sensitivity to triazolam in the elderly. *N Engl J Med*. 1991;324(24):1691–1698.

33. Sanger DJ. The pharmacology and mechanisms of action of new generation, non-benzodiazepine hypnotic agents. *CNS Drugs*. 2004;18(Suppl 1):9–15; discussion 41, 43–15.

34. Fick DM, Mion LC, Beers MH, L Waller J. Health outcomes associated with potentially inappropriate medication use in older adults. *Res Nurs Health*. 2008;31(1):42–51.

35. Ascione F. Evaluating the scientific literature. In: *Principles of Scientific Literature Evaluation: Critiquing Clinical Drug Trials*. Washington, DC: American Pharmaceutical Association; 2001:1–23.

36. Forest J, McGovern Kupiec, L. Evidence-based decision making: introduction and formulating good clinical questions. *Procter & Gamble. Dental Continuing Education Courses*. https://www.dentalcare.com/en-us/professional-education/ce-courses/ce311/levels-of-evidence. Published 2019. Accessed October 7, 2019.

37. US Food and Drug Administration. Certain prescription insomnia medicines: new boxed warning due to risk of serious injuries caused by sleepwalking, sleep driving and engaging in other activities while not fully awake. https://www.fda.gov/safety/medical-product-safety-information/certain-prescription-insomnia-medicines-new-boxed-warning-due-risk-serious-injuries-caused. Published 2019. Updated April 30, 2019. Accessed October 8, 2019.

38. Wang PS, Bohn RL, Glynn RJ, Mogun H, Avorn J. Hazardous benzodiazepine regimens in the elderly: effects of half-life, dosage, and duration on risk of hip fracture. *Am J Psychiatry*. 2001;158(6):892–898.

39. Pary R, Sarai SK, Micchelli A, Lippmann S. Anxiety disorders in older patients. *Prim Care Companion CNS Disord*. 2019;21(1).

40. Mackenzie CS, El-Gabalawy R, Chou KL, Sareen J. Prevalence and predictors of persistent versus remitting mood, anxiety, and substance disorders in a national sample of older adults. *Am J Geriatr Psychiatry*. 2014;22(9):854–865.

41. Stein DJ, Scott KM, de Jonge P, Kessler RC. Epidemiology of anxiety disorders: from surveys to nosology and back. *Dialogues Clin Neurosci*. 2017;19(2):127–136.

42. Tom SE, Wickwire EM, Park Y, Albrecht JS. Nonbenzodiazepine sedative hypnotics and risk of fall-related injury. *Sleep*. 2016;39(5):1009–1014.

43. Gunja N. The clinical and forensic toxicology of Z-drugs. *J Med Toxicol*. 2013a;9(2):155–162.

44. Salzman C. The APA Task Force report on benzodiazepine dependence, toxicity, and abuse. *Am J Psychiatry*. 1991;148(2):151–152.

45. Rickels K, Rynn M. Pharmacotherapy of generalized anxiety disorder. *J Clin Psychiatry.* 2002;63(Suppl 14):9–16.
46. Markota M, Rummans TA, Bostwick JM, Lapid MI. Benzodiazepine use in older adults: dangers, management, and alternative therapies. *Mayo Clin Proc.* 2016;91(11):1632–1639.
47. Tannenbaum C, Martin P, Tamblyn R, Benedetti A, Ahmed S. Reduction of inappropriate benzodiazepine prescriptions among older adults through direct patient education: the EMPOWER cluster randomized trial. *JAMA Intern Med.* 2014;174(6):890–898.
48. Bloom HG, Ahmed I, Alessi CA, et al. Evidence-based recommendations for the assessment and management of sleep disorders in older persons. *J Am Geriatr Soc.* 2009;57(5):761–789.
49. Morin CM, Vallieres A, Guay B, et al. Cognitive behavioral therapy, singly and combined with medication, for persistent insomnia: a randomized controlled trial. *JAMA.* 2009;301(19):2005–2015.
50. Morin CM, Colecchi C, Stone J, Sood R, Brink D. Behavioral and pharmacological therapies for late-life insomnia: a randomized controlled trial. *JAMA.* 1999;281(11):991–999.
51. Organon/Merck. Remeron prescribing information. https://www.drugs.com/pro/remeron.html. Published 2014. Updated December 3, 2018. Accessed May 25, 2019.
52. Pernix Therapeutics. Silenor prescribing information. https://www.drugs.com/pro/silenor.html. Published 2014. Updated January 1, 2018. Accessed May 25, 2019.
53. Sateia MJ, Buysse DJ, Krystal AD, Neubauer DN, Heald JL. Clinical practice guideline for the pharmacologic treatment of chronic insomnia in adults: an American Academy of Sleep Medicine clinical practice guideline. *J Clin Sleep Med.* 2017;13(2):307–349.
54. Garfinkel D, Zisapel N, Wainstein J, Laudon M. Facilitation of benzodiazepine discontinuation by melatonin: a new clinical approach. *Arch Intern Med.* 1999;159(20):2456–2460.
55. Takeda. Rozerem prescribing information. https://www.drugs.com/pro/rozerem.html#s-34090-1. Published 2018. Updated December 1, 2018. Accessed May 25, 2019.
56. Zammit G, Erman M, Wang-Weigand S, Sainati S, Zhang J, Roth T. Evaluation of the efficacy and safety of ramelteon in subjects with chronic insomnia. *J Clin Sleep Med.* 2007;3(5):495–504.
57. Roth T, Seiden D, Sainati S, Wang-Weigand S, Zhang J, Zee P. Effects of ramelteon on patient-reported sleep latency in older adults with chronic insomnia. *Sleep Med.* 2006;7(4):312–318.
58. Hall J, Kellett S, Berrios R, Bains MK, Scott S. Efficacy of cognitive behavioral therapy for generalized anxiety disorder in older adults: systematic review, meta-analysis, and meta-regression. *Am J Geriatr Psychiatry.* 2016;24(11):1063–1073.
59. Litwin H, Erlich B, Dunsky A. The complex association between fear of falling and mobility limitation in relation to late-life falls: a SHARE-based analysis. *J Aging Health.* 2018;30(6):987–1008.
60. Bristol-Myers S. BuSpar prescribing information. *Drugs.com.* https://www.drugs.com/pro/buspar.html#s-34068-7. Published 2010. Updated November 1, 2018. Accessed May 25, 2019.
61. Flores B, Schatzberg A. Mirtazapine In: Schatzberg A, Nemeroff, C, eds. *Textbook of Psychopharmacology.* Third ed. Washington, DC: American Psychiatric Publishing; 2004:341–347.
62. Pfizer, Inc. Effexor XR prescribing information. 2018, https://www.drugs.com/pro/effexor-xr.html#s-34068-7. Accessed May 27, 2019.
63. Eli Lilly and Company. Cymbalta Prescribing Information. 2016; https://www.drugs.com/pro/cymbalta.html#s-34068-7. Accessed May 26, 2019.
64. Griffin CE 3rd, Kaye AM, Bueno FR, Kaye AD. Benzodiazepine pharmacology and central nervous system-mediated effects. *Ochsner J.* 2013;13(2):214–223.

65. Federico A, Tamburin S, Maier A, et al. Multifocal cognitive dysfunction in high-dose benzodiazepine users: a cross-sectional study. *Neurol Sci.* 2017;38(1):137–142.

66. Gunja N. In the zzz zone: the effects of Z-drugs on human performance and driving. *J Med
Toxicol.* 2013b;9(2):163–171.

67. Centers for Disease Control and Prevention. Traumatic Brain injury–related emergency department visits, hospitalizations, and deaths—United States, 2007 and 2013. https://www.
cdc.gov/mmwr/volumes/66/ss/ss6609a1.htm?s_cid=ss6609a1_e. Published 2017.

68. Burns E, Kakara R. Deaths from falls among persons aged ≥65 years—United States,
2007–2016. *Morb Mortal Wkly Rep 2018.* 2018;67(18):509–514.

69. Centers for Disease Control and Prevention. Injury prevention and control. https://www.
cdc.gov/injury/wisqars/index.html. Published 2019. Updated March 21, 2019. Accessed
May 10, 2019.

70. de Vries OJ, Peeters G, Elders P, et al. The elimination half-life of benzodiazepines and fall
risk: two prospective observational studies. *Age Ageing.* 2013;42(6):764–770.

71. van Strien AM, Koek HL, van Marum RJ, Emmelot-Vonk MH. Psychotropic medications,
including short acting benzodiazepines, strongly increase the frequency of falls in elderly.
Maturitas. 2013;74(4):357–362.

72. Bakken MS, Engeland A, Engesaeter LB, Ranhoff AH, Hunskaar S, Ruths S. Risk of hip
fracture among older people using anxiolytic and hypnotic drugs: a nationwide prospective cohort study. *Eur J Clin Pharmacol.* 2014;70(7):873–880.

73. Johnson B, Streltzer J. Risks associated with long-term benzodiazepine use. *Am Fam
Physician.* 2013;88(4):224–226.

74. He Q, Chen X, Wu T, Li L, Fei X. Risk of dementia in long-term benzodiazepine users: evidence from a meta-analysis of observational studies. *J Clin Neurol.* 2019;15(1):9–19.

75. Zhong G, Wang Y, Zhang Y, Zhao Y. Association between benzodiazepine use and dementia: a meta-analysis. *PLoS One.* 2015;10(5):e0127836.

76. Gallacher J, Elwood P, Pickering J, Bayer A, Fish M, Ben-Shlomo Y. Benzodiazepine use
and risk of dementia: evidence from the Caerphilly Prospective Study (CaPS). *J Epidemiol
Community Health.* 2012;66(10):869–873.

CHAPTER 5

The Central Benzodiazepine Receptor

MICHAEL H. OSSIPOV

HIGHLIGHTS

- Benzodiazepines act at an allosteric binding site of the γ-aminobenzoic acid (GABA) type A (GABA$_A$) receptor and enhance GABA-mediated opening of the calcium ion channel, which mediates neuronal hyperpolarization.
- GABA$_A$ receptors consist of five subunits, representing different combinations drawn from a total of 19 subunit components: α(1–6), β(1–3), γ(1–3), δ, ε, θ, π, and ρ(1–3).
- GABA$_A$ receptors consisting of different subunit configurations are differentially expressed throughout the brain.
- It may be possible to design compounds selective for certain subunit configurations, thus selecting for activity of GABA$_A$ receptors in certain parts of the brain to target a narrow psychopharmacologic profile.
- Drugs acting at the benzodiazepine binding site may be agonists, which enhance the inhibitory effect of GABA via the receptor; antagonists, which block the effect of benzodiazepine site agonists; and inverse agonists, which reduce the hyperpolarization and neuronal inhibition normally produced by GABA via the receptor.

INTRODUCTION

Benzodiazepines are a chemical class of sedative-hypnotic drugs that have been used clinically for decades. The prototypic benzodiazepine, chlordiazeoxide (Librium®) was approved by the US Food and Drug in 1960 for the relief of anxiety. Diazepam

(Valium®) was approved in 1962 and is indicated for management of anxiety, skeletal muscle spasm, and acute alcohol withdrawal and as an adjunct in convulsive disorders. There are currently 14 different benzodiazepines, differing in rates on onset, half-life, and duration of action. In general, the benzodiazepines have been considered to be safe and well-tolerated, and deaths from overdose are rare (Tesar, 1990). In fact, when they were first introduced, they were touted as a safe replacement for barbiturates, which were associated with high incidences of nonzedical use, physiologic dependence, and overdose (Cheng et al, 2018; Wafford, 2005).

A well-known instance of attempted suicide with diazepam was when Admiral Robert McFarlane was caught up in a political scandal in 1987 and ingested 25 to 30 tablets of diazepam and was still conscious when the ambulance appeared (Schachter and Gerstenzang, 1987). In a different case report, two patients ingested 500 and 2000 mg of diazepam in suicide attempts and were in a moderately deep coma but recovered and were discharged within 48 hours (Greenblatt et al., 1978). Yet behind this seemingly benign façade lurks considerable danger. In combination with alcohol or opiates, benzodiazepines can be deadly. This is best exemplified by the tragic case of Karen Ann Quinlan, a young lady who, after ingesting benzodiazepines with alcohol, fell into a coma and remained in a persistent vegetative state for nearly 10 years (Fine, 2005). Additionally, as with alcohol and barbiturates, withdrawal from benzodiazepines is serious and, in some cases, can lethal (Lann and Molina, 2009). Prolonged use is also associated with some significant changes in physiology. In this chapter, we explore the central benzodiazepine receptor that gives these compounds such a range in behavior. It is also important to note that although the benzodiazepines are well known to act within the central nervous system (CNS), these drugs also act on different receptors at noncentral sites. These peripheral benzodiazepine receptors, also referred to as translocator protein or tryptophan-rich sensory protein are found in mammalian tissue and are especially prominent in mitochondria and immune cells. The peripheral benzodiazepine receptors are discussed in Chapter 6 of this volume.

BENZODIAZEPINE RECEPTOR—STRUCTURE

The benzodiazepines do not act at a specific central benzodiazepine receptor, per se, but rather they modulate the activity of the $GABA_A$ receptor. Benzodiazepines selectively bind to an allosteric modulatory site on the $GABA_A$ receptor, which enhances the activity of the endogenous ligand GABA, the most abundant inhibitory neurotransmitter in the CNS *vide infra*. The $GABA_A$ receptor is a ligand-gated ion channel that is activated by GABA, causing the opening of a chloride (Cl^-) ion channel that hyperpolarized the neurons and creates inhibitory post-synaptic potentials. Benzodiazepines, by binding to an allosteric modulatory site, increase the frequency of channel opening induced by GABA (Sieghart, 1992, 1994; Rudolph and Knoflach, 2011; Wafford, 2005).

The $GABA_A$ receptor is made up of five protein subunits arranged in a circular formation and forming a central pore (Figure 5.1) (Sieghart, 1992, 1994; Rudolph and

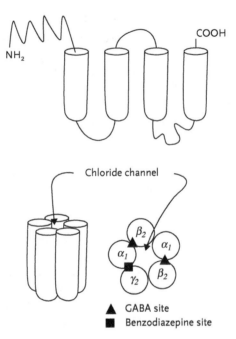

Figure 5.1 Schematic representation of the GABA$_A$ receptor composed of five subunits, each with four helical transmembrane domains and an intracellular loop. Each GABA$_A$ receptor consists of five subunits arranged in a circular pattern to form a central chloride channel. The GABA recognition site is formed between the α and β subunits, and the benzodiazepine site is formed between the α and γ subunits.

Knoflach, 2011; Wafford, 2005). Binding of GABA to the recognition site on the receptor causes a conformational change opening the pore and allowing the flow of Cl⁻ through the pore. Each protein subunit has a molecular weight of about 50 KDa, and consists of approximately 450 amino acid residues. Approximately one-half of the protein chain forms the hydrophilic extracellular N-terminal, which may contain a recognition site for GABA. The GABA$_A$ receptor belongs to the cysteine loop-type ligand-gated ion channel superfamily, which share a highly conserved region of 13 amino acids between two cysteine residues connected by a disulfide bond N-terminal, forming the loop. An intracellular loop between the third and fourth transmembrane domains that participates in phosphorylation-mediated modulation of the receptor (Sieghart, 1992, 1994; Rudolph and Knoflach, 2011; Wafford, 2005).

Whereas a GABA$_A$ receptor consists of 5 subunits, there are 19 different subunits available, identified as α(1–6), β(1–3), γ(1–3), δ, ε, θ, π, and ρ(1–3), thus creating a potential for a myriad of receptor isoforms, each with different pharmacologic profiles; however, the actual number of different isotypes of the GABA receptor that occur in nature is uncertain (Mortensen et al., 2012). Receptors with different subunit compositions can be differentially expressed in the CNS, effectively meaning that different brain regions can be differentially sensitive to GABA or to its modulator, because of these differences. For example, some subunits are broadly expressed throughout the

CNS, others have a somewhat restricted distribution, and the α6 subunit is expressed only on cerebellar granule neurons.

Most GABA$_A$ receptors consist of two α subunits, two β subunits, and one γ subunit (Mortensen et al., 2012). An electrophysiologic study where HEK cells were transfected with complementary DNA to generate different isoforms of the GABA$_A$ receptor, it was found that GABA had the lowest potency at those expressing the α2 or α3 subunits and the highest potency for those containing the α6 subunit. Notably, ranges in potency for GABA among these isoforms ranged as high as 175-fold. Affinities for different isoforms of the GABA receptors are summarized in Table 5.1 (Mortensen et al., 2012).

The GABA$_A$ receptors occur at postsynaptic sites, where the release of GABA from a nerve terminal results in opening of chloride channels and hyperpolarization of the postsynaptic neuron. This phasic inhibition event occurs rapidly and is measured in milliseconds. There are also extrasynaptic GABA receptors that respond to ambient levels of GABA and maintain a persistent inhibitory tone (Farrant and Nusser, 2005). Receptors that include the δ subunit in their structure are only found at extrasynaptically (Clarkson, 2012; Mortensen et al., 2012). These GABA$_A$ receptor subtypes are highly sensitive to neurosteroids, and dysfunction of these receptors may be linked to reduced

Table 5.1 GABA POTENCY AND MAXIMAL CURRENTS AT DIFFERENT SUBUNIT COMPOSITIONS

Subunit Composition	EC$_{50}$	Maximum Current (pA)	CNS Distribution
α1β3γ2S	2.1μM	3367±662	Widespread
α2β3γ2S	13.4μM	3056±435	Widespread
α3β3γ2S	12.5μM	3776±305	Thalamic and hypothalamic nuclei, locus coeruleus, dentate granule cells
α4β3γ2S	2.1μM	2574±292	Thalamus
α5β3γ2S	1.4μM	2446±445	Hippocampus
α6β3γ2S	0.17μM	2446±445	Cerebellum and cochlear granule cells
α1β1γ2S	10.9μM	3575±799	
α1β2γ2S	6.6μM	2230±193	Widespread
α4β3	0.97μM	328±67	Thalamus
α4β3δ	1.7μM	1224±264	Thalamus
α6β3	0.076μM	490±125	Cerebellar granule cells
α6β3δ	0.17μM	706±148	Cerebellar granule cells
α1β2	1.7μM	1863±333	Widespread
α3β3	4.5μM	3924±288	Thalamic and hypothalamic nuclei, locus coeruleus
α1β2δ	3.7μM	398±147	Hippocampus
α4β2δ	0.91μM	1544±263	Hippocampus
α3β3θ	3.4μM	1680±508	Hypothalamic nuclei, locus coeruleus
α3β3ε	0.86μM	811±300	Hypothalamic nuclei, locus coeruleus

Note: Subunits in the shaded area are found only at extrasynaptic sites.

seizure thresholds and certain anxiety disorders (Sigel and Steinmann, 2012; Farrant and Nusser, 2005; Maguire, 2005).

Endogenous modulators of the $GABA_A$ receptor are neurosteroids and the endogenous cannabinoid 2-arachidonoyl glycerol, and there are numerous small molecules that modulate the receptor as well. It is believed that the diversity of compounds that can interact with the $GABA_A$ receptor is due to the numerous pockets, or cavities, that form in the transmembrane portions of the $GABA_A$ receptor subunits (Sigel and Steinmann, 2012; Ernst, 2005). Computational modeling indicates that the $GABA_A$ different subunits of the $GABA_A$ receptors contain form numerous cavities with different conformations such that they act as binding sites for different classes of drugs that can alter functioning of the $GABA_A$ receptor (Sigel and Steinmann, 2012; Ernst, 2005). Thus far, different sites that are selective for the endogenous substrates 2-arachidonoyl glycerol and neurosteroids, as well as sites selective for benzodiazepines, ethyl alcohol, barbiturates, and general anesthetics have been identified (Sigel and Steinmann, 2012; Ernst, 2005). Occupation of one of these cavities by a substrate causes changes in receptor conformation and can enhance binding of GABA to the receptor and/or alter the characteristics of the channel to remain open longer or more frequently (Sigel and Steinmann, 2012; Ernst, 2005). Consequently, benzodiazepines and other substances such as alcohol are in a position to synergize each other's effects at the GABA receptor.

Benzodiazepine Modulation of the $GABA_A$ Receptor

Although there are many possible configurations, most $GABA_A$ receptors consist of two α1, two β2, and a single γ2 subunit (Sharkey and Czajkowski, 2008). The benzodiazepine binding site is situated at the interface between the α and γ subunits in a manner analogous to the GABA binding site between the α and β subunits. Because of this arrangement, a single α1 subunit makes up part of both the GABA and benzodiazepine binding sites (Sharkey and Czajkowski, 2008). The result is that the GABA and the benzodiazepine binding sites are physically linked, so that occupation of one of the sites can alter the configuration of the other site, thus allowing for the allosteric modulation of the GABA receptor by the benzodiazepine binding site (Figure 5.1).

Benzodiazepine Agonism

The benzodiazepines are not agonists in the strict sense of the word, as their binding to the allosteric site does not directly produce an effect. Rather, binding to the benzodiazepine binding site by an agonist induces a conformational shift resulting in enhanced current in response to activation by GABA (Figure 5.2). There are numerous ligands that are capable of interacting with the benzodiazepine binding site. Agonists, such as diazepam, potentiate currents induced by GABA and are positive modulators. So-called inverse agonists perform the opposite effect by inhibiting GABA-induced currents and thus are negative modulators (Oakley and Jones, 1980; Macdonald et al., 1992).

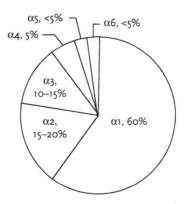

α5, <5%

α6, <5%

α4, 5%

α3, 10–15%

α2, 15–20%

α1, 60%

Figure 5.2 Schematic representation of the effects of GABA and benzodiazepine modulators on current. GABA opens the chloride channel, allowing inward flow of negatively charged chloride ions and causing hyperpolarization. Benzodiazepines (positive allosteric modulators) enhance GABA activity, increasing the hyperpolarization due to GAB but do not open the chloride channels alone. Benzodiazepine site antagonists neither enhance nor diminish the effect of GABA. Negative allosteric modulators, or "inverse agonists", reduce the effect of GABA on the chloride channel, resulting in decreased level of hyperpolarization (see Rudolph and Knoflach, 2011).

Antagonists (e.g., flumazenil) bind to the benzodiazepine site but produce no effect on currents, and are "zero" modulators (Braestrup et al., 1982), *vide infra*.

Early studies performed with isolated cultured embryonic chick spinal cord neurons measured conduction changes indicative of an increase in permeability to chloride ions in response to the iontophoretic or injected presence of GABA (Choi, 1977). Chlordiazepoxide produced a concentration-dependent augmentation of the responses to GABA and enhanced synaptic potentials mediated by GABA (Choi, 1977). Importantly, chlordiazepoxide alone did not have any effect on the neurons. Combined with studies showing that diazepam binds to selective sites in the brain but is not displaced by GABA or by GABA antagonists, it was suggested that benzodiazepines bind to a modulating site that can modify the coupling between occupation of the receptor by GABA and the opening of the chloride channels (Choi, 1977). In electrophysiologic studies performed with tissue cultured mammalian spinal cord neurons, chlordiazepoxide, or diazepam dose-dependently augmented the response elicited by GABA (MacDonald and Barker, 1978). These studies also showed that benzodiazepines act by modulating the effect of GABA at its receptor and not by a direct action at the GABA binding site. Benzodiazepines increase the frequency of chloride channel opening but do not increase conductance, nor are they able to open chloride channels by themselves (Rudolph and Knoflach, 2011). Thus, the effect of benzodiazepines is self-limited, in that the conductance of the Cl⁻ channel in the presence of both benzodiazepines and GABA is not higher than that which can be achieved with GABA alone (Rudolph and Knoflach, 2011). This is in contrast to the barbiturates, which can enhance Cl⁻ conductance even in the absence of GABA (Rudolph and Knoflach, 2011) and may help explain the more favorable therapeutic index (i.e., 10-fold) of benzodiazepines as compared to barbiturates (Sieghart, 1992; Guina and Merrill, 2018).

Benzodiazepine Antagonism

The fact that benzodiazepines are allosteric modulators of the GABA receptor, acting through a specific modulatory site on that receptor, presents some unique challenges. Typically, when examining agonist/antagonist activities at a receptor site, an antagonist, which binds at the receptor without activating the receptor, can block the activity of endogenous ligands and produce an effect opposite of that of the agonist. That is, an antagonist produces an effect opposite of the agonist. For example, the commonly used β-blockers block the effect of circulating epinephrine, preventing increased blood pressure and heart rate. However, blocking an allosteric modulatory site could simply produce no effect, since the modulator itself does not produce an effect of its own, but enhances that of an endogenous ligand. The midazobenzodiazepine derivative, Ro 15-1788, is the first reported antagonist for the benzodiazepine modulatory site. Electrophysiologic studies showed that Ro 15-1788 at doses of up to 10 mg/kg, i.v. had no effects on segmental dorsal root potentials, polysynaptic ventral root reflexes, and Renshaw cell responses to antidromic stimulation of the ventral roots, but it blocked the responses to several benzodiazepines (meclonazepam, diazepam, midazolam) or to zopiclone, a nonbenzodiazepine agonist acting at the benzodiazepine binding site, at a dose of 1 mg/kg, i.v. (Polc et al., 1981). In contrast, the effects of phenobarbital on these spinal cord responses were not affected by Ro 15-1788, which is consistent with a separate allosteric modulatory site for the barbiturates. In addition, Ro 15-1788 blocked the reductions of spontaneous multiunit activity in several regions of the rat brain in response to midazolam but had no effect alone or on the responses to phenobarbital (Polc et al., 1981). Similar results were seen with regard to electroencephalogram (EEG) patterns in rats. These studies showed that Ro 15-1788 acts as an antagonist of benzodiazepine activity through an interaction at the benzodiazepine modulatory site. In a randomized clinical trial, Ro 15-1788 prevented the impairment, cognitive, psychomotor, and subjective effects of orally administered diazepam (Darragh et al., 1982). This compound was developed as flumazenil for the rapid reversal of conscious sedation in patients receiving benzodiazepines and for the reversal of toxic doses of benzodiazepines, for example, as in drug overdose (Flumazenil in Intravenous Conscious Sedation With Diazepam Multicenter Study Group, 1992).

A seemingly counterintuitive use of flumazenil is in the treatment of withdrawal from benzodiazepines in individuals who have become tolerant and dependent on these drugs (Quaglio et al., 2012; Hood et al., 2014). If we look at an analogous situation, individuals who are dependent on opiates will develop withdrawal symptoms if given the opiate antagonist naloxone (Stitzer et al., 1991). While a single bolus infusion of flumazenil (e.g., 1 mg in five minutes) produces signs of benzodiazepine withdrawal in tolerant individuals, multiple slow infusions of low doses of flumazenil actually reduces the appearance of withdrawal symptoms in individuals who use benzodiazepines chronically and then discontinue use (Quaglio et al., 2012). This seemingly paradoxical use of a benzodiazepine antagonist is due to the allosteric modulatory relationship between benzodiazepines and the $GABA_A$ receptor. Chronic exposure to benzodiazepines causes alterations in the benzodiazepine modulatory site on the $GABA_A$ receptor resulting in an uncoupling between the benzodiazepine and GABA binding sites and a loss of the allosteric enhancement of GABA by benzodiazepines, along with a possible downregulation of benzodiazepine receptors (Quaglio et al., 2012; Ali and Olsen, 2001). It is possible that the degree to which uncoupling occurs could impact the manifestation of withdrawal severity. In studies with cultured neurons, this uncoupling was demonstrated by a reduced sensitivity of GABA-activated chloride channels to enhancement by benzodiazepines (Ali and Olsen, 2001). Cell culture studies performed with Sf9 cells transfected to express the $GABA_A$ receptor suggest that chronic exposure to benzodiazepines changes the conformation of the $GABA_A$ receptor such that it favors internalization into the cell and uncoupling of the GABA and benzodiazepine binding sites (Ali and Olsen, 2001). This altered conformation is rapidly normalized by flumazenil, restoring the $GABA_A$ receptor to the normal condition (Ali and Olsen, 2001). In addition, it was also shown that chronic exposure to benzodiazepines can cause changes in the relative levels of $GABA_A$ receptor subunits, decreasing the levels of those that are sensitive to benzodiazepines with subunits that are less sensitive or insensitive to benzodiazepines (see Ali and Olsen, 2001). It is remarkable that these effects can all be reversed, or normalized, by a single short exposure to the benzodiazepine antagonist flumazenil.

In a blinded, placebo-controlled clinical trial, individuals who were identified as abusing flunitrazepam ($N=18$) or lormetazepam for ≥9 months were treated with flumazenil or placebo infusions (Gerra et al., 1993). Patients receiving flumazenil had significantly lower withdrawal scores when compared to those on placebo. Patients in the flumazenil-treated group reported improved family relationships, attentiveness, and mood perceptions (Gerra et al., 1993). This study showed the potential for the use of a benzodiazepine antagonist in managing withdrawal from chronic use of benzodiazepines.

Reverse Agonism

The testing of structural modifications made to ethyl β-carboline-3-carboxylate, an antagonist at the benzodiazepine recognition site, led to the discovery of inverse agonists, or negative modulators of the $GABA_A$ receptor (Braestrup et al., 1982). It was found in Braestrup's study that methyl 6,7-dimethoxy-4-ethyl- β-carboline-3-carboxylate caused convulsions in mice and rats, as did a related compound, methyl β-carboline-3-carboxylate. Convulsions occurred at doses at which these compounds bound to the benzodiazepine site. Convulsions were blocked not only by benzodiazepines and barbiturates but also by the benzodiazepine antagonist Ro 15-1788. Moreover, it was found that whereas benzodiazepines enhance binding of GABA to the $GABA_A$ receptor, these compounds reduced the binding affinity for GABA. It appears that these inverse agonists bind preferentially to the conformation with a closed chloride channel and lock the channel in a configuration that reduces the likelihood of its opening in response to GABA. Thus, the inverse agonists block the inhibitory effect of GABA on neurons (Braestrup et al., 1982). Animal studies have suggested that partial inverse agonists, or negative allosteric modulators, especially those acting at selective subtypes, may be useful in managing inflammatory and neuropathic pain, cognitive impairment (e.g., Alzheimer's and Downs syndromes), and recovery from stroke (Rudolph and Knoflach, 2011).

The fluoroquinolone carboxylic acid derivatives, which include ciprofloxacin, levofloxacin, norfloxacin, and ofloxacin, are common antibiotics used for a wide range of infections (Kamath, 2013; Unseld et al., 1990). These drugs are associated with CNS-related adverse events such as dizziness, headache, insomnia, restlessness, and visual impairment, which can be treated with benzodiazepines (Kamath, 2013; Unseld et al., 1990). Competition binding studies showed that ciprofloxacin, norfloxacin, and ofloxacin all displaced $[^3\text{H}]$-flunitrazepam in a concentration-dependent manner in a range of 10 μM to 1,000 μM (Unseld et al., 1990). In EEG studies conducted with healthy volunteers, ciprofloxacin caused changes in EEG profile similar to those elicited by flumazenil, and flumazenil intensified those produced by ciprofloxacin (Unseld et al., 1990). These changes were reversed by midazolam. Based on these and other studies, it appears that the fluoroquinolones fit the profile of a benzodiazepine antagonist/partial inverse agonists (Kamath, 2013; Unseld et al., 1990).

RECEPTOR SUBTYPE COMPOSITION MAY ALTER BENZODIAZEPINE EFFECTS

There are six isoforms of the α subunit and three of the γ subunit. The benzodiazepine binding site is formed at the interface between the α and γ subunits. In addition, the γ2 subunit is required to form a classical benzodiazepine binding site; consequently, the potential combinations of α/β/γ subunits forming functional benzodiazepine site is somewhat limited (Fritschy and Mohler, 1995). The development of transgenic mouse models, including knock-outs or point mutations of genes coding for different GABA$_A$ subunit subtypes and the development of selective ligands for different subtypes have allowed for some detailed examination of these different receptor subunit compositions in response to modulators (Cheng et al., 2018). The different subtypes of the α subunits have been found to be differentially expressed in the CNS (Cheng et al., 2018; Fritschy and Mohler, 1995). An immunohistochemical survey performed in the rat brain found that the α1 subtype is widely expressed throughout the brain, whereas the α2, α3, and α5 subtypes had more limited distributions (Fritschy and Mohler, 1995). The α4 and α6 subtypes were not included, as they represent less than 10% of immunoprecipitated GABA$_A$ receptors. GABA$_A$ receptors consisting of αl/β2,3/γ2, α2/β2,3/γ2, α3/β2,3/γ2, and α5/β2,3/γ2 are the most abundant and widespread triplets found. Notably, every brain region was found to express a unique pattern of neurons expressing the different subtype combinations, underlining the complexity and remarkable diversity of GABA-mediated neurotransmission (Fritschy and Mohler, 1995), which carries with it the potential for different effects of benzodiazepines at these different regions.

Animal studies performed either with transgenic mouse models or selective ligands have shown that different subtypes of the α subunit can be associated with different psychopharmacological effects of benzodiazepines. The relative abundance of the α subunit

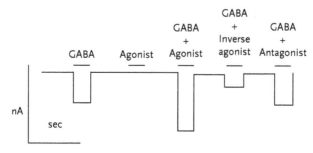

Figure 5.3 Representation of the relative abundance of α subunit subtypes (see Rudolph and Knoflach, 2011).

subtypes is represented in Figure 5.3. For example, mice with point mutations of the α1 subunit were resistant to benzodiazepine-induced sedation, and benzodiazepines that do not bind to sites that include the α1 subunit (e.g., TPA123, TPA023, L-838,417) show anxiolytic activity with no sedation in animal models (Cheng et al., 2018). The compound MRK-409, a partial agonist at α2-, α3-, and α5-expressing receptors but with minor activity at α1-containing sites, was anxiolytic without sedation in animal models but showed sedation in clinical trials. It was reasoned that even a little activity at α1 was sufficient to produce sedation. In contrast, TPA023B, which is a partial agonist at $GABA_A$ receptors expressing α2 or α3 and antagonist at α1 was anxiolytic without sedation in clinical trials (see Cheng et al., 2018). The psychopharmacological effects of benzodiazepines at different subtypes are summarized in Table 5.2.

Addiction liability and abuse potential are believed to depend in part on activation of reward circuitry involving mesolimbic pathways and dopaminergic mechanisms of the ventral tegmental area (VTA; Heikkinen et al., 2009). Benzodiazepines disinhibit dopaminergic transmission in the VTA, which explains their addiction/abuse liability. Selective benzodiazepine site partial agonists without activity at α1 sites, such as TPA023, show very little abuse liability (see Cheng et al., 2018). Although the α2 and α3 subtypes are critical for the anxiolytic properties of benzodiazepines, these subtypes are also implicated with a minor role in addiction liability. It is possible, therefore, that

Table 5.2 RELATIVE CONTRIBUTIONS OF A SUBUNITS TO THE PSYCHOPHARMACOLOGIC PROPERTIES OF BENZODIAZEPINES

Property	α1	α2	α3	α5
Sedation	++++	0/+	0/+	0/+
Addiction	++++	++	++	0/+
Anxiolysis	0/+	++++	++++	++
Myorelaxation	++	++++	++	++
Anticonvulsive	++++	+++	++	0/+
Amnesia	++++	0/+	0/+	++++

Notes: 0/+ None/negligible; ++ Minor; +++ Moderate; ++++ Significant.

benzodiazepines that have no antagonistic activity at α1 and are partial α2 or α3 agonists could have limited abuse potential. Development of antagonists at the α1 subtype is currently under consideration as a novel pharmacotherapeutic strategy for the treatment of alcohol addiction (Orrico et al., 2017; Holtyn et al., 2017).

Tolerance represents a complex phenomenon, in part because it develops differently, or not at all, to different psychopharmacologic properties of benzodiazepines. For example, tolerance develops fairly rapidly to sedative and anticonvulsant effects of benzodiazepines but not to their anxiolytic or amnesic effects (Cheng et al., 2018). Differences in the role of coupling and of receptor downregulation among the receptors expressing different α subtypes are still needed for a better understanding of this property.

SUMMARY

Benzodiazepines gained popularity in the 1970s and 1980s, in large part because they were safer than the barbiturates. However, with growing use came the awareness that they, too, can be associated with tolerance, physiologic dependence, and abuse. Moreover, the safety profile of benzodiazepines can be reduced when used in combination with other sedatives. The pharmacology of benzodiazepines in due to a positive allosteric modulation of the $GABA_A$ receptor. The realization that the $GABA_A$ receptor is composed of variations of subunit combinations, together with the discovery that the subunits themselves have different subtypes led to investigations into the role of the subtypes in different aspects of the psychopharmacology of benzodiazepines. It seems that the possibility exists for the development of safer benzodiazepine-like drugs, with reduced, if not totally absent, abuse liability and tolerance development.

REFERENCES

Ali, N.J., Olsen, R.W., 2001. Chronic benzodiazepine treatment of cells expressing recombinant GABA(A) receptors uncouples allosteric binding: studies on possible mechanisms. J Neurochem. 79, 1100–1108. https://doi.org/10.1046/j.1471-4159.2001.00664.x

Braestrup, C., Schmiechen, R., Neef, G., Nielsen, M., Petersen, E.N., 1982. Interaction of convulsive ligands with benzodiazepine receptors. Science. 216, 1241–1243.

Cheng, T., Wallace, D.M., Ponteri, B.B., Tuli, M., 2018. Valium without dependence? Individual GABAA receptor subtype contribution toward benzodiazepine addiction, tolerance, and therapeutic effects. NDT. 14, 1351–1361. https://doi.org/10.2147/NDT.S164307

Choi, D.W., Farb, D.H., Fischbach, G.D., 1977. Chlordiazepoxide selectively augments GABA action in spinal cord cell cultures. Nature. 269, 342–344. https://doi.org/10.1038/269342a0

Clarkson, A.N., 2012. Perisynaptic GABA receptors: the overzealous protector. Adv Pharmacol Sci. 2012, 1–8. https://doi.org/10.1155/2012/708428

Darragh, A., Lambe, R., Kenny, M., Brick, I., Taaffe, W., O'Boyle, C., 1982. RO 15-1788 antagonises the central effects of diazepam in man without altering diazepam bioavailability. Br J Clin Pharmacol. 14, 677–682.

Ernst, M., Bruckner, S., Boresch, S., Sieghart, W., 2005. Comparative models of GABAa receptor extracellular and transmembrane domains: important insights in pharmacology and function. Mol Pharmacol. *68*, 1291–1300. https://doi.org/10.1124/mol.105.015982

Fine, R.L., 2005. From Quinlan to Schiavo: medical, ethical, and legal issues in severe brain injury. Proc (Bayl Univ Med Cent). *18*, 303–310. https://doi.org/10.1080/08998280.2005.11928086

Flumazenil in Intravenous Conscious Sedation With Diazepam Multicenter Study Group, 1992. Reversal of central benzodiazepine effects by flumazenil after intravenous conscious sedation with diazepam and opioids: report of a double-blind multicenter study. Clin Ther. *14*, 910–923.

Fritschy, J.-M., Mohler, H., 1995. GABA$_A$-receptor heterogeneity in the adult rat brain: Differential regional and cellular distribution of seven major subunits. J Comp Neurol. *359*, 154–194. https://doi.org/10.1002/cne.903590111

Gerra, G., Marcato, A., Caccavari, R., Fertonani-Affini, G., Fontanesi, B., Zaimovic, A., Avanzini, P., Delsignore, R., 1993. Effectiveness of flumazenil (RO 15-1788) in the treatment of benzodiazepine withdrawal. Curr Therapeut Res. *54*, 580–587. https://doi.org/10.1016/S0011-393X(05)80679-4

Greenblatt, D.J., Woo, E., Allen, M.D., Orsulak, P.J., Shader, R.I., 1978. Rapid recovery from massive diazepam overdose. JAMA. *240*, 1872–1874.

Guina, J., Merrill, B., 2018. Benzodiazepines I: upping the care on downers: the evidence of risks, benefits and alternatives. J Clin Med. *7*, 17. https://doi.org/10.3390/jcm7020017

Heikkinen, A.E., Möykkynen, T.P., Korpi, E.R., 2009. Long-lasting modulation of glutamatergic transmission in VTA dopamine neurons after a single dose of benzodiazepine agonists. Neuropsychopharmacology. *34*, 290–298. https://doi.org/10.1038/npp.2008.89

Holtyn, A.F., Tiruveedhula, V.V.N.P.B., Stephen, M.R., Cook, J.M., Weerts, E.M., 2017. Effects of the benzodiazepine GABAA α1-preferring antagonist 3-isopropoxy-β-carboline hydrochloride (3-ISOPBC) on alcohol seeking and self-administration in baboons. Drug Alcohol Depend. *170*, 25–31. https://doi.org/10.1016/j.drugalcdep.2016.10.036

Hood, S.D., Norman, A., Hince, D.A., Melichar, J.K., Hulse, G.K., 2014. Benzodiazepine dependence and its treatment with low dose flumazenil: benzodiazepine dependence and its treatment. Br J Clin Pharmacol. *77*, 285–294. https://doi.org/10.1111/bcp.12023

Kamath, A., 2013. Fluoroquinolone induced neurotoxicity: a review J Adv Pharm Ed Res. *3*(1), 16–19.

Lann, M.A., Molina, D.K., 2009. A fatal case of benzodiazepine withdrawal. Am J Forensic Med Pathol. *30*, 177–179. https://doi.org/10.1097/PAF.0b013e3181875aa0

Macdonald, R., Barker, J.L., 1978. Benzodiazepines specifically modulate GABA-mediated postsynaptic inhibition in cultured mammalian neurones. Nature. *271*, 563–564. https://doi.org/10.1038/271563a0

Macdonald, R.L., Twyman, R.E., Ryan-Jastrow, T., Angelotti, T.P., 1992. Regulation of GABAA receptor channels by anticonvulsant and convulsant drugs and by phosphorylation. Epilepsy Res Suppl. *9*, 265–277.

Maguire, J.L., Stell, B.M., Rafizadeh, M., Mody, I., 2005. Ovarian cycle-linked changes in GABA(A) receptors mediating tonic inhibition alter seizure susceptibility and anxiety. Nat Neurosci. *8*, 797–804. https://doi.org/10.1038/nn1469

Mortensen, M., Patel, B., Smart, T.G., 2012. GABA potency at GABA$_A$ receptors found in synaptic and extrasynaptic zones. Front Cell Neurosci. *6*. https://doi.org/10.3389/fncel.2012.00001

Oakley, N.R., Jones, B.J., 1980. The proconvulsant and diazepam-reversing effects of ethyl-beta-carboline-3-carboxylate. Eur J Pharmacol. *68*, 381–382. https://doi.org/10.1016/0014-2999(80)90538-5

Orrico, A., Martí-Prats, L., Cano-Cebrián, M.J., Granero, L., Polache, A., Zornoza, T., 2017. Pre-clinical studies with D-penicillamine as a novel pharmacological strategy to treat alcoholism: updated evidences. Front Behav Neurosci. *11*. https://doi.org/10.3389/fnbeh.2017.00037

Polc, P., Laurent, J.-P., Scherschlicht, R., Haefely, W., 1981. Electrophysiological studies on the specific benzodiazepine antagonist Ro 15-1788. Naunyn-Schmiedeberg's Arch. Pharmacol. *316*, 317–325. https://doi.org/10.1007/BF00501364

Quaglio, G., Pattaro, C., Gerra, G., Mathewson, S., Verbanck, P., Des Jarlais, D.C., Lugoboni, F., 2012. High dose benzodiazepine dependence: Description of 29 patients treated with flumazenil infusion and stabilised with clonazepam. Psychiatry Res. *198*, 457–462. https://doi.org/10.1016/j.psychres.2012.02.008

Rudolph, U., Knoflach, F., 2011. Beyond classical benzodiazepines: novel therapeutic potential of GABAA receptor subtypes. Nat Rev Drug Discov. *10*, 685–697. https://doi.org/10.1038/nrd3502

Schachter, J., Gerstenzang, J., 1987, February 10. McFarlane Tried suicide, police believe. Los Angeles Times. https://www.latimes.com/archives/la-xpm-1987-02-10-mn-2292-story.html. Accessed October 19, 2019.

Sharkey, L.M., Czajkowski, C., 2008. Individually monitoring ligand-induced changes in the structure of the $GABA_A$ receptor at benzodiazepine binding site and non-binding-site interfaces. Mol Pharmacol. *74*, 203–212. https://doi.org/10.1124/mol.108.044891

Sieghart, W., 1992. $GABA_A$ receptors: ligand-gated Cl– ion channels modulated by multiple drug-binding sites. Trends Pharmacol Sci. *13*, 446–450. https://doi.org/10.1016/0165-6147(92)90142-S

Sieghart, W., 1994. Pharmacology of benzodiazepine receptors: an update. J Psychiatry Neurosci. *19*, 24–29.

Sigel, E., Steinmann, M.E., 2012. Structure, function, and modulation of GABA A receptors. J Biol Chem. *287*, 40224–40231. https://doi.org/10.1074/jbc.R112.386664

Stitzer, M.L., Wright, C., Bigelow, G.E., June, H.L., Felch, L.J., 1991. Time course of naloxone-precipitated withdrawal after acute methadone exposure in humans. Drug Alcohol Depend. *29*, 39–46. https://doi.org/10.1016/0376-8716(91)90020-y

Tesar, G.E., 1990. High-potency benzodiazepines for short-term management of panic disorder: the U.S. experience. J Clin Psychiatry. *51*(Suppl), 4–10; discussion 50–53.

Unseld, E., Ziegler, G., Gemeinhardt, A., Janssen, U., Klotz, U., 1990. Possible interaction of fluoroquinolones with the benzodiazepine-GABAA- receptor complex. Brit J Clin Pharmacol. *30*, 63–70. https://doi.org/10.1111/j.1365-2125.1990.tb03744.x

Wafford, K.A., 2005. $GABA_A$ receptor subtypes: any clues to the mechanism of benzodiazepine dependence? Curr Opinion Pharmacol. *5*, 47–52. https://doi.org/10.1016/j.coph.2004.08.006

CHAPTER 6

Benzodiazepine Receptors in the Periphery

ROBERT B. RAFFA

HIGHLIGHTS

- There are γ-aminobutyric acid type A (GABA$_A$) receptors located in the periphery.
- Benzodiazepines (BZDs) and other BZD receptor agonists (BzRAs) bind to specific sites on these receptors, which are termed peripheral BZD receptors (PBRs); they are also known as TSPO (translocator protein or tryptophan-rich sensory protein).
- Peripheral BZD receptors are extensively located throughout the periphery and in notably high concentrations in mitochondria and immune cells.
- Little is known about the consequences of long-term use of BZDs (i.e., more than 2–4 weeks) on PBR activity.
- Almost nothing is known about the contribution of PBRs to the development of BZD physical dependence or to BZD withdrawal phenomena.

BENZODIAZEPINES AND Z-DRUGS: WHAT'S IN A NAME?

The classification of a chemical substance (whether drug, exploratory research compound, or any other ligand) as a BZD is, strictly speaking, based solely on its molecular structure.[1] Specifically, it is classified based on a particular arrangement of a heterocyclic ring linked to a benzene ring that forms a core structural motif. Since there are several locations along the core structure that allow for chemical modification (e.g., addition of substituent groups, such as methyl, ethyl, etc.), variations in chemical substituents superimposed upon the core structure result in structurally related yet unique members of the family of BZD compounds.[2] Consequently, each member of the family has its own chemical (and pharmacologic) features and characteristics.[3]

Following the discovery that multiple chemical moieties that have the BZD chemical structural motif have notable utility (good efficacy and safety profile) in the clinical management of acute anxiety conditions,[4] the term *benzodiazepine* slowly became synonymous with this class of anxiolytic drugs. That is, the definition of BZD transitioned from a chemical one to a sort of clinical one. When basic science research discovered the underlying molecular basis for the anti-anxiety (anxiolytic) effect produced by these structurally related compounds (viz., allosteric modulation of the central $GABA_A$ receptor complex[5]), it became common to refer to the site on the $GABA_A$ receptor complex to which these drugs and compounds bind as the *BZD receptor*.[6] This nomenclature turned out to be premature and unfortunate, because it was subsequently found that some compounds that lacked the classic BZD structural motif also had anxiolytic activity—and produced the effect by the same mechanism, namely, by binding to site(s) on the central $GABA_A$ receptor complex and allosterically modulating its activity.[7] In short order, several more drugs that have the same mechanism of action and pharmacologic effects as the BZDs, but different chemical structures, were discovered.[8] Because of the similarities in general mechanism of action (binding to a site on the $GABA_A$ complex), and some shared pharmacologic effects, such compounds, irrespective of the nature of their chemical structures, are sometimes called—mistakenly—BZDs. To further confuse things, because the earliest of such drugs had generic names that began with the letter Z (such as zolpidem and zaleplon, and the more recent zopiclone),[9] these drugs have become colloquially known as the Z-drugs. This terminology muddies the water for several reasons, including that subsequent such drugs have names that do not start with the letter Z (e.g., eszopiclone).

The proper designation for this pharmacologic class is not BZDs, because there are non-BZDs that act in the same way, nor is Z-drugs appropriate, since this is artefactual because it is based on the naming of specific drugs. A current compromise is based on the shared pharmacologic mechanism of action[10]: BzRA. Thus, a drug can be a BZD BzRA or a non-BZD BzRA (such as the Z-drugs). In either case, it will produce the same pharmacologic effects.[11] We will herein use terminology that best makes a particular point, but most often, BzRA.

It should be noted that as discussed in previous chapters (e.g., Chapter 3 and Chapter 5) of this volume), the $GABA_A$ receptor is a large pentameric protein that functions as a ligand-gated ion channel. It includes multiple binding sites to which several categories of substances bind (Figure 6.1). It is thus commonly termed the $GABA_A$ receptor complex. This chapter refers to substances that bind to a common site defined in the pharmacologic sense—that is, competitive binding inhibition by the same substance—in this case, flumazenil.

WHY BZRAS: TOTO, I'VE A FEELING WE'RE NOT IN KANSAS ANYMORE

For many years, the conditions for which BzRAs are currently used were treated with barbiturates or meprobamate.[12,13] The barbiturates represented a significant advance

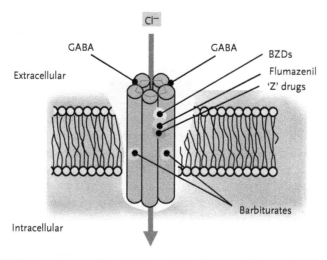

Figure 6.1 Multiple categories of drugs bind to multiple distinguishable sites (or subsites) on the GABA$_A$ receptor complex. Binding to each site results in a shared effect (i.e., the allosteric modulation of GABA-induced Cl$^-$ influx), but nuances in the individual details mechanism of this action (e.g., on the magnitude vs. rate of influx) and the specifics of the consequent individual clinical effects (e.g., relative anxiolysis vs. sedation vs. muscle relaxation, etc.).

at the time but were far from ideal. Since they are nonselective central nervous system (CNS) depressants, they cause a host of off-target, adverse effects.[14] In contrast, the BzRAs are generally far more selective in their action than the barbiturates (anxiolytic vs. generalized depressant) and, in general, produce less (or at least less severe) adverse effects on alertness, sleep patterns, and respiration, with fewer metabolic drug interactions, much wider therapeutic window, etc. than the barbiturates.[3] They represented a clear advance along a trajectory of improved therapeutic efficacy and safety (i.e., generally more specific for anxiety with fewer or less severe side effects).[15] In a similar manner, the non-BZD BzRAs represent a continuation of the trajectory (efficacy and safety), and represent an advance over the BZDs, for the same reasons as well as greater efficacy for insomnia, although the differences might not yet result in sufficient safety.[16] We thus do not minimize the contributions made by the BZDs and the non-BZD BzRA drugs. However, like all drugs, they are not devoid of problems.

ANXIOLYTIC MECHANISM OF ACTION: LOOKING UNDER THE HOOD

The molecular mechanism by which the BZDs, as well as the non-BZD BzRAs, produce their anxiolytic action is now well-known in great detail and excellent reviews are available.[3,10,17,18] BzRAs bind to specific sites on the large GABA$_A$ receptor complex, which are distinct from the sites to which GABA binds. The differentiation of the binding sites, plus meeting other pharmacologic requirements for characterization as a receptor, gives rise to the term *BZD receptor*. The binding of a BzRA to its receptor in the absence of endogenous GABA tone at the $GABA_A$ receptor does not produce an effect by itself; rather, such binding enhances the action of GABA at the $GABA_A$ receptor (GABA-induced Cl^- influx).[19] It does so allosterically, that is, at a distance separated from the site where GABA binds.[20] Since the binding of GABA to the $GABA_A$ receptor produces an increase in influx of Cl^- ions across neuronal membranes, the binding of BzRAs to BZD receptors magnifies GABA-induced Cl^- influx,[17,21,22] which results in an increase in the magnitude of the negative resting transmembrane potential difference.[23] That is, it hyperpolarizes the neuron and raises the threshold before a neuron will respond by firing an action potential. The neurons will still respond to a stimulus, but a larger stimulus will be required. The clinical impact is that the neurons will be less hypersensitive, which translates into an anxiolytic effect. The current Z-drugs and other BzRAs (as well as any future BzRAs) act in the same way. They bind to BZD receptors and allosterically enhance GABA-induced influx of Cl^-.[3] Hence, all BzRAs produce their anti-anxiety therapeutic effect in the same way—allosteric enhancement of the hyperpolarizing action of the inhibitory neurotransmitter GABA at $GABA_A$ receptors in the brain.[24]

BZRAS: CURIOUS

For most patients who are prescribed BzRAs, the most commonly experienced adverse effects are drowsiness, fatigue, muscle weakness, or ataxia.[25] And the majority of the adverse experiences are relatively mild in most patients most of the time. However, a complete list of adverse effects experienced by patients prescribed BzRAs is quite extensive.[25]

From a basic science point of view, the extensiveness of the list, and in particular the diversity of the effects, is at first puzzling. How is it, for example, that a BzRA interacting with receptors at a central $GABA_A$ receptor complex produces constipation, hypotension, urinary retention, dry mouth, and elevated transaminase and alkaline phosphatase?[25] The answer is that there are also $GABA_A$ receptors located in the periphery and that BzRAs bind to these sites and to peripheral BzRA receptors.

BZRA WITHDRAWAL SIGNS: CURIOUSER AND CURIOUSER

As is true for almost all drugs, some degree of tolerance and physical dependence develop to the use of BzRAs.[26,27] These phenomena are normal physiological processes and are not usually a clinical concern (might not even be observed or manifested). Tolerance and physical dependence are normal physiological adaptations to almost any drug (viz., compensatory responses usually opposite to the drug-induced effect).[28-30] However, on discontinuation of the drug, or during the interdose intervals of short-acting drugs, physical dependence is manifested as withdrawal symptoms. The symptoms can be experienced by some patients no matter how short a duration of exposure to the drug; it becomes an ever-increasing problem with increased duration and dose of drug administration. So although for the overwhelming majority of patients who use BzRAs for a short term, tolerance and physical dependence are normal and not problematic per se; the two phenomena can contribute to a physiological feedback loop of cues that can make it difficult to stop taking BzRAs without experiencing troubling, or even disabling, negative medical and quality-of-life symptomatology.[31–34]

Normally, withdrawal symptoms result from the body's now unopposed (drug no longer present) compensatory mechanism. Therefore, they are usually easily recognizable as generally opposite to the effects produced by the administered drug. It is to be expected, for example, that anxiety would be withdrawal symptom associated with anxiolytic drugs, since anxiety is opposite to the drug-induced anxiolytic effect.[35,36] Somewhat perplexing, however, is that withdrawal from BzRAs can give rise to a bewildering array of symptoms that are difficult to reconcile with BzRA-induced anti-anxiety effect.

A particularly curious aspect of BzRA withdrawal symptoms relates to the time course. Some of the symptoms persist a perplexingly long time, clearly exceeding the time that the drug has presumably been eliminated from the body, although some sequestration in a nonobvious body compartment cannot be excluded. Further, the duration of symptoms is not always correlated to the dose of BzRA or to the duration of its use. Thus, these symptoms do not appear to be residual adverse effects, but rather appear to be unusually protracted withdrawal symptoms. This is not at all typical for withdrawal from most other drugs.

Just as it is difficult to reconcile some of the adverse effects that are produced by BzRA use, there is currently no good understanding of the mechanistic processes that can explain the protracted withdrawal symptoms that sometimes follows discontinuation of use. The fact that there is such a broad spectrum of BzRA withdrawal symptoms and that not all of the symptoms are experienced by all of the patients (indeed, only a subset of patients experience a subset of symptoms) challenges our current understanding of BzRA action. Some plausible pharmacologic explanations are long-term changes in the number of $GABA_A$ receptors or BzRA binding sites (up- or downregulation or an effect on promoters of BZD receptor protein synthesis or degradation) or changes in the transduction of signaling. It might also be the consequence of some change in the drug's ADME (absorption, distribution, metabolism, elimination), or even of some change in $GABA_A$ receptor composition, function, or subtype arrangement. A recently recognized possibility is that it might involve peripheral BzRA binding sites.[37]

BZRA PHARMACOLOGY: RECONSIDERED

As described previously, BZDs are distinct chemically from the so-called Z-drugs (e.g., zaleplon, zolpidem, and zopiclone),[38] but because they are similar pharmacologically,[39] they operate in a similar manner (i.e., as BzRAs). Although the Z-drugs lack the distinctive BZD chemical structure, they act as agonists at BZD receptors, which allosterically modulate the $GABA_A$ receptor complex.[17,40]

GABA is the major inhibitory neurotransmitter that mediates inhibitory transmissions at most brain neurons.[41,42] Cellular levels of GABA are held in tight steady state with the major CNS excitatory neurotransmitter glutamate through the negative feedback controls in the Krebs cycle that regulate their mutual cellular levels.[43] GABA produces its effects because of its binding to (affinity) and activation of (intrinsic efficacy) GABA receptors, of which three types have been identified (designated by subscripts): $GABA_A$, ionotropic receptor (of which there are multiple subtypes), $GABA_B$, a metabotropic receptor, and $GABA_C$, which is not believed to be relevant to the topic of anxiolysis. [44] The $GABA_A$ receptor is a ligand-gated ion channel (ionotropic) type receptor, which means that activation by an endogenous agonist (i.e., GABA), exogenous agonist, or positive allosteric modulator (e.g., BZDs or Z-drugs) results in an increase neuronal Cl^- influx as the mechanism of signal transduction.[45] Increased Cl^- influx hyperpolarizes the neuron (increases the magnitude of the negative transmembrane resting potential difference), rendering it less likely to fire (i.e., initiate an action potential) in response to excess stimulation (analogous to anxiety at the clinical level). Hence, chemical ligands that enhance $GABA_A$ receptor functionality (influx of Cl^-) are clinically anti-anxiety agents. BzRAs are such ligands. They bind in a stereospecific and saturable manner to BZD receptors that are located throughout the brain and throughout the periphery (the latter are discussed subsequently).[46]

Most $GABA_A$ receptors are a pentameric composite of subunits designated α, β, and γ.[44] Since there are at least six different α-subunits, four different β-subunits, and three different γ-subunits, there is a large number of possible subunit combinations, which results in a potential for multiple $GABA_A$ receptors, each with a different and distinct electrophysiological and pharmacological profile. Benzodiazepine receptors are one of several allosteric modulatory sites located on these $GABA_A$ receptor complexes.[46] Thus BzRAs bind to not just one $GABA_A$ receptor, but rather to the multiple subtypes, and they potentiate the inhibitory effects of GABA at each subtype of receptor located throughout the brain.[47-49] Viewed in this context, the BzRAs have much less specificity than the early in vitro radioligand binding studies conducted using the predominant subtype suggested. They have no intrinsic activity at the GABA-binding site. Furthermore, at the BZD binding site, ligands can act in one of several possible ways: as full agonists, as partial agonists, as neutral antagonists, or as inverse agonists (full or partial).[50-53] Thus depending on the compound, GABAergic transmission may be enhanced, reduced, or not affected by the binding activity.[46] The BzRAs act as agonists (full or partial); the best-known BZD receptor antagonist (or weak partial agonist) is flumazenil.[44]

PERIPHERAL BENZODIAZEPINE RECEPTORS: REALLY?

All the pieces necessary to understand the anxiolytic mechanism of action of BZDs have been in place for many years. GABA was reported to be present in the brains of multiple species in 1950.[54,55] Benzodiazepine receptors were demonstrated in the CNS of rats in 1977 using high-affinity tritiated diazepam binding (with a note added in proof that "the benzodiazepine receptor in human brain corresponds to that of rat brain in affinity, stereospecificity and regional distribution" (p. 851).[56] The localization of BZD receptors throughout the brain, including human brain, has subsequently been extensively described.[14, 56-61] However it was not recognized at first that these receptors, GABA$_A$ receptors, and anxiolytic action of BZDs are related.[62] This was because of some mismatch between brain regional distribution of GABA$_A$ and BZD receptors[63] and that some substances that increased GABA (e.g., amino-oxyacetate) are not anxiolytic.[64] However, the pharmacology of GABA, GABA$_A$ receptors, and the molecular basis for the anxiolytic action of BzRAs is now well understood, as previously described.

In the publication that demonstrated the BZD receptor in the brain, it is stated that "benzodiazepine binding in rat kidney, liver, and lung . . . differs fundamentally from that in cortex" (p. 851).[56] The actual data were published subsequently. It was meant to dismiss any importance of the non-CNS receptors to the anxiolytic effect of BZDs. In retrospect, although correct regarding the anxiolytic effect of BzRAs, it obfuscated understanding some of the adverse events related to BzRAs and to their protracted withdrawal symptoms (discussed later in this chapter).

PERIPHERAL GABA AND GABA$_A$ RECEPTORS

Although GABA was already believed to be a major neurotransmitter in the vertebrate CNS prior to 1979 and it was known to be an inhibitory neurotransmitter in the peripheral nervous system of certain invertebrates, in 1979 GABA was demonstrated in the vertebrate peripheral nervous system using light and electron microscopic autoradiographic techniques.[65,66] In the same year, it was demonstrated in a screen of selected peripheral organs of the rat that GABA is generally present outside the CNS of vertebrates.[67] Various physiological actions of GABA mediated via GABA$_A$ receptors that are located in the periphery were subsequently described.[68-72] Given the presence of peripheral GABA and GABA$_A$ receptors, it was reasonable to search for peripheral BZD receptors.

PERIPHERAL BENZODIAZEPINE RECEPTORS: UNDER THE RADAR

Peripheral BZD receptors were identified early during the history of BZD receptor research, but interest in the peripheral sites was understandably secondary to the interest focused on the central, particularly brain, sites. Specific attention to the peripheral sites began to emerge during the 1980s and 1990s.[37,73-76] Due to the seeming disconnect from BZD-induced anxiolytic effect, there was some drift in terminology that in a way obfuscated making a connection between BzRA use and peripheral adverse effects or the peripheral manifestations of withdrawal resulting from discontinuation of BzRAs. Specifically, the peripheral BZD binding site (receptor, PBR) has at various times, and for various reasons, been termed the $\omega3$ receptor,[77,78] mitochondrial BZD receptor, peripheral benzodiazepine binding (or acceptor) site, p-site, and mitochondrial diazepam binding inhibitor (DBI), and, more recently, it has become commonly known as translocator protein or tryptophan-rich sensory protein (TSPO). The original terminology of PBR will be used herein.

Although the functions of the sites have not yet been fully elucidated, they may be involved in steroid biochemistry, cell proliferation, apoptosis, and immunomodulatory effects. Recently, a study that reported the results of six healthy subjects undergoing positron emission tomography scans dramatically revealed that the sites are widespread throughout the body, associated with mitochondria (the cell's energy organelles) and immune cells.[79]

The PBR was discovered by serendipity. During the course of radioligand binding experiments to identify and characterize high-affinity diazepam binding sites in brain, peripheral tissues were used as controls since the anxiolytic and anticonvulsant effects of BZDs were thought to be mediated by receptors located exclusively in the CNS. But diazepam binding sites were detected in the control peripheral tissues.[80] Of the initial compounds that were used in rats, the rank order of binding potency to PBR was Ro5-4865 (4'-chlorodiazepam) > diazepam ≥ flunitrazepam >>> clonazepam (dissociation constants from 6 nM for Ro5-4864 to >10 μM for clonazepam). This the reverse order of binding of these compounds to the central BZD receptor, suggesting some distinction in the receptors.[81]

PBRS: WHERE AND WHY

The PBR is found in virtually all mammalian tissues[82] and in multiple species.[83-90] The density is highest in endocrine tissue[91-93]; it is found in greatest abundance in the outer membrane of mitochondria[94-98] and on red blood cells (which do not contain mitochondria).[99] PBRs are located in adrenal glands (high in the cortex, low in the medulla),[85,92] salivary glands,[85] cardiovascular system,[100,101] epithelium, liver,[85,97] testes,[92] and kidney (distal convoluted tubule, and ascending loop of Henle).[80,81,102,103] In an interesting twist, PBRs are also relatively abundant within the CNS (particularly glial cells)[101]; in fact PBRs exceed the density of central BZD receptor in some areas.[75,81]

PBR-specific ligands elicit multiple dose-dependent physiological effects such as inhibition of mitochondrial respiration,[94,104,105] enhanced prolactin-stimulated mitogenesis[106] and effects on cardiovascular tissues, and stimulation or inhibition of cell growth.[107-110] Two very nice early reviews of PBRs are Parola et al.[76] and Woods and Williams.[111] The PBR are thought to be involved to some uncertain extent in steroidogenesis (although this has recently been questioned),[112] mitochondrial respiration, calcium channel modulation, heme metabolism, cell proliferation and differentiation, and immunomodulation.[111]

PBRS: STRUCTURE

The complimentary DNA for PBR has been cloned from various species including humans.[113] There is a high degree of conserved primary coding sequence among the PBRs of the various species (but only about 30% sequence homology)[101] The human PBR gene (TSPO) is located on chromosome 22. The PBRs are heterotrimer receptors that are composed of three protein components: ANT (a 30 kDa adenine-nucleotide transporter), IBP (an 18 kDa isoquinoline-binding protein), and VDAC (a 32 kDa

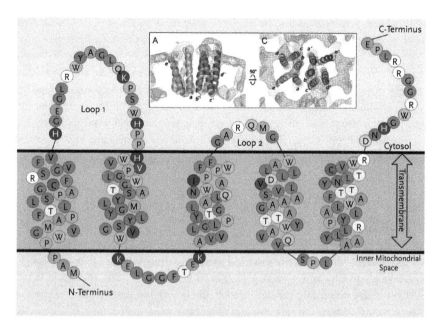

Figure 6.2 Schematic of a topological model of the human peripheral PBR (through the outer mitochondrial membrane). Cytosolic loop 1 and loop 2 are the binding sites for small molecule ligands such as benzodiazepines. *Inset:* View of the TSPO dimer, perpendicular and parallel to the membrane plane.

From Austin et al.[114] Used with permission.

voltage-dependent anion channel).[101] The PBR is a rather large complex, consisting of several molecules of IBP typically conjugated with ANT and VDAC molecules. A variety of additional molecules can be associated with the core proteins (Figure 6.2).[101,114]

Ro5 4864 and other BZDs appear to bind to all three components of the PBR complex (ANT, IBP, VDAC), whereas PK 11195 [1-(2-chlorophenyl)-N-methyl-N-(1-methyl-propyl)-3-isoquinolinecarboxamide] appears to bind more selectively to the IBP component of the PBR complex. Several endogenous ligands for PBRs have been identified.[101] Of possible particular relevance to BZD use and discontinuation is DBI and triakontatetraneuropeptide, a posttranslational product of DBI.[101] The implication of the endogenous PBR ligands is that they are regulators of PBR activity, and therefore administration or discontinuation of exogenous ligands (viz., BZD therapies) might interfere with or disrupt normal endogenous homeostatic control of PBR function. In humans, DBI (or, more precisely, DBI-like immunoreactivity) is found in highest concentration in liver and kidney and also throughout the CNS.[101]

PBRS: ARE THEY RELEVANT?

The PBRs are pharmacologically distinct from the central BZD receptors associated with the anxiolytic action of BzRAs, including insensitivity to GABA.[73–75,80,81] And the

PBR in humans have generally low affinity binding for BZD drugs,[99,115–119] particularly when measured under conditions designed to approximate the in vitro cerebral environment.[120] But these are all measurements of acute exposure. The binding following chronic administration is unknown. It seems reasonable to assume that significant changes would occur in PBR affinity and transduction (second-messenger coupling) during chronic administration and during withdrawal. Given the large number and very wide distribution of PBRs in the periphery and in the CNS, it seems reasonable to speculate that PBRs may play a significant role in explaining some of the unusual adverse effects of BzRAs as well as some of the unusual reported protracted withdrawal symptoms.[75,81]

DISCONTINUANCE AND WITHDRAWAL

With continued administration, almost all drugs (and other bioactive molecules) begin to elicit a progressive and increasingly large compensatory response that works in opposition to the direct drug-induced effect.[29] The observable external manifestation of this physiologic adjustment is a development of tolerance, the progressive decrease in drug-induced effect with each subsequent administration of drug.[121] Development of tolerance to BzRAs should not generally be a concern if they are properly prescribed for a short term (i.e., 2–4 weeks).[122] Nevertheless, when BzRAs are prescribed for durations that exceed this time and, rarely, less than this time,[123] development of tolerance is manifested in a negative way upon abrupt cessation of drug use. In this situation, compensatory mechanisms are unopposed, and symptoms opposite to the drug-induced effects are experienced (i.e., withdrawal symptoms).[124] Withdrawal symptoms are disagreeable or dysphoric and contribute to craving (i.e., a perceived want or need to take BzRA despite no true medical need or a desire to reinitiate taking the drug to avoid the unpleasant effects of not taking it).[125] Although detailed advice about how to effectively taper from BZD therapy is readily available,[126] some patients report serious, protracted symptoms.[127] A physiologic explanation for this phenomenon is lacking. The enigmatic PBR seems a likely candidate.

CONCLUSION AND PERSPECTIVE

PBRs, distinct from the traditional BZD receptor, are widely distributed throughout peripheral tissues and are also quite prevalent (despite the nomenclature) in the CNS. The fact that neither the basic pharmacology nor the effects mediated by PBRs are fully known is viewed in the context of the subject of this book not as a weakness, but rather a reason for believing that they might be a key for unlocking the mystery of unexplained adverse effects and the protracted withdrawal syndrome experienced by some patients while taking or discontinuing taking BzRAs.

REFERENCES

1. Archer GA, Sternbach LH. Chemistry of benzodiazepines. *Chem Rev.* 1968;68(6):747–784.
2. Information. NCfB. PubChem Compound Database; CID=134664. https://pubchem. ncbi.nlm.nih.gov/compound/134664. Accessed March 2, 2019.
3. Griffin CE 3rd, Kaye AM, Bueno FR, Kaye AD. Benzodiazepine pharmacology and central nervous system-mediated effects. *Ochsner J.* 2013;13(2):214–223.
4. Wick JY. The history of benzodiazepines. *Consult Pharm.* 2013;28(9):538–548.
5. Tallman JF, Paul SM, Skolnick P, Gallager DW. Receptors for the age of anxiety: pharmacology of the benzodiazepines. *Science.* 1980;207(4428):274–281.
6. Olsen RW. GABA-benzodiazepine-barbiturate receptor interactions. *J Neurochem.* 1981;37(1):1–13.
7. Lippa AS, Coupet J, Greenblatt EN, Klepner CA, Beer B. A synthetic non-benzodiazepine ligand for benzodiazepine receptors: a probe for investigating neuronal substrates of anxiety. *Pharmacol Biochem Behav.* 1979;11(1):99–106.
8. Lloyd KG, Depoortere H, Manoury P, et al. Non-benzodiazepine anxiolytics: potential activity of phenylpiperazines without 3H-diazepam displacing action. *Clinical Neuropharmacology.* 1984;7:896–897.
9. Perrault G, Morel E, Sanger DJ, Zivkovic B. Differences in pharmacological profiles of a new generation of benzodiazepine and non-benzodiazepine hypnotics. *Eur J Pharmacol.* 1990;187(3):487–494.
10. Campo-Soria C, Chang Y, Weiss DS. Mechanism of action of benzodiazepines on GABAA receptors. *Br J Pharmacol.* 2006;148(7):984–990.
11. Nutt DJ, Malizia AL. New insights into the role of the GABA(A)-benzodiazepine receptor in psychiatric disorder. *Br J Psychiatry.* 2001;179:390–396.
12. Laties VG, Weiss B. A critical review of the efficacy of meprobamate (miltown, equanil) in the treatment of anxiety. *J Chronic Dis.* 1958;7(6):500–519.
13. Berger FM. The similarities and differences between meprobamate and barbiturates. *Clin Pharmacol Ther.* 1963;4:209–233.
14. Stewart SH, Westra HA. Benzodiazepine side-effects: from the bench to the clinic. *Curr Pharm Des.* 2002;8(1):1–3.
15. Lopez-Munoz F, Ucha-Udabe R, Alamo C. The history of barbiturates a century after their clinical introduction. *Neuropsychiatr Dis Treat.* 2005;1(4):329–343.
16. Brandt J, Leong C. Benzodiazepines and Z-Drugs: An Updated Review of Major Adverse Outcomes Reported on in Epidemiologic Research. *Drugs R D.* 2017;17(4):493–507.
17. Gielen MC, Lumb MJ, Smart TG. Benzodiazepines modulate GABAA receptors by regulating the preactivation step after GABA binding. *J Neurosci.* 2012;32(17):5707–5715.
18. Poisbeau P, Gazzo G, Calvel L. Anxiolytics targeting GABAA receptors: Insights on etifoxine. *World J Biol Psychiatry.* 2018;19(Supp 1):S36–S45.
19. Macdonald RL, Olsen RW. GABAA receptor channels. *Annu Rev Neurosci.* 1994;17:569–602.
20. Ticku MK. Benzodiazepine-GABA receptor-ionophore complex: current concepts. *Neuropharmacology.* 1983;22(12B):1459–1470.
21. Costa E, Guidotti A. Molecular mechanisms in the receptor action of benzodiazepines. *Annu Rev Pharmacol Toxicol.* 1979;19:531–545.
22. Watanabe M, Fukuda A. Development and regulation of chloride homeostasis in the central nervous system. *Front Cell Neurosci.* 2015;9:371.
23. Cardozo D. An intuitive approach to understanding the resting membrane potential. *Adv Physiol Educ.* 2016;40(4):543–547.

24. Sanger DJ. The pharmacology and mechanisms of action of new generation, non-benzodiazepine hypnotic agents. *CNS Drugs.* 2004;*18*(Suppl 1):9–15; discussion 41, 43–15.

25. Gudex C. Adverse effects of benzodiazepines. *Soc Sci Med.* 1991;*33*(5):587–596.

26. Greenblatt DJ, Shader RI. Dependence, tolerance, and addiction to benzodiazepines: clinical and pharmacokinetic considerations. *Drug Metab Rev.* 1978;*8*(1):13–28.

27. Vinkers CH, Olivier B. Mechanisms underlying tolerance after long-term benzodiazepine use: a future for subtype-selective GABA(A) receptor modulators? *Adv Pharmacol Sci.* 2012;*2012*:416864.

28. Hodding GC, Jann M, Ackerman IP. Drug withdrawal syndromes: a literature review. *West J Med.* 1980;*133*(5):383–391.

29. Siegel S, Baptista MA, Kim JA, McDonald RV, Weise-Kelly L. Pavlovian psychopharmacology: the associative basis of tolerance. *Exp Clin Psychopharmacol.* 2000;*8*(3):276–293.

30. Siegel S. Drug Tolerance, Drug Addiction, and Drug Anticipation. *Cur Dir Psychol Sci.* 2005;*14*(6):296–300.

31. Roy-Byrne PP, Hommer D. Benzodiazepine withdrawal: overview and implications for the treatment of anxiety. *Am J Med.* 1988;*84*(6):1041–1052.

32. Onyett SR. The benzodiazepine withdrawal syndrome and its management. *J R Coll Gen Pract.* 1989;*39*(321):160–163.

33. Fluyau D, Revadigar N, Manobianco BE. Challenges of the pharmacological management of benzodiazepine withdrawal, dependence, and discontinuation. *Ther Adv Psychopharmacol.* 2018;*8*(5):147–168.

34. Higgitt A, Fonagy P, Lader M. The natural history of tolerance to the benzodiazepines. *Psychol Med Monogr Suppl.* 1988;*13*:1–55.

35. Petursson H. The benzodiazepine withdrawal syndrome. *Addiction.* 1994;*89*(11):1455–1459.

36. Ashton H. Protracted withdrawal syndromes from benzodiazepines. *J Subst Abuse Treat.* 1991;*8*(1-2):19–28.

37. McEnery MW, Snowman AM, Trifiletti RR, Snyder SH. Isolation of the mitochondrial benzodiazepine receptor: association with the voltage-dependent anion channel and the adenine nucleotide carrier. *Proc Natl Acad Sci U S A.* 1992;*89*(8):3170–3174.

38. Bond A, Lader M. Anxiolytics and Sedatives. In: Verster J, Brady K, Galanter M, Conrod P, eds. *Drug Abuse and Addiction in Medical Illness.* New York, NY: Springer; 2012.

39. Drover DR. Comparative pharmacokinetics and pharmacodynamics of short-acting hypnosedatives: zaleplon, zolpidem and zopiclone. *Clin Pharmacokinet.* 2004;*43*(4):227–238.

40. Gavish M, Snyder SH. Benzodiazepine recognition sites on GABA receptors. *Nature.* 1980;*287*(5783):651–652.

41. Mody I, Pearce RA. Diversity of inhibitory neurotransmission through GABA(A) receptors. *Trends Neurosci.* 2004;*27*(9):569–575.

42. Fritschy JM, Panzanelli P. GABAA receptors and plasticity of inhibitory neurotransmission in the central nervous system. *Eur J Neurosci.* 2014;*39*(11):1845–1865.

43. Duncan NW, Wiebking C, Northoff G. Associations of regional GABA and glutamate with intrinsic and extrinsic neural activity in humans-a review of multimodal imaging studies. *Neurosci Biobehav Rev.* 2014;*47*:36–52.

44. Barnard E, Skolnick P, Olsen R, et al. International Union of Pharmacology. XV. subtypes of γ-aminobutyric acid(A) receptors: classification on the basis of subunit structure and receptor function. *Pharmacol Rev.* 1998;*50*(2):291–314.

45. Tietz EI, Chiu TH, Rosenberg HC. Regional GABA/benzodiazepine receptor/chloride channel coupling after acute and chronic benzodiazepine treatment. *Eur J Pharmacol.* 1989;*167*(1):57–65.

46. Sieghart W. Pharmacology of benzodiazepine receptors: an update. *J Psychiatr Neurosci.* 1994;*19*(1):24–29.
47. Costa E, Guidotti A, Mao CC, Suria A. New concepts on the mechanism of action of benzodiazepines. *Life Sci.* 1975;*17*(2):167–185.
48. Haefely W, Kulcsar A, Mohler H. Possible involvement of GABA in the central actions of benzodiazepines. *Psychopharmacol Bull.* 1975;*11*(4):58–59.
49. Haefely W. Pharmacology of benzodiazepine antagonists. *Pharmacopsychiatry.* 1985;*18*(1):163–166.
50. Haefely W, Martin JR, Schoch P. Novel anxiolytics that act as partial agonists at benzodiazepine receptors. *Trends Pharmacol Sci.* 1990;*11*(11):452–456.
51. Cole BJ, Hillmann M, Seidelmann D, Klewer M, Jones GH. Effects of benzodiazepine receptor partial inverse agonists in the elevated plus maze test of anxiety in the rat. *Psychopharmacology (Berl).* 1995;*121*(1):118–126.
52. TenBrink RE, Im WB, Sethy VH, Tang AH, Carter DB. Antagonist, partial agonist, and full agonist imidazo[1,5-a]quinoxaline amides and carbamates acting through the GABAA/benzodiazepine receptor. *J Med Chem.* 1994;*37*(6):758–768.
53. Braestrup C, Nielsen M, Honore T, Jensen LH, Petersen EN. Benzodiazepine receptor ligands with positive and negative efficacy. *Neuropharmacology.* 1983;*22*(12B):1451–1457.
54. Awapara J, Landua AJ, Fuerst R, Seale B. Free gamma-aminobutyric acid in brain. *J Biol Chem.* 1950;*187*(1):35–39.
55. Roberts E, Frankel S. gamma-Aminobutyric acid in brain: its formation from glutamic acid. *J Biol Chem.* 1950;*187*(1):55–63.
56. Möhler H, Okada T. Benzodiazepine receptor: demonstration in the central nervous system. *Science.* 1977;*198*(4319):849–851.
57. Squires RF, Brastrup C. Benzodiazepine receptors in rat brain. *Nature.* 1977;*266*(5604):732–734.
58. Enna SJ, Snyder SH. A simple, sensitive and specific radioreceptor assay for endogenous GABA in brain tissue. *J Neurochem.* 1976;*26*(1):221–224.
59. Nelson H, Mandiyan S, Nelson N. Cloning of the human brain GABA transporter. *FEBS Lett.* 1990;*269*(1):181–184.
60. Perry TL, Berry K, Hansen S, Diamond S, Mok C. Regional distribution of amino acids in human brain obtained at autopsy. *J Neurochem.* 1971;*18*(3):513–519.
61. McCormick DA. GABA as an inhibitory neurotransmitter in human cerebral cortex. *J Neurophysiol.* 1989;*62*(5):1018–1027.
62. Braestrup C, Squires RF. Brain specific benzodiazepine receptors. *Br J Psychiatry.* 1978;*133*:249–260.
63. Beaumont K, Chilton WS, Yamamura HI, Enna SJ. Muscimol binding in rat brain: association with synaptic GABA receptors. *Brain Res.* 1978;*148*(1):153–162.
64. Cook L, Sepinwall J. Behavioral analysis of the effects and mechanisms of action of benzodiazepines. *Adv Biochem Psychopharmacol.* 1975(14):1–28.
65. Jessen KR. GABA and the enteric nervous system. A neurotransmitter function? *Mol Cell Biochem.* 1981;*38*(Pt 1):69–76.
66. Jessen KR, Mirsky R, Dennison ME, Burnstock G. GABA may be a neurotransmitter in the vertebrate peripheral nervous system. *Nature.* 1979;*281*(5726):71–74.
67. Gerber JC 3rd, Hare TA. Gamma-aminobutyric acid in peripheral tissue, with emphasis on the endocrine pancreas: presence in two species and reduction by streptozotocin. *Diabetes.* 1979;*28*(12):1073–1076.
68. MacNaughton WK, Pineau BC, Krantis A. gamma-Aminobutyric acid stimulates electrolyte transport in the guinea pig ileum in vitro. *Gastroenterology.* 1996;*110*(2):498–507.
69. Tsai LH, Tsai W, Wu JY. Action of myenteric GABAergic neurons in the guinea pig stomach. *Neurochem Int.* 1993;*23*(2):187–193.

70. Erdo SL, Mione MC, Amenta F, Wolff JR. Binding of [3H]-muscimol to GABAA sites in the guinea-pig urinary bladder: biochemical assay and autoradiography. *Br J Pharmacol.* 1989;96(2):313–318.

71. Krantis A, Harding RK. GABA-related actions in isolated in vitro preparations of the rat small intestine. *Eur J Pharmacol.* 1987;141(2):291–298.

72. Chintagari NR, Liu L. GABA receptor ameliorates ventilator-induced lung injury in rats by improving alveolar fluid clearance. *Crit Care.* 2012;16(2):R55.

73. Regan JW, Yamamura HI, Yamada S, Roeske WR. Renal benzodiazepine binding increases during deoxycorticosterone/salt hypertension in rats. *Eur J Pharmacol.* 1980;67(1):167–168.

74. Regan JW, Yamamura HI, Yamada S, Roeske WR. High affinity [3H]flunitrazepam binding: characterization, localization, and alteration in hypertension. *Life Sci.* 1981;28(9):991–998.

75. Marangos PJ, Patel J, Boulenger JP, Clark-Rosenberg R. Characterization of peripheral-type benzodiazepine binding sites in brain using [3H]Ro 5-4864. *Mol Pharmacol.* 1982;22(1):26–32.

76. Parola AL, Yamamura HI, Laird HE 3rd. Peripheral-type benzodiazepine receptors. *Life Sci.* 1993;52(16):1329–1342.

77. Langer SZ, Arbilla S, Tan S, et al. Selectivity for omega-receptor subtypes as a strategy for the development of anxiolytic drugs. *Pharmacopsychiatry.* 1990;23(Suppl 3):103–107.

78. Langer SZ, Arbilla S. Imidazopyridines as a tool for the characterization of benzodiazepine receptors: a proposal for a pharmacological classification as omega receptor subtypes. *Pharmacol Biochem Behav.* 1988;29(4):763–766.

79. Endres CJ, Coughlin JM, Gage KL, Watkins CC, Kassiou M, Pomper MG. Radiation dosimetry and biodistribution of the TSPO ligand 11C-DPA-713 in humans. *J Nuclear Med.* 2012;53(2):330–335.

80. Braestrup C, Squires RF. Specific benzodiazepine receptors in rat brain characterized by high-affinity (3H)diazepam binding. *Proc Natl Acad Sci U S A.* 1977;74(9):3805–3809.

81. Schoemaker H, Boles RG, Horst WD, Yamamura HI. Specific high-affinity binding sites for [3H]Ro 5-4864 in rat brain and kidney. *J Pharmacol Exp Ther.* 1983;225(1):61–69.

82. Wang JK, Taniguchi T, Spector S. Structural requirements for the binding of benzodiazepines to their peripheral-type sites. *Mol Pharmacol.* 1984;25(3):349–351.

83. Le Fur G, Perrier ML, Vaucher N, et al. Peripheral benzodiazepine binding sites: effect of PK 11195, 1-(2-chlorophenyl)-N-methyl-N-(1-methylpropyl)-3-isoquinolinecarboxamide. I. In vitro studies. *Life Sci.* 1983;32(16):1839–1847.

84. Le Fur G, Guilloux F, Rufat P, et al. Peripheral benzodiazepine binding sites: effect of PK 11195, 1-(2-chlorophenyl)-N-methyl-(1-methylpropyl)-3 isoquinolinecarboxamide. II. In vivo studies. *Life Sci.* 1983;32(16):1849–1856.

85. Anholt RR, De Souza EB, Oster-Granite ML, Snyder SH. Peripheral-type benzodiazepine receptors: autoradiographic localization in whole-body sections of neonatal rats. *J Pharmacol Exp Ther.* 1985;233(2):517–526.

86. Peterson CL, Duerson KC, Buckley AR, Putnam CW, Russell DH, Laird HE 2nd. Embryological development of peripheral benzodiazepine binding sites in the chick liver. *Proc West Pharmacol Soc.* 1988;31:263–264.

87. Eshleman AJ, Murray TF. Differential binding properties of the peripheral-type benzodiazepine ligands [3H]PK 11195 and [3H]Ro 5-4864 in trout and mouse brain membranes. *J Neurochem.* 1989;53(2):494–502.

88. Lesouhaitier O, Feuilloley M, Lihrmann I, et al. Localization of diazepam-binding inhibitor-related peptides and peripheral type benzodiazepine receptors in the frog adrenal gland. *Cell Tissue Res.* 1996;283(3):403–412.

89. Snyder MJ, Van Antwerpen R. Evidence for a diazepam-binding inhibitor (DBI) benzodiazepine receptor-like mechanism in ecdysteroidogenesis by the insect prothoracic gland. *Cell Tissue Res.* 1998;294(1):161–168.

90. Betti L, Giannaccini G, Nigro M, Dianda S, Gremigni V, Lucacchini A. Studies of peripheral benzodiazepine receptors in mussels: comparison between a polluted and a nonpolluted site. *Ecotoxicol Environ Saf.* 2003;54(1):36–42.

91. Verma A, Snyder SH. Peripheral type benzodiazepine receptors. *Annu Rev Pharmacol Toxicol.* 1989;29:307–322.

92. De Souza EB, Anholt RR, Murphy KM, Snyder SH, Kuhar MJ. Peripheral-type benzodiazepine receptors in endocrine organs: autoradiographic localization in rat pituitary, adrenal, and testis. *Endocrinology.* 1985;116(2):567–573.

93. Fares F, Bar-Ami S, Brandes JM, Gavish M. Gonadotropin- and estrogen-induced increase of peripheral-type benzodiazepine binding sites in the hypophyseal-genital axis of rats. *Eur J Pharmacol.* 1987;133(1):97–102.

94. Hirsch JD, Beyer CF, Malkowitz L, Loullis CC, Blume AJ. Characterization of ligand binding to mitochondrial benzodiazepine receptors. *Mol Pharmacol.* 1989;35(1):164–172.

95. Anholt RR, Pedersen PL, De Souza EB, Snyder SH. The peripheral-type benzodiazepine receptor. Localization to the mitochondrial outer membrane. *J Biol Chem.* 1986;261(2):576–583.

96. O'Beirne GB, Williams DC. The subcellular location in rat kidney of the peripheral benzodiazepine acceptor. *Eur J Biochem.* 1988;175(2):413–421.

97. O'Beirne GB, Woods MJ, Williams DC. Two subcellular locations for peripheral-type benzodiazepine acceptors in rat liver. *Eur J Biochem.* 1990;188(1):131–138.

98. Antkiewicz-Michaluk L, Guidotti A, Krueger KE. Molecular characterization and mitochondrial density of a recognition site for peripheral-type benzodiazepine ligands. *Mol Pharmacol.* 1988;34(3):272–278.

99. Olson JM, Ciliax BJ, Mancini WR, Young AB. Presence of peripheral-type benzodiazepine binding sites on human erythrocyte membranes. *Eur J Pharmacol.* 1988;152(1-2):47–53.

100. Doble A, Benavides J, Ferris O, et al. Dihydropyridine and peripheral type benzodiazepine binding sites: subcellular distribution and molecular size determination. *Eur J Pharmacol.* 1985;119(3):153–167.

101. Veenman L, Gavish M. The peripheral-type benzodiazepine receptor and the cardiovascular system. Implications for drug development. *Pharmacol Ther.* 2006;110(3):503–524.

102. Gehlert DR, Yamamura HI, Wamsley JK. Autoradiographic localization of "peripheral" benzodiazepine binding sites in the rat brain and kidney using [3H]RO5-4864. *Eur J Pharmacol.* 1983;95(3-4):329–330.

103. Gehlert DR, Yamamura HI, Wamsley JK. Autoradiographic localization of "peripheral-type" benzodiazepine binding sites in the rat brain, heart and kidney. *Naunyn Schmiedebergs Arch Pharmacol.* 1985;328(4):454–460.

104. Beavis AD. On the inhibition of the mitochondrial inner membrane anion uniporter by cationic amphiphiles and other drugs. *J Biol Chem.* 1989;264(3):1508–1515.

105. Larcher JC, Vayssiere JL, Le Marquer FJ, et al. Effects of peripheral benzodiazepines upon the O2 consumption of neuroblastoma cells. *Eur J Pharmacol.* 1989;161(2-3):197–202.

106. Laird HE 2nd, Gerrish KE, Duerson KC, Putnam CW, Russell DH. Peripheral benzodiazepine binding sites in Nb 2 node lymphoma cells: effects on prolactin-stimulated proliferation and ornithine decarboxylase activity. *Eur J Pharmacol.* 1989;171(1):25–35.

107. Clarke GD, Ryan PJ. Tranquillizers can block mitogenesis in 3T3 cells and induce differentiation in Friend cells. *Nature.* 1980;287(5778):160–161.

108. Wang JK, Morgan JI, Spector S. Benzodiazepines that bind at peripheral sites inhibit cell proliferation. *Proc Natl Acad Sci U S A.* 1984;81(3):753–756.

109. Ishiguro K, Taft WC, DeLorenzo RJ, Sartorelli AC. The role of benzodiazepine receptors in the induction of differentiation of HL-60 leukemia cells by benzodiazepines and purines. *J Cell Physiol.* 1987;*131*(2):226–234.

110. Ikezaki K, Black KL. Stimulation of cell growth and DNA synthesis by peripheral benzodiazepine. *Cancer Lett.* 1990;*49*(2):115–120.

111. Woods MJ, Williams DC. Multiple forms and locations for the peripheral-type benzodiazepine receptor. *Biochem Pharmacol.* 1996;*52*(12):1805–1814.

112. Selvaraj V, Stocco DM. The changing landscape in translocator protein (TSPO) function. *Trends Endocrinol Metab.* 2015;*26*(7):341–348.

113. Bonsack F, Sukumari-Ramesh S. TSPO: an evolutionarily conserved protein with elusive functions. *Int J Mol Sci.* 2018;*19*(6).

114. Austin CJ, Kahlert J, Kassiou M, Rendina LM. The translocator protein (TSPO): a novel target for cancer chemotherapy. *Int J Biochem Cell Biol.* 2013;*45*(7):1212–1216.

115. Moingeon P, Dessaux JJ, Fellous R, et al. Benzodiazepine receptors on human blood platelets. *Life Sci.* 1984;*35*(20):2003–2009.

116. O'Beirne GB, Williams DC. Binding of benzodiazepines to blood platelets from various species. *Biochem Pharmacol.* 1984;*33*(9):1568–1571.

117. Valtier D, Malgouris C, Gilbert JC, et al. Binding sites for a peripheral type benzodiazepine antagonist ([3H]PK 11195) in human iris. *Neuropharmacology.* 1987;*26*(6):549–552.

118. Mihara S, Fujimoto M. High-affinity binding sites for PK 11195, but not for RO5-4864, in porcine aortic smooth muscle. *Life Sci.* 1989;*44*(22):1713–1720.

119. Broaddus WC, Bennett JP Jr. Peripheral-type benzodiazepine receptors in human glioblastomas: pharmacologic characterization and photoaffinity labeling of ligand recognition site. *Brain Res.* 1990;*518*(1-2):199–208.

120. Kalk NJ, Owen DR, Tyacke RJ, et al. Are prescribed benzodiazepines likely to affect the availability of the 18 kDa translocator protein (TSPO) in PET studies? *Synapse.* 2013;*67*(12):909–912.

121. Ramsay DS, Woods SC. Biological consequences of drug administration: implications for acute and chronic tolerance. *Psychol Rev.* 1997;*104*(1):170–193.

122. Baldwin DS, Aitchison K, Bateson A, et al. Benzodiazepines: risks and benefits: a reconsideration. *J Psychopharmacol.* 2013;*27*(11):967–971.

123. Lembke A, Papac J, Humphreys K. Our other prescription drug problem. *N Engl J Med.* 2018;*378*(8):693–695.

124. Pétursson H. The benzodiazepine withdrawal syndrome. *Addiction.* 1994;*89*(11):1455–1459.

125. Robinson TE, Berridge KC. The neural basis of drug craving: an incentive-sensitization theory of addiction. *Brain Res Brain Res Rev.* 1993;*18*(3):247–291.

126. Ashton CH. *The Ashton Manual: Benzodiazepines: How They Work and How to Withdraw.* https://www.benzoinfo.com/ashtonmanual/. Revised 2002, with 2011, 2012, and 2013 supplements.

127. Meret-Carmen M. *Repairing the Benzo Blunder: a Mosaic of Recovery.* Bend, OR: Moonglade Press; 2017.

CHAPTER 7

Drug Withdrawal

A Modern Motivational View and Neurobiological Substrates

GEORGE F. KOOB

HIGHLIGHTS

- A motivational component of alcohol and drug withdrawal is conceptualized as a major motivational factor that drives compulsive drug taking.
- The negative emotional state (hyperkatifeia) that is associated with alcohol and drug withdrawal sets up a new source of motivation for drug seeking, termed *negative reinforcement*.
- Neurobiological substrates for such hyperkatifeia include within-system decreases in reward function in the basal ganglia and between-system increases in the activity of brain stress systems in the extended amygdala.
- Benzodiazepines may be unique from other drugs of abuse, in that they tap largely into the withdrawal/negative affect stage of the addiction cycle via between-system neuroadaptations.

ADDICTION

Alcohol and substance use disorders can be defined as a compulsion to seek and take a drug, the loss of control in limiting intake, and the emergence of a negative emotional state when access to the drug is prevented (Koob et al., 1998). A heuristic framework for alcohol and substance use disorders has been conceptualized that consists of a three-stage cycle—*binge/intoxication, withdrawal/negative affect*, and *preoccupation/*

anticipation—that provides a starting point for exploring the modern concept of drug withdrawal. Under this framework, alcohol and substance use disorders represent dysregulation in three functional domains (incentive salience/habits, negative emotional states, and executive function) that are mediated by three major neurocircuitry elements (basal ganglia, extended amygdala, and prefrontal cortex, respectively; Koob and Le Moal, 1997).

Opioids and alcohol are classic drugs of addiction, and the pattern that is present in humans varies highly but is also parochial. In opioid use disorder, there is an evolving pattern of use that includes intense initial intoxication that is associated with intravenous or smoked drug intake, the development of profound tolerance, and the consequent escalation of intake. Abstinence results in profound dysphoria, physical discomfort, and somatic signs of withdrawal. Intense preoccupation with obtaining opioids (craving) then develops, often preceding somatic signs of withdrawal. This craving is linked to stimuli that are associated with obtaining the drug and stimuli that are associated with withdrawal and internal and external states of stress. A pattern develops in which the drug must be administered to avoid the severe dysphoria and discomfort that are associated with abstinence (Koob et al., 2019).

In alcohol use disorder (AUD), a somewhat different pattern of drug taking develops that depends on the severity of the disorder. The initial intoxication is less intense than opioids, and the pattern of drug taking is often characterized by binges of alcohol intake that can be daily episodes or prolonged days of heavy drinking. A binge is currently defined by the U.S. National Institute on Alcohol Abuse and Alcoholism as consuming five standard drinks for males and four standard drinks for females in a 2-hour period or obtaining a blood alcohol level of 0.08 g%. Alcoholism or AUD is characterized by a severe emotional and somatic withdrawal syndrome and intense craving for the drug that is often driven by both negative emotional states and positive emotional states. Many individuals with AUD continue with such a binge/withdrawal pattern for extended periods; for others, the pattern evolves into an opioid-like substance use disorder, in which individuals must have alcohol available at all times to avoid the consequences of abstinence (Koob et al., 2019).

Nicotine addiction (or tobacco use disorder) is different from opioids and alcohol and associated with virtually no binge-like behavior in the binge/intoxication stage of the addiction cycle. Tobacco smokers and now nicotine vapers who use electronic cigarettes presumably engage in self-administration for the pleasurable and psychostimulant effects of nicotine but not in a binge-like fashion. Historically, cigarette smokers who meet the criteria for substance use disorder in the moderate to severe range likely smoke throughout the waking hours and experience negative emotional states (dysphoria, irritability, and intense craving) during abstinence. The pattern of intake is one of highly titrated intake of the drug during waking hours (Koob et al., 2019).

For psychostimulants, such as cocaine and amphetamines, the pattern of intake that is most associated with substance use disorder is one of repeated binges that can last hours or days, often followed by a crash that is characterized by extreme dysphoria and inactivity. Intense craving and anxiety occur later and are driven by both environmental cues that signal availability of the drug and internal states that are often linked to negative emotional states and stress (Koob et al., 2019).

Marijuana follows a pattern that is similar to nicotine, with a significant intoxication stage. As chronic use continues, individuals begin to show a pattern of chronic intoxication during waking hours. Marijuana withdrawal is long in onset and protracted because of the long half-life of Δ^9-tetrahydrocannaninol (Δ^9-THC) and is characterized by dysphoria, irritability, and sleep disturbances. Marijuana craving is most likely linked to both cues and internal states that are associated with negative emotional states and stress, similar to other drugs of abuse but again with a longer onset because of the relatively long half-life (Koob et al., 2019).

The pattern of benzodiazepine addiction (or sedative, hypnotic, or anxiolytic use disorder) can derive from several sources, including recreational use, medication treatment gone awry, or self-medication gone awry (O'Brien, 2005). The latter scenario is associated with a common progression of misuse. With long-term therapeutic administration or self-medication, upon the cessation of use, a benzodiazepine withdrawal syndrome is manifest, characterized by symptoms that include anxiety, depressed mood, sleep disturbances, tremor, shakiness, and headache and can include somatic symptoms of anxiety, depersonalization, derealization, hypersensitivity to touch, pain, muscular aches, and twitches (Khong et al., 2004; O'Brien, 2005). Subjects report feeling unable to cope without the drug, unsuccessful attempts to cut back or stop drug use, and feeling uncomfortable when not taking the drug (O'Brien, 2005). As with other drugs of abuse, benzodiazepines with a long half-life may have a longer onset of hyperkatifeia-like withdrawal that is less intense and more prolonged, whereas benzodiazepines with a short half-life induce opposite withdrawal effects. For example, abuse potential appears to vary with pharmacokinetic parameters (Mintzer and Griffiths, 2005), but more data are needed to confirm a pharmacokinetic hyperkatifeia hypothesis with benzodiazepines.

From a dynamic perspective, excessive drug taking in the binge/intoxication stage drives an allostatic-like process, in which the break with reward homeostasis triggers compensatory responses in the brain reward and stress systems to generate the withdrawal/negative affect stage and preoccupation/anticipation stage (Koob and Le Moal, 1997). The three stages feed into each other, become more intense, and ultimately lead to the pathological state of substance use disorder (Koob and Le Moal, 1997; Figure 7.1). Particularly with opioids, alcohol, and benzodiazepines, the termination of drug taking inevitably leads to negative emotional states of acute and protracted withdrawal in the withdrawal/negative affect stage, which generates a second motivational drive from negative reinforcement. Protracted abstinence incorporates residual elements of negative emotional states and cue and contextual craving to form the preoccupation/anticipation stage. Opioid, psychostimulant, alcohol, marijuana, and sedative-hypnotic use disorders are now considered spectrum disorders as described by the *Diagnostic and Statistical Manual of Mental Disorders*, fifth edition (American Psychiatric Association, 2013), which provides a framework for the intensity of symptoms with regard to the number of symptoms that are presented. The spectrum framework also emphasizes that an individual can enter the addiction cycle at different stages. For example, with opioid, alcohol, and benzodiazepine use disorders, individuals may start with recreational use of the drug and progress to the withdrawal/negative affect stage as negative reinforcement evolves (Koob et al., 2019). However, possibly different from preconceptions

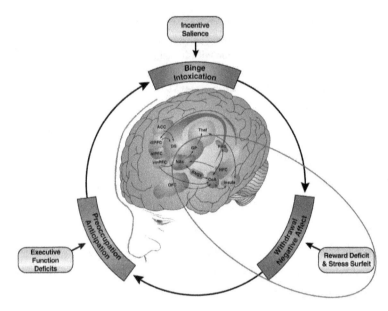

Figure 7.1 Conceptual framework for neurobiological bases of substance use disorders. See text.
Abbreviations: ACC, anterior cingulate cortex; BNST, bed nucleus of the stria terminalis; CeA, central nucleus of the amygdala; DS, dorsal striatum; dlPFC, dorsolateral prefrontal cortex; GP, globus pallidus; HPC, hippocampus; NAC, nucleus accumbens; OFC, orbitofrontal cortex; Thal, thalamus; vlPFC, ventrolateral prefrontal cortex; vmPFC, ventro-medial prefrontal cortex.
Modified from Koob and Volkow (2010).

about addiction, much substance use develops because negative reinforcement may be the initial starting point either via self-medication or chronic pain (Ballantyne et al., 2019). The focus of this chapter is on drug withdrawal and symptoms that are associated with the withdrawal/negative affect stage. Notably, however, the focus is not on physical or somatic signs of withdrawal but rather negative emotional and motivational signs of withdrawal, sometimes termed *hyperkatifeia* (Shurman and Koob, 2010). The relationship with emotional pain and the neurobiological circuits that are engaged to produce negative emotional states that drive negative reinforcement are explored later in this chapter.

WHAT IS WITHDRAWAL? DEFINITIONS

Withdrawal is historically defined as abstinence or removal from chronic drug use, usually characterized by signs and symptoms that are opposite to the acute effects of the drug (Koob et al., 2019). Somatic or physical symptoms of withdrawal are defined as physical/body symptoms that are associated with drug withdrawal (Koob, 2019a; Table 7.1). Motivational symptoms of withdrawal are defined as symptoms of withdrawal that are associated with negative emotional states (Koob, 2019a; Table 7.2).

Table 7.1 SOMATIC WITHDRAWAL SIGNS

Opioid withdrawal

Rats	Humans
Weight loss	Weight loss
Diarrhea	Diarrhea
Escape attempts	Yawning
Wet dog shakes	Lacrimation
Abdominal constrictions	Rhinorrhea
Facial fasciculations	Perspiration
Teeth chattering	Gooseflesh
Salivation	Tremor
Ptosis	Dilated pupils
Abnormal posture	Anorexia
Penile grooming	Nausea
Erection/ejaculation	Emesis
Irritability	Hyperthermia
	Increased blood pressure

Alcohol withdrawal

Rats	Humans
Hyperactivity	Tremor
Tail tremors	Increased heart rate
Tail stiffness	Increased blood pressure
Akinesia	Increased body temperature
Spastic rigidity	Anorexia
Convulsions	Convulsions
	Hyperthermia
	Delirium tremens

Table 7.2 MOTIVATIONAL WITHDRAWAL SIGNS

Rats	Humans
Elevated reward thresholds	Anhedonia or hypohedonia
Irritability	Irritability
Anxiety-like responses[a]	Anxiety
Conditioned place aversion	Dysphoria

[a]Responses in the elevated plus maze, open field test, probe burying test, marble burying test, light–dark test, etc.

Withdrawal from drugs of abuse is one symptom of what is defined symptomatically as substance use disorder in the *Diagnostic and Statistical Manual of Mental Disorders*, fifth edition, and *International Statistical Classification of Diseases and Related Health Problems*, 10th revision (World Health Organization, 1992) and is historically focused on what were defined as physical symptoms of withdrawal and reflected by signs and symptoms of a physical nature that are usually opposite to the acute effects of the drug itself. For example, with opioids, pupillary dilation is a telltale sign of opioid withdrawal, whereas pupillary constriction is a telltale sign of opioid intoxication. Similarly for alcohol, sympathetic-like responses, such as hyperthermia, indicate withdrawal, whereas hypothermia characterizes acute intoxication (see Table 7.1). However, these somatic measures are basically a red herring for the more motivational measures of withdrawal from the perspective of negative reinforcement, drug-seeking, and craving that are associated with acute and protracted abstinence. Nevertheless, the somatic signs of withdrawal are useful as an index of dependence, in which more motivational measures generally have an earlier onset at lower doses.

Here, the manifestation of a withdrawal syndrome after the cessation of chronic drug administration is defined in terms of motivational aspects of dependence, such as the emergence of a negative emotional state (e.g., dysphoria, anxiety, and irritability—all incorporated in the term *hyperkatifeia*; see following discussion) when access to the drug is prevented, rather than physical signs of dependence. Indeed, some have argued that the development of such a negative affective state can define dependence as it relates to addiction:

> The notion of dependence on a drug, object, role, activity or any other stimulus-source requires the crucial feature of negative affect experienced in its absence. The degree of dependence can be equated with the amount of this negative affect, which may range from mild discomfort to extreme distress, or it may be equated with the amount of difficulty or effort required to do without the drug, object, etc. (Russell, 1976)

Rather than focusing on the physical signs of dependence, the conceptual framework herein focuses on motivational aspects of alcohol and substance use disorders. The emergence of a negative emotional state (dysphoria, anxiety, irritability) when access to the drug is prevented is associated with the transition from drug use to substance use disorder (Koob and Le Moal, 2001).

OPPONENT PROCESS

An overarching hypothesis to explain tolerance and withdrawal falls within the realm of counteradaptations, and such a counteradaptation hypothesis fits well with the motivational component of withdrawal. Counteradaptations were initially hypothesized to explain the physiological (physical, somatic) effects of opioid withdrawal in the domain of body temperature (Martin, 1968; Himmelsbach, 1943) but were later expanded to the hedonic domain. Here, the initial acute effects of a drug are opposed or counteracted by homeostatic changes in systems that mediate the primary effects of the drug (Poulos and Cappell, 1991; Siegel, 1975; Solomon and Corbit, 1974). Termed *opponent-process theory* (Solomon and Corbit, 1973, 1974; Solomon, 1980; Koob and Bloom, 1988; Hoffman and Solomon, 1974; D'Amato, 1974), it was applied not only to drugs of abuse but also to many hedonic breaks with homeostasis, including fear conditioning, tonic immobility, ulcer formation, eating disorders, jogging, peer separation, glucose preference, and even skydiving (Solomon, 1980; Solomon and Corbit, 1973, 1974; Hoffman and Solomon, 1974).

Opponent process theory argues that the brain contains many affective control mechanisms that serve as an emotional immunization system that counteracts or opposes departures from emotional neutrality or equilibrium, regardless of whether they are aversive or pleasant (Solomon and Corbit, 1974). This theory is basically a negative feed-forward control construct that is designed to keep mood in homeostatic balance, even with strong perturbations, or what has been termed *allostatic load* (McEwen and Stellar, 1993; McEwen, 2000). First, an unconditioned arousing stimulus triggers a primary affective process, termed the *a-process*, an unconditional reaction that translates the intensity, quality, and duration of the stimulus (e.g., the first, initial use of a drug). Second, as a consequence of the *a-process*, the opposing *b-process* is evoked after a short delay, thus defining the opponent process. The *b-process* was hypothesized to provide a negative signal, subtracting the impact of the already existing *a-process*. These two responses are consequently and temporally linked (*a* triggers *b*) and were hypothesized to depend on different neurobiological mechanisms, but such neurobiological mechanisms that were presumed to be distinct were later shown to exhibit both within- and between-system neuroadaptations (see following discussion). The *b-process* has a longer latency, but some data show that it may appear soon after stimulus onset in the course of the stimulus action (Larcher et al., 1998). The *b-process* also has more inertia than the *a-process*, slower recruitment, and a more sluggish decay (Solomon and Corbit, 1974). Thus, at a given time point, the impact on affect will simply be the algebraic sum of these opposite influences, yielding the net product of the opponent process over time (Solomon, 1980).

A further argument is that with repetition of the stimulus, the dynamics or net product is a result of a progressive increase in the *b-process*. In other words, the *b-process* itself is sensitized with repeated drug use and appears progressively more rapidly after the unconditioned stimulus onset. It then persists longer after its initial, intended action (the unconditioned effect) and eventually masks the unconditioned effect (*a-process*), resulting in what has been termed *apparent tolerance* (Laulin et al., 1999; Colpaert, 1996). Indeed, data indicate that if the development of the *b-process* is blocked, then tolerance does not develop. Under this framework, the unconditioned effect of the drug does not change with repeated drug administration but rather the development of the *b-process* reflects the development of a negative emotional withdrawal symptoms, masked to some extent by the hedonic properties of the unconditioned stimulus. However, in the case of drugs of abuse, as the neurobiological opponent *b-process* grows, it takes the form of an aversive negative emotional state with such symptoms as dysphoria, anxiety, alexithymia, irritability, sleep disturbances, subjective feelings of unease, and simply not feeling hedonically normal.

This hyperemotional state, termed hyperkatifeia, sensitizes with repeated drug exposure and withdrawal and shows parallels to the greater sensitivity to physical pain, termed hyperalgesia, that is associated with withdrawal from chronic opioids and alcohol (Shurman et al., 2010; Koob, 2019b). In terms of the motivation for drug seeking, a new source of acquired motivation is generated, termed negative reinforcement (Ahmed and Koob, 2005). Negative reinforcement can be defined as an increase in the probability of a response that is produced by the removal of an aversive event. Here, negative reinforcement becomes the source of motivation for drug seeking as the individual works to reduce, terminate, or prevent the negative emotional state or the hyperkatifeia of drug withdrawal. As a result, a greater quantity and more frequent use of the previously rewarding drug is needed to maintain or approach euthymia.

Thus, the argument of this chapter is that there are elements of drug withdrawal and repeated, chronic drug intake that are expressed in common elements across different drugs of abuse (see Table 7.2). A further hypothesis is that subjects misregulate intake by taking more drug to alleviate hyperkatifeia, which paradoxically drives more hyperkatifeia. (Koob and Le Moal, 1997). Under this framework, substance use is compulsively escalated or renewed (in relapse) via negative reinforcement mechanisms because it transiently prevents or relieves the negative emotional symptoms or hyperkatifeia. This compulsive drug seeking then defends a hedonic set point that gradually gains allostatic load and shifts from a homeostatic hedonic state to an allostatic hedonic state (Koob and Le Moal, 2001; Figure 7.2).

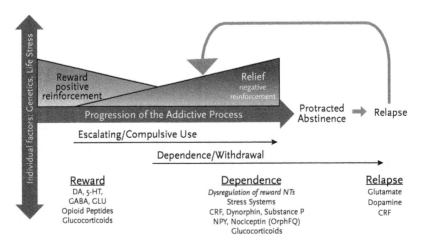

Figure 7.2 Figurative representation of the role of positive and negative reinforcement in alcohol and substance use disorders. Addiction begins with positive reinforcement, but negative reinforcement dominates as the disorder progresses. Negative reinforcement drives continued drug use, and residual conditioned reinforcement drives relapse. Different neurotransmitters/neuromodulators are engaged in the progression of addiction.

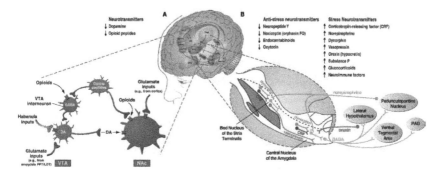

Figure 7.3 Neural circuitry associated with the negative emotional state of the *withdrawal/negative affect* stage. (A) Extended amygdala and within-system neuroadaptations. Note the loss of dopamine and opioid peptide function in VTA-nucleus accumbens circuitry, with a hypothesized contribution of the habenula that suppresses VTA neuron activity (*Inset*). (B) Extended amygdala and between-system neuroadaptations. Note the gain of stress neurotransmitter and neuromodulator function and loss of anti-stress neurotransmitter and neuromodulator function throughout the neurocircuitry of the extended amygdala (*Inset*). The extended amygdala is composed of several basal forebrain structures, including the bed nucleus of the stria terminalis, central nucleus of the amygdala, and possibly a transition area in the medial portion (shell) of the nucleus accumbens.

Abbreviations: ACC, anterior cingulate cortex; BNST, bed nucleus of the stria terminalis; CeA, central nucleus of the amygdala; DS, dorsal striatum; dlPFC, dorsolateral prefrontal cortex; GP, globus pallidus; HPC, hippocampus; NAC, nucleus accumbens; OFC, orbitofrontal cortex; Thal, thalamus; vlPFC, ventrolateral prefrontal cortex; vmPFC, ventromedial prefrontal cortex.

Adapted from Koob (2008) and George and Koob (2013).

HEDONIC OPPONENT PROCESS IN HUMANS AND ANIMAL MODELS

A key common element of all drugs of abuse is the dysregulation of brain reward function that is associated with the cessation of chronic drug administration. Rapid acute tolerance and opponent-process-like actions against the hedonic effects of cocaine have been reported in humans who smoke coca paste (Van Dyke and Byck, 1982) and subjects who receive intravenous cocaine (Breiter et al., 1997). Thus, in opponent-process theory, tolerance and dependence are inextricably linked, in which the hedonic effects of the drug subside, and the *b-process* emerges as an aversive negative emotional state (Solomon and Corbit, 1974). The *b-process* gets progressively larger over time, in effect contributing to or producing more complete tolerance to the initial euphoric effects of the drug.

Hedonic-like opponent processes generalize to animal models of addiction (Koob and Le Moal, 2005). All major drugs of abuse produce elevations of reward thresholds, measured by intracranial self-stimulation during withdrawal, and these effects are particularly dramatic in animal models of extended access to drugs of abuse. With extended access, animals escalate their drug intake and exhibit parallel elevations of intracranial self-stimulation reward thresholds. Such elevations have been observed with extended access to cocaine (Ahmed et al., 2002), methamphetamine (Jang et al., 2013), heroin (Kenny et al., 2006), and nicotine (Harris et al., 2011).

Several lines of evidence, ranging from a factor analysis of responses on self-reports and neuropsychological tests in humans with AUD to a connectome imaging study in mice, have validated the importance of the hyperkatifeia construct as a key stage in the development and maintenance of alcohol and substance use disorders. In an attempt to translate the research domain framework to a clinical framework, a study was performed with the goal of translating and reverse translating knowledge that has been derived from animal models of alcohol and substance use disorders to the human condition via measures of neurobiological processes that are orthologous in animals and humans and that are shared in alcohol and substance use disorders (Kwako et al., 2016). Thus, the hypothesis was that measures of three neuroscience-based functional domains (incentive salience, negative emotionality, and executive function) can capture many of the effects of inheritance and early exposure that lead to trait vulnerability that is shared across different addictive disorders. A further hypothesis under test was that measures of these domains in a general framework of an Addictions Neuroclinical Assessment have the possibility to transform the assessment and nosology of addictive disorders and can be informative for staging disease progression. A subhypothesis was that a focus on negative emotionality and stress may serve as a bridge to a reformulation of the addiction nosology to better capture individual differences in patients for whom the withdrawal/negative affect stage drives compulsive drug taking (Kwako and Koob, 2017). Using the Addictions Neuroclinical Assessment, five subdomains of negative emotional states that can be operationally measured in human laboratory settings and paralleled by animal models were outlined (Kwako et al., 2016). In a subsequent study, the three neurofunctional domains that were proposed to be critical for the addiction cycle (incentive salience, negative emotionality, and executive function) were validated using a factor analysis of a deeply phenotyped clinical sample (Kwako et al., 2019). Clinical, behavioral, and self-report measures of addiction, personality, cognition, behavior, and exposure to early life stress were collected as part of a screening and natural history study of AUD in 454 individuals who represented the spectrum of alcohol use and AUD. A three-factor model generally demonstrated a good fit with the assessment measures, and the factors closely aligned with the Addictions Neuroclinical Assessment domains of Incentive Salience, Negative Emotionality, and Executive Function.

A connectome imaging study using a hypothesis-free analysis of combined resting-state functional magnetic resonance imaging diffusion tractography showed that μ-opioid receptor gene (*Oprm1*) inactivation produced dramatic changes in aversion/pain-related connectivity rather than reward connectivity (Mechling et al., 2016). The authors argued that these results may reflect stronger inhibitory μ-opioid receptor tone or a developmental influence on negative affect neurocircuits, at least under resting-state conditions. Behavioral modifications in *Oprm1* mutant mice with regard to pain and emotional and reward-related behaviors correlated predominantly with alterations within reward/aversion pathways (Kieffer and Gaveriaux-Ruff, 2002). Examinations of alterations of hub status and direct statistical intergroup comparisons indicated a reshaping of networks that are known to process information of negative valence. Such structures as the periaqueductal gray, hippocampus, amygdala, cingulate cortex, median raphe, and habenula were components of such a negative valence network (Mechling et al., 2016).

Consistent with the connectome results, neurochemistry and neurocircuitry studies have shown that neuroadaptations that mediate hyperkatifeia have a focal point in the extended amygdala. The extended amygdala comprises several basal forebrain structures, including the bed nucleus of the stria terminalis, central nucleus of the amygdala, sublenticular substantia innominata, and a transition zone in the shell of the nucleus accumbens (Heimer and Alheid, 1991). Lesions of the central nucleus of the amygdala blocked the development of morphine withdrawal-induced conditioned place aversion but had less of an effect on somatic signs of withdrawal (Watanabe et al., 2002).

WITHIN- AND BETWEEN-SYSTEM NEUROADAPTATIONS IN DRUG WITHDRAWAL

A conceptual framework that was adopted to explain the neural systems that are argued to mediate hyperkatifeia and drive the motivational component of opponent processes of excessive drug use involved the within-system downregulation of brain reward circuitry and between-system recruitment of brain stress circuitry, all within the extended amygdala (Koob and Bloom, 1988; Koob and Le Moal, 2008; Koob, 2019b). Within-system neuroadaptations were defined as the process by which the primary cellular response element to the drug within a given neurochemical circuit itself adapts to neutralize the effects of the drug. In contrast, between-system neuroadaptations were defined as a circuitry change, in which another circuit (i.e., stress or antireward circuits) is activated by reward circuits. Persistence of the opposing effects after removal of the drug is reflected by the negative emotional withdrawal syndrome that is described above.

Within-System Neuroadaptations

For opioids, one source of within-system neuroadaptations involves elements of opioid receptor function that mediate tolerance to opioids, and this tolerance would extend to the rewarding effects of the drug. G proteins that are activated through the μ-opioid receptor modulate the activity of several second messengers and cellular effectors, which may generate both short- and long-term neuroadaptations that are relevant to tolerance at the molecular and cellular levels. Other molecular/cellular events, in addition to G-protein signaling cascades, contribute to μ-opioid receptor signaling, including receptor desensitization, receptor internalization, transcriptional changes, and structural changes, such as dendritic spine remodeling (Al-Hasani and Bruchas, 2011; Sugiura et al., 2009; Williams et al., 2013). Tolerance at the cellular level may be the sum of these multiple events (Cahill et al., 2016).

For alcohol, within-system neuroadaptations include alterations of neurotransmitter systems that are known to be modulated by the acute effects of alcohol. Two key neurotransmitter systems are γ-aminobutyric acid (GABA) and glutamate.

Chronic alcohol decreases GABA receptor function, with multiple effects on GABA receptor subunits with some of the most consistent being downregulation of the α1 subunit and upregulation of the α4 subunit (Mhatre et al., 1993; Devaud et al., 1997). Alcohol withdrawal is characterized by a hyperglutamatergic state. Competitive glutamate receptor antagonists can reverse the anxiogenic-like effects of alcohol withdrawal (Gatch et al., 1999). Chronic acamprosate, a glutamate modulator and Food and Drug Administration–approved treatment for AUD, blocks alcohol deprivation effect-induced drinking in rodents (Heyser et al., 1998) and blocks increases in glutamate in the brain in humans (Hermannn et al., 2012; Umhau et al., 2010).

For benzodiazepines, chronic treatment reduces the function of $GABA_A$ receptors (Bateson, 2002). Thus, a within-system neuroadaptation that is hypothesized for benzodiazepines involves a decrease in GABAergic function via numerous adaptations that occur at the level of the $GABA_A$ receptor (i.e., downregulation, desensitization, allosteric uncoupling, and subsensitivity, among others; Licata and Rowlett, 2008; Bateson, 2002). Additionally, similar to alcohol, pharmacological and molecular studies implicate an excitatory glutamatergic compensatory response to the benzodiazepine-induced enhancement of inhibition. Excitatory glutamatergic mechanisms become more sensitive, and this sensitivity is reflected by glutamatergic overactivity upon withdrawal (Stephens, 1995; Licata and Rowlett, 2008; Tsuda et al., 1999). For example, anxiety-like responses in rats during benzodiazepine withdrawal are associated with enhanced α-amino-3-hydroxy-5-methylisoxazole-4-propionic acid receptor–mediated glutamatergic transmission in the hippocampus (Das et al., 2008). Evidence also indicates a reduction of synaptic GluN1/GluN2B receptors and the preservation of GluN1/GluN2A receptors in the hippocampus during benzodiazepine withdrawal (Das et al., 2010).

The repeated administration or extended-access self-administration of most drugs of abuse produces a compromised dopamine system during acute withdrawal that in humans extends into protracted abstinence. For psychostimulants, both presynaptic and postsynaptic components of the dopamine system in the striatum are downregulated in stimulant users (Ashok et al., 2017). For opioids, early studies showed that precipitated opioid withdrawal was associated with decreases in extracellular dopamine levels in the nucleus accumbens (Pothos et al., 1991) and that the mesolimbic dopamine system was compromised, with decreases in dopamine neuron firing and extracellular dopamine levels during opioid withdrawal (Rossetti et al., 1992; Diana, 2011).

In humans, positron emission tomography studies showed lower baseline dopamine D_2 receptor availability in the striatum in subjects with opioid, psychostimulant, and alcohol use disorders compared with controls (Wang et al., 1997; Ashok et al., 2017). One mechanism to explain the hypodopaminergic state is that opioids, psychostimulants, and alcohol produce the activation of dynorphin, particularly in the shell of the nucleus accumbens, triggered by a cascade of molecular events that involve cyclic adenosine monophosphate to dynorphin activation (Carlezon et al., 2000; Chavkin and Koob, 2016), also see below.

Note that unlike most other drugs of abuse, the acute administration of benzodiazepine-type drugs does not increase extracellular dopamine levels in the nucleus accumbens in animal models (Licata and Rowlett, 2008). Thus, there is little evidence of changes in dopamine that are associated with benzodiazepine withdrawal in the context of an opponent-process construct. This leads to the hypothesis that hyperkatifeia-like effects that are observed during benzodiazepine withdrawal draw more from between-system neuroadaptations with the recruitment of brain stress systems than via the suppression of reward systems.

Between-System Neuroadaptations

For between-system neuroadaptations, the recruitment of brain stress systems, including corticotropin-releasing factor (CRF), norepinephrine, hypocretin, and dynorphin, among others, is a major key substrate that is responsible for the aversive stimulus effects of drug withdrawal that drive compulsive-like drug seeking (Koob and Bloom, 1988).

For opioids, early work showed that the antagonism of CRF receptors and noradrenergic receptors in the extended amygdala blocked the aversive stimulus effects of drug withdrawal (Koob, 2015). The administration of a CRF_1/CRF_2 peptide receptor antagonist in the central nucleus of the amygdala blocked precipitated conditioned place aversion that was produced by opioid withdrawal (Heinrichs et al., 1995). The blockade of noradrenergic function in the bed nucleus of the stria terminalis also blocked opioid withdrawal-induced place aversions (Delfs et al., 2000; Watanabe et al., 2003). These same neuropharmacological systems that are implicated in the aversive effects of drug withdrawal are also implicated in compulsive drug taking and seeking that are associated with extended-access intravenous self-administration in animal models. CRF receptor antagonists also dose-dependently decreased compulsive-like drug intake in rats with extended access to psychostimulants, opioids, nicotine, and alcohol (Koob, 2017). Similarly, benzodiazepine withdrawal is associated with higher CRF messenger RNA activity in the bed nucleus of the stria terminalis, paraventricular nucleus of the hypothalamus, and cortex (Skelton et al., 2004). Anxiety-like responses that are associated with benzodiazepine withdrawal can be blocked by systemic administration of CRF antagonists in rats (Skelton et al., 2007).

Brain stress systems are not limited to CRF (Koob, 2015). Multiple neurotransmitter systems converge on the extended amygdala to meet the needs of an organism to respond to an acute stressor but also to sustain a response to a chronic stressor (such as the cycle of repeated binge–withdrawal in alcohol and substance use disorders). Other modulatory brain neurotransmitter systems that have pro-stress actions also converge on the extended amygdala and include norepinephrine, serotonin, vasopressin, substance P, hypocretin (orexin), and dynorphin, all of which may contribute to negative emotional states that are associated with drug withdrawal or protracted abstinence (Koob, 2008). κ-opioid receptor agonists (administered systemically) and dynorphins (administered intracerebrally) produce aversive-like effects in both animals and humans (Shippenberg et al., 2007) and have been hypothesized to mediate negative emotional states that are associated with drug withdrawal (Chavkin and Koob, 2016). High compulsive-like drug intake that is associated with extended access to and dependence on methamphetamine, heroin, and alcohol is blocked by both systemic and intracerebral κ-opioid receptor antagonist administration. Two sites for these actions are the shell of the nucleus accumbens and amygdala, suggesting a κ-opioid receptor–dynorphin contribution within the extended amygdala to negative emotional states (Chavkin and Koob, 2016). High compulsive-like alcohol drinking in dependent rats during withdrawal can also be blocked by a β-adrenergic receptor antagonist, α1 adrenergic receptor antagonist, κ-opioid receptor antagonist, vasopressin-1b receptor antagonist, glucocorticoid receptor antagonist, and neuroimmune system antagonist (Koob, 2008, 2017). High compulsive-like heroin intake in the model of extended-access self-administration was blocked by a substance P antagonist and hypocretin-2 antagonist (Barbier et al., 2013; Schmeichel et al., 2015; see Figure 7.2). Serotonin systems have been hypothesized to be activated during benzodiazepine withdrawal and contribute to the anxiety-like effects that are observed in animal models (Andrews and File, 1993).

Similarly, one may hypothesize that the vulnerability to drive allostasis in alcohol and substance use disorders may not only derive from the activation of pro-stress neurotransmitter systems but also from anti-stress neurotransmitter systems. Anti-stress neurotransmitter systems may serve as neuroadaptive buffers to the pro-stress actions that are described above. Neurotransmitter/neuromodulatory systems that are implicated in anti-stress actions include neuropeptide Y (NPY), nociceptin, and endocannabinoids. Neuropeptide Y has powerful orexigenic and anxiolytic effects and has been hypothesized to act in opposition to the actions of CRF in alcohol and substance use disorders (Heilig and Koob, 2007). The activation of NPY in the central nucleus of the amygdala has opposite effects to CRF, in which NPY, injected into the brain, blocks the increase in GABA release in the central nucleus of the amygdala that is produced by alcohol, blocks high compulsive-like alcohol administration, and blocks the transition to excessive drinking with the development of dependence (Gilpin et al., 2003, 2008, 2011; Thorsell et al., 2005a, 2005b, 2007). Nociceptin has anti-stress-like effects in animals (Ciccocioppo et al., 2003; Martin-Fardon et al., 2010). Nociceptin and synthetic nociception receptor agonists have effects on GABA synaptic activity in the central nucleus of the amygdala that are similar to NPY and can block high alcohol consumption in a genetically selected line of rats that is known to be hypersensitive to stressors (Economidou et al., 2008). Evidence also implicates endocannabinoids in the regulation of affective states, in which reductions of cannabinoid CB_1 receptor signaling produce anxiogenic-like behavioral effects (Serrano and Parsons, 2011). Blocking endocannabinoid clearance can also block some drug-seeking behaviors (Scherma et al., 2008; Adamczyk et al., 2009; Forget et al., 2009). Thus, endocannabinoids may play a protective role in preventing drug dependence by buffering the stress activation that is associated with withdrawal (see Figure 7.2).

CONCLUSION

In summary, drug withdrawal, conceptualized from the perspective of the hyperkatifeia domain, remains a key part of alcohol and substance use disorders and could be argued in moderate to severe alcohol and substance use disorders to be the key factor that motivates sustained drug seeking. Such hyperkatifeia is mediated by a multidetermined neurocircuitry that compromises within-system neurochemical systems that are involved in the rewarding effects of drugs and promotes the activation of pro-stress neuromodulators that combine with a weakening or inadequate anti-stress response. Different drugs of abuse interact with the different stages of the addiction cycle with varying emphasis, with psychostimulants classically entering during the binge/intoxication stage and alcohol entering during any of the three stages of the addiction cycle (depending on subject age, genetic history, and social context). Benzodiazepines likely enter the addiction cycle via between-system neuroadaptations in the brain stress systems during the withdrawal/negative affect stage when considering the relatively sparse evidence of benzodiazepine actions on midbrain dopamine systems. Altogether, these neurocircuitry, neurochemical, and molecular changes lead to negative emotional states that set up an allostatic hedonic load that drives negative reinforcement. Under this framework, strong multidetermined buffers, if activated and sufficient to allow the reward and pro-stress systems to recover, may help return the organism to homeostasis.

REFERENCES

Adamczyk P, McCreary AC, Przegalinski E, Mierzejewski P, Bienkowski P, Filip M. The effects of fatty acid amide hydrolase inhibitors on maintenance of cocaine and food self-administration and on reinstatement of cocaine-seeking and food-taking behavior in rats. Journal of Physiology and Pharmacology, 2009, 60: 119–125.

Ahmed SH, Kenny PJ, Koob GF, Markou A. Neurobiological evidence for hedonic allostasis associated with escalating cocaine use. Nature Neuroscience, 2002, 5: 625–626.

Ahmed SH, Koob GF. The transition to drug addiction: a negative reinforcement model based on an allostatic decrease in reward function. Psychopharmacology, 2005, 180: 473–490.

Al-Hasani R, Bruchas MR. Molecular mechanisms of opioid receptor-dependent signaling and behavior. Anesthesiology, 2011, 115: 1363–1381.

American Psychiatric Association. Diagnostic and Statistical Manual of Mental Disorders, 5th ed. Washington DC: American Psychiatric Publishing; 2013.

Andrews N, File SE. Increased 5-HT release mediates the anxiogenic response during benzodiazepine withdrawal: a review of supporting neurochemical and behavioural evidence. Psychopharmacology, 1993, 112: 21–25.

Ashok AH, Mizuno Y, Volkow ND, Howes OD. Association of stimulant use with dopaminergic alterations in users of cocaine, amphetamine, or methamphetamine: a systematic review and meta-analysis. JAMA Psychiatry, 2017, 74: 511–519.

Ballantyne JC, Sullivan MD, Koob GF. Refractory dependence on opioid analgesics. Pain, 2019, 60: 2655–2660.

Barbier E, Vendruscolo LF, Schlosburg JE, Edwards S, Juergens N, Park PE, Misra KK, Cheng K, Rice KC, Schank J, Schulteis G, Koob GF, Heilig M. The NK1 receptor antagonist L822429 reduces heroin reinforcement. Neuropsychopharmacology, 2013, 38: 976–984.

Bateson AN. Basic pharmacologic mechanisms involved in benzodiazepine tolerance and withdrawal. Curr Pharmaceut Design, 2002, 8: 5–21.

Breiter HC, Gollub RL, Weisskoff RM, Kennedy DN, Makris N, Berke JD, Goodman JM, Kantor HL, Gastfriend DR, Riorden JP, Mathew RT, Rosen BR, Hyman SE. Acute effects of cocaine on human brain activity and emotion. Neuron, 1997, 19: 591–611.

Cahill CM, Walwyn W, Taylor AMW, Pradhan AAA, Evans CJ. Allostatic mechanisms of opioid tolerance beyond desensitization and downregulation. Trends in Pharmacological Science, 2016, 37: 963–976.

Carlezon WA Jr, Nestler EJ, Neve RL. Herpes simplex virus-mediated gene transfer as a tool for neuropsychiatric research. Critical Reviews in Neurobiology, 2000, 14: 47–67.

Chavkin C, Koob GF. Dynorphin, dysphoria and dependence: the stress of addiction. Neuropsychopharmacology, 2016, 41: 373–374.

Ciccocioppo R, Economidou D, Fedeli A, Massi M. The nociceptin/orphanin FQ/NOP receptor system as a target for treatment of alcohol abuse: a review of recent work in alcohol-preferring rats. Physiology and Behavior, 2003, 79: 121–128.

Colpaert FC. System theory of pain and of opiate analgesia: no tolerance to opiates. Pharmacological Reviews, 1996, 48: 355–402.

D'Amato MR. Derived motives. Annual Review of Psychology, 1974, 25: 83–106.

Das P, Lilly SM, Zerda R, Gunning WT 3rd, Alvarez FJ, Tietz EI. Increased AMPA receptor GluR1 subunit incorporation in rat hippocampal CA1 synapses during benzodiazepine withdrawal. Journal of Comparative Neurology, 2008, 511: 832–846.

Das P, Zerda R, Alvarez FJ, Tietz EI. Immunogold electron microscopic evidence of differential regulation of GluN1, GluN2A, and GluN2B, NMDA-type glutamate receptor subunits in rat hippocampal CA1 synapses during benzodiazepine withdrawal. Journal of Comparative Neurology, 2010, 518: 4311–4328.

Delfs JM, Zhu Y, Druhan JP, Aston-Jones G. Noradrenaline in the ventral forebrain is critical for opiate withdrawal-induced aversion. Nature, 2000, 403: 430–434.

Devaud LL, Fritschy JM, Sieghart W, Morrow AL. Bidirectional alterations of GABAA receptor subunit pepetide levels in rat cortex during chronic ethanol consumption and withdrawal. Journal of Neurochemistry, 1997, 69: 126–130.

Diana M. The dopamine hypothesis of drug addiction and its potential therapeutic value. Front Psychiatry, 2011, 2: 64.

Economidou D, Hansson AC, Weiss F, Terasmaa A, Sommer WH, Cippitelli A, Fedeli A, Martin-Fardon R, Massi M, Ciccocioppo R, Heilig M. Dysregulation of nociceptin/orphanin FQ activity in the amygdala is linked to excessive alcohol drinking in the rat. Biological Psychiatry, 2008, 64: 211–218.

Forget B, Coen KM, Le Foll B. Inhibition of fatty acid amide hydrolase reduces reinstatement of nicotine seeking but not break point for nicotine self-administration: comparison with CB1 receptor blockade. Psychopharmacology, 2009, 205: 613–624.

Gatch MB, Wallis CJ, Lal H. Effects of NMDA antagonists on ethanol-withdrawal induced "anxiety" in the elevated plus maze, Alcohol, 1999, 19: 207–211.

George O, Koob GF. Control of craving by the prefrontal cortex. Proceedings of the National Academy of Sciences USA, 2013, 110: 4165–4166.

Gilpin NW, Misra K, Herman MA, Cruz MT, Koob GF, Roberto M. Neuropeptide Y opposes alcohol effects on gamma-aminobutyric acid release in amygdala and blocks the transition to alcohol dependence. Biological Psychiatry, 2011, 69: 1091–1099.

Gilpin NW, Misra K, Koob GF. Neuropeptide Y in the central nucleus of the amygdala suppresses dependence-induced increases in alcohol drinking. Pharmacology Biochemistry and Behavior, 2008, 90: 475–480.

Gilpin NW, Stewart RB, Murphy JM, Li TK, Badia-Elder NE. Neuropeptide Y reduces oral ethanol intake in alcohol-preferring (P) rats following a period of imposed ethanol abstinence. Alcoholism: Clinical and Experimental Research, 2003, 27: 787–794.

Harris AC, Pentel PR, Burroughs D, Staley MD, Lesage MG. A lack of association between severity of nicotine withdrawal and individual differences in compensatory nicotine self-administration in rats. Psychopharmacology, 2011, 217: 153–166.

Heilig M, Koob GF. A key role for corticotropin-releasing factor in alcohol dependence. Trends in Neurosciences, 2007, *30*: 399–406.

Heimer L, Alheid G. Piecing together the puzzle of basal forebrain anatomy. In: Napier TC, Kalivas PW, Hanin I, eds. *The Basal Forebrain: Anatomy to Function* (Advances in Experimental Medicine and Biology, Vol 295). New York, NY: Plenum Press; 1991: 1–42.

Heinrichs SC, Menzaghi F, Schulteis G, Koob GF, Stinus L. Suppression of corticotropin-releasing factor in the amygdala attenuates aversive consequences of morphine withdrawal. Behavioural Pharmacology, 1995, *6*: 74–80.

Hermann D, Weber-Fahr W, Sartorius A, Hoerst M, Frischknecht U, Tunc-Skarka N, Perreau-Lenz S, Hansson AC, Krumm B, Kiefer F, Spanagel R, Mann K, Ende G, Sommer WH. Translational magnetic resonance spectroscopy reveals excessive central glutamate levels during alcohol withdrawal in humans and rats. Biologial Psychiatry, 2012, *71*: 1015–1021.

Heyser CJ, Schulteis G, Durbin P, Koob GF. Chronic acamprosate eliminates the alcohol deprivation effect while having limited effects on baseline responding for ethanol in rats. Neuropsychopharmacology, 1998, *18*: 125–133.

Himmelsbach CK. Can the euphoric, analgetic, and physical dependence effects of drugs be separated? IV. With reference to physical dependence. Federation Proceedings, 1943, 2: 201–203.

Hoffman HS, Solomon RL. An opponent-process theory of motivation: III. Some affective dynamics in imprinting. Learning and Motivation, 1974, *5*: 149–164.

Jang CG, Whitfield T, Schulteis G, Koob GF, Wee S. A dysphoric-like state during early withdrawal from extended access to methamphetamine self-administration in rats. Psychopharmacology, 2013, *225*: 753–763.

Kenny PJ, Chen SA, Kitamura O, Markou A, Koob GF. Conditioned withdrawal drives heroin consumption and decreases reward sensitivity. Journal of Neuroscience, 2006, *26*: 5894–5900.

Khong E, Sim MG, Hulse G. Benzodiazepine dependence. Australian Family Physician, 2004, 33: 923–926.

Kieffer BL, Gaveriaux-Ruff C. Exploring the opioid system by gene knockout. Progress in Neurobiology, 2002, *66*: 285–306.

Koob GF. A role for brain stress systems in addiction. Neuron, 2008, *59*: 11–34.

Koob GF. The dark side of emotion: the addiction perspective. European Journal of Pharmacology, 2015, *753*: 73–87.

Koob GF. Antireward, compulsivity, and addiction: seminal contributions of Dr. Athina Markou to motivational dysregulation in addiction. Psychopharmacology, 2017, *234*: 1315–1332

Koob GF. Animal models of substance use disorders: motivational perspective. In: Johnson B, ed. *Addiction Medicine: Science and Practice.* 2nd ed. New York, NY: Elsevier; 2020a.

Koob GF. Neurobiology of opioid addiction: opponent process, hyperkatifeia, and negative reinforcement. Biological Psychiatry, 2020b, 87: 44–53.

Koob GF, Arends MA, McCracken M, Le Moal M. *Neurobiology of Addiction: Vol. 1. Introduction to Addiction.* New York, NY: Elsevier; 2019.

Koob GF, Bloom FE. Cellular and molecular mechanisms of drug dependence. Science, 1988, 242: 715–723.

Koob GF, Le Moal M. Drug abuse: hedonic homeostatic dysregulation. Science, 1997, 278: 52–58.

Koob GF, Le Moal M. Drug addiction, dysregulation of reward, and allostasis. Neuropsychopharmacology, 2001, *24*: 97–129.

Koob GF, Le Moal M. Plasticity of reward neurocircuitry and the "dark side" of drug addiction. Nature Neuroscience, 2005, 8: 1442–1444.

Koob GF, Le Moal M. Addiction and the brain antireward system. Annual Review of Psychology, 2008, 59: 29–53.

Koob GF, Sanna PP, Bloom FE. Neuroscience of addiction. Neuron, 1998, 21: 467–476.

Koob GF, Volkow ND. Neurocircuitry of addiction. Neuropsychopharmacology Reviews, 2010, 35: 217–238, erratum: 1051.

Kwako L, Koob GF. Neuroclinical framework for the role of stress in addiction. Chronic Stress, 2017, 1: 1–14.

Kwako LE, Momenan R, Litten RZ, Koob GF, Goldman D. Addictions neuroclinical assessment: a neuroscience-based framework for addictive disorders. Biological Psychiatry, 2016, 80: 179–189.

Kwako LE, Schwandt ML, Ramchandani VA, Diazgranados N, Koob GF, Volkow ND, Blanco C, Goldman D. Neurofunctional domains derived from deep behavioral phenotyping in alcohol use disorder. American Journal of Psychiatry, 2019, 176: 744–753.

Larcher A, Laulin JP, Celerier E, Le Moal M, Simonnet G. Acute tolerance associated with a single opiate administration: involvement of N-methyl- -aspartate-dependent pain facilitatory systems. Neuroscience, 1998, 84: 583–589.

Laulin JP, Celerier E, Larcher A, Le Moal M, Simonnet G. Opiate tolerance to daily heroin administration: an apparent phenomenon associated with enhanced pain sensitivity. Neuroscience, 1999, 89: 631–636.

Licata SC, Rowlett JK. Abuse and dependence liability of benzodiazepine-type drugs: GABAA receptor modulation and beyond. Pharmacology Biochemistry and Behavior, 2008, 90: 74–89.

Martin WR, A homeostatic and redundancy theory of tolerance to and dependence on narcotic analgesics. In: Wikler A, ed. The Addictive States. Baltimore, MD: Williams and Wilkins; 1968: 206–225.

Martin-Fardon R, Zorrilla EP, Ciccocioppo R, Weiss F. Role of innate and drug-induced dysregulation of brain stress and arousal systems in addiction: Focus on corticotropin-releasing factor, nociceptin/orphanin FQ, and orexin/hypocretin. Brain Research, 2010, 1314: 145–161.

McEwen BS. Allostasis and allostatic load: implications for neuropsychopharmacology. Neuropsychopharmacology, 2000, 22: 108–124.

McEwen BS, Stellar E. Stress and the individual: mechanisms leading to disease. Archives of Internal Medicine, 1993, 153: 2093–2101.

Mechling AE, Arefin T, Lee HL, Bienert T, Reisert M, Ben Hamida S, Darcq E, Ehrlich A, Gaveriaux-Ruff C, Parent MJ, Rosa-Neto P, Hennig J, von Elverfeldt D, Kieffer BL, Harsan LA. Deletion of the mu opioid receptor gene in mice reshapes the reward-aversion connectome. Proceedings of the National Academy of Science USA, 2016, 113: 11603–11608.

Mhatre MC, Pena G, Sieghart W, Ticku MK. Antibodies specific for GABA_A receptor alpha subunits reveal that chronic alcohol treatment down-regulates α-subunit expression in rat brain regions. Journal of Neurochemistry, 1993, 61: 1620–1625.

Mintzer MZ, Griffiths RR. An abuse liability comparison of flunitrazepam and triazolam in sedative drug abusers. Behavioral Pharmacology, 2005, 16: 579–584.

O'Brien CP. Benzodiazepine use, abuse, and dependence. Journal of Clinical Psychiatry, 2005, 66(Suppl 2): 28–33.

Pothos E, Rada P, Mark GP, Hoebel BG. Dopamine microdialysis in the nucleus accumbens during acute and chronic morphine, naloxone-precipitated withdrawal and clonidine treatment. Brain Research, 1991, 566: 348–350.

Poulos CX, Cappell H. Homeostatic theory of drug tolerance: a general model of physiological adaptation. Psychological Reviews, 1991, 98: 390–408.

Rossetti ZL, Hmaidan Y, Gessa GL. Marked inhibition of mesolimbic dopamine release: a common feature of ethanol, morphine, cocaine and amphetamine abstinence in rats. European Journal of Pharmacology, 1992, 221: 227–234.

Russell MAH. What is dependence? In: Edwards G, ed. *Drugs and Drug Dependence*. Lexington, MA: Lexington Books; 1976: 182–187.

Scherma M, Fadda P, Le Foll B, Forget B, Fratta W, Goldberg SR, et al. The endocannabinoid system: a new molecular target for the treatment of tobacco addiction. CNS Neurological Disorders Drug Targets, 2008, 7: 468–481.

Schmeichel BE, Barbier E, Misra KK, Contet C, Schlosburg JE, Grigoriadis D, Williams JP, Karlsson C, Pitcairn C, Heilig M, Koob GF, Vendruscolo LF. Hypocretin receptor 2 antagonism dose-dependently reduces escalated heroin self-administration in rats. Neuropsychopharmacology, 2015, 40: 1123–1129.

Serrano A, Parsons LH. Endocannabinoid influence in drug reinforcement, dependence and addiction-related behaviors. Pharmacology and Therapeutics, 2011, 132: 215–241.

Shippenberg TS, Zapata A, Chefer VI. Dynorphin and the pathophysiology of drug addiction. Pharmacology and Therapeutics, 2007, 116: 306–321.

Shurman J, Koob GF, Gutstein HB. Opioids, pain, the brain, and hyperkatifeia: a framework for the rational use of opioids for pain. Pain Medicine, 2010, 11: 1092–1098.

Siegel S. Evidence from rats that morphine tolerance is a learned response. Journal of Comparative and Physiological Psychology, 1975, 89: 498–506.

Skelton KH, Gutman DA, Thrivikraman KV, Nemeroff CB, Owens MJ. The CRF1 receptor antagonist R121919 attenuates the neuroendocrine and behavioral effects of precipitated lorazepam withdrawal. Psychopharmacology (Berl), 2007, 192: 385–396.

Skelton KH, Nemeroff CB, Owens MJ. Spontaneous withdrawal from the triazolobenzodiazepine alprazolam increases cortical corticotropin-releasing factor mRNA expression. Journal of Neuroscience, 2004, 24: 9303–9312.

Solomon RL. The opponent-process theory of acquired motivation: the costs of pleasure and the benefits of pain. American Psychologist, 1980, 35: 691–712.

Solomon RL, Corbit JD. An opponent-process theory of motivation: II. Cigarette addiction. Journal of Abnormal Psychology, 1973, 81: 158–171.

Solomon RL, Corbit JD. An opponent-process theory of motivation: 1. Temporal dynamics of affect. Psychological Reviews, 1974, 81: 119–145.

Stephens DN. A glutamatergic hypothesis of drug dependence: extrapolations from benzodiazepine receptor ligands. Behavioral Pharmacology, 1995, 6: 425–446.

Sugiura H, Tanaka H, Yasuda S, Takemiya T, Yamagata K. Transducing neuronal activity into dendritic spine morphology: new roles for p38 MAP kinase and N-cadherin. Neuroscientist, 2009, 15: 90–104.

Thorsell A, Rapunte-Canonigo V, O'Dell L, Chen SA, King A, Lekic D, Koob GF, Sanna PP. Viral vector-induced amygdala NPY overexpression reverses increased alcohol intake caused by repeated deprivations in Wistar rats. Brain, 2007, 130: 1330–1337.

Thorsell A, Slawecki CJ, Ehlers CL. Effects of neuropeptide Y and corticotropin-releasing factor on ethanol intake in Wistar rats: interaction with chronic ethanol exposure. Behavioural Brain Research, 2005a, 161: 133–140.

Thorsell A, Slawecki CJ, Ehlers CL. Effects of neuropeptide Y on appetitive and consummatory behaviors associated with alcohol drinking in Wistar rats with a history of ethanol exposure. Alcoholism: Clinical and Experimental Research, 2005b, 29: 584–590.

Tsuda M, Shimizu N, Suzuki T. Contribution of glutamate receptors to benzodiazepine withdrawal signs. Japanese Journal of Pharmacology, 1999, 81: 1–6.

Umhau JC, Momenan R, Schwandt ML, Singley E, Lifshitz M, Doty L, Adams LJ, Vengeliene V, Spanagel R, Zhang Y, Shen J, George DT, Hommer D, Heilig M. Effect of acamprosate on magnetic resonance spectroscopy measures of central glutamate in detoxified alcohol-dependent individuals: a randomized controlled experimental medicine study. Archives of General Psychiatry, 2010, 67: 1069–1077.

Van Dyke C, Byck R. Cocaine. Scientific American, 1982, 246: 128–141.

Wang GJ, Volkow ND, Fowler JS, Logan J, Abumrad NN, Hitzemann RJ, Pappas NS, Pascani K. Dopamine D2 receptor availability in opiate-dependent subjects before and after naloxone-precipitated withdrawal. Neuropsychopharmacology, 1997, 16: 174–182.

Watanabe T, Nakagawa T, Yamamoto R, Maeda A, Minami M, Satoh M. Involvement of noradrenergic system within the central nucleus of the amygdala in naloxone-precipitated morphine withdrawal-induced conditioned place aversion in rats. Psychopharmacology, 2003, 170: 80–88.

Watanabe T, Yamamoto R, Maeda A, Nakagawa T, Minami M, Satoh M. Effects of excitotoxic lesions of the central or basolateral nucleus of the amygdala on naloxone-precipitated withdrawal-induced conditioned place aversion in morphine-dependent rats. Brain Research, 2002, 958: 423–428.

Williams JT, Ingram SL, Henderson G, Chavkin C, von Zastrow M, Schulz S, Koch T, Evans CJ, Christie MJ. Regulation of μ-opioid receptors: desensitization, phosphorylation, internalization, and tolerance. Pharmacological Reviews, 2013, 65: 223–254.

World Health Organization. International Statistical Classification of Diseases and Related Health Problems. 10th revision. Geneva, Switzerland: World Health Organization; 1992.

CHAPTER 8

Benzodiazepine Withdrawal

Clinical Aspects

STEVEN L. WRIGHT

HIGHLIGHTS

- Benzodiazepines and related compounds cause a wide range of adverse reactions, including withdrawal.
- Withdrawal symptoms can be categorized as psychological, neurophysiologic, and somatic, which may be prolonged and misdiagnosed.
- Deprescribing is recommended when there is loss of efficacy, any major side effect, or use for four or more weeks.
- Discontinuation should involve support, adjunctive approaches, and a tapering process led by patients and may require 12 to 18 months or more for completion.

> Climate is what you expect,
> Weather is what you get.
> —Mark Twain

INTRODUCTION

Adverse outcomes from benzodiazepine (BZD) use have been known for more than 50 years. After becoming available, they rapidly supplanted the more dangerous barbiturates and meprobamate, which have a lower therapeutic index and a greater risk for overdose death.[1,2] Even so, it was only a year after the 1960 launch of chlordiazepoxide that major withdrawal reactions, including life-threatening seizures, were reported.[3] This was followed by identification of an expanding array of sometimes severe adverse effects that early clinicians did not expect—consequences that today's practitioners need to address, including withdrawal.

Terri S. was 54 years old when she realized something had to change. Fifteen years on BZDs for sleep and 10 years on opioids for pain, "the medications stopped working. I wanted my life back." Functionally disabled, she "needed a walker, was losing short-term memory, and lost the ability to perform in [her] PhD program." Most of her help came from friends, family, and "BZD survivors," as many who are severely affected call themselves. She found little advice from her physicians and only limited help from her pharmacist. Taking medications as prescribed, she had entered a dystopian world without good professional guidance.

Unfortunately, this is a story heard far too often.

> "Where is the medical support?
> Why do I feel I am on my own?"
> —Terri S.

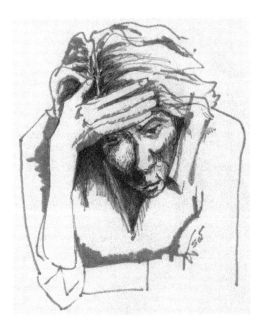

© Susan Wright

Some, like Terri, recognize when BZD receptor agonists (BzRAs: BZDs, Z-drugs, other sedative hypnotics) cause problems and seek assistance to discontinue. Others are unaware and associate BzRA use with relief even when they are actually the source of problems. They, as well as their prescribers, may believe these medications are necessary and that symptoms are due to other medical conditions. This is a real challenge, but while continued BzRA prescribing can improve patients' lives in the short term, trouble may loom ahead as use continues.

BACKGROUND

BzRA exposure results in complex neuroadaptations that begin with the very first exposure to any of these agents. Downregulation of the number and function of the γ-aminobutyric acid (GABA) type A $(GABA_A)$–BZD receptor complex causes decreased GABAergic (*viz.*, affecting the inhibitory neurochemical GABA) responses over time.[4,5] As delineated in the fifth edition of the *Diagnostic and Statistical Manual of Mental Disorders* (DSM-5), this results in tolerance seen clinically as (i) the need for an increased amount of drug to achieve a particular effect and/or (ii) a diminished effect with continued use of the same amount of the agent.[6]

BzRA exposure also results in opponent processes, notably compensatory glutamatergic (excitatory) potentiation.[5,7] This may be amplified by discontinuous BzRA use, a type of hypersensitization termed *kindling*.[5,7] Multiple central nervous system loci as well as the hypothalamic-pituitary-adrenal axis are involved.[8–10] Genetics, oxidative stress, polyvagal mechanisms, and the peripheral-type BZD receptors are all implicated, but insufficiently studied.[11–15] Taken together, these and perhaps other mechanisms, result in a withdrawal syndrome when BzRAs are discontinued.[16–18]

Physiologic dependence encompasses both tolerance and withdrawal.[19] The term *dependence* by itself, however, is used to mean *addiction* by the *International Classification of Diseases*, 10th revision, clinical modification; the World Health Organization; and often in the literature.[20] This is confusing, since medications like antihypertensives are associated with physiologic dependence but are not addiction-prone.[21] Physiologic dependence as a criterion is not required to make the diagnosis of the disease of addiction, which instead is best characterized behaviorally as substance-related compulsion, loss of control, and continued use despite adverse consequences.[6,20,22] Substance use disorder (SUD) and addiction are used interchangeably. Adopted in 2013, the DSM-5 argues that SUD is the preferred nomenclature, citing that it has a more neutral tone and because of uncertainty about the definition of addiction. The DSM-5 also replaced the diagnostic category "abuse" in the fourth edition with "mild SUD." Eleven criteria in DSM-5 delineate SUD along a continuum: mild (2–3 criteria), moderate (4–5 criteria), and severe ($\geq$6 criteria).[6]

Multiple meanings of such terminology challenge our understanding and interpretation of older and even more recent literature. For purposes of this chapter, *addiction* and *SUD* have equivalent meaning. *Dependence* by itself is avoided, as this may confuse physiologic dependence with addiction. Instead, *physiologic dependence* is employed as the broad category that finds its expression in tolerance and withdrawal with both physical and psychological symptomatology. *Abuse* is replaced with *nonmedical use* (*i.e.*, use for a reason other than medically indicated; *e.g.*, euphoria) and *misuse* (*i.e.*, medical use for the prescribed reason but used inappropriately; *e.g.*, double-dosing for anxiety).

True addiction or BzRA use disorder (BUD) occurs but is quite unusual.[23] Clinically, BUD is uniquely different from the experience of the vast majority of patients who struggle with these agents.[18,23] The latter do not meet criteria for BUD but do experience physiologic dependence. For them, the DSM-5 criterion "a persistent desire or unsuccessful efforts to cut down" is not applicable, for instance, because it is not the consequence of craving but is rather due to the challenges of withdrawal itself. Even most nonmedical BzRA users are not addicted to these drugs but use them to amplify or temper effects of other addiction-prone substances, which is problematic in and of itself but is not BUD per se.[24-26]

Physiologic dependence to BzRAs is observed clinically in anywhere from 20% to 100% of users.[9,21,27-34] Differences among studies can, at least in part, be explained by type, dosage, and/or duration of BzRA use; speed of discontinuation; and threshold criteria used.[21] Previous attribution of anxiety and insomnia to pseudo-withdrawal symptoms, for example, is now understood to describe features of the syndrome itself, not simply re-emergence of the underlying conditions.[16,21,35] Neuropharmacologic adaptation occurs upon initiation, and its clinical expression can occur after as little as a few days of use at normally prescribed or even lower dosages.[19,36-38] Because clinical expression of physiologic dependence frequently develops within four weeks of BzRA exposure, *long term* appropriately designates any timeframe extending beyond this period. The literature, on the other hand, must be interpreted in light of variable definitions for "long term" that range anywhere from one month to several years, most commonly six months.[39]

WITHDRAWAL SYMPTOMS

Many patients experience only mild adverse manifestations upon discontinuation; for others, it is much worse. Research is insufficient, but it is estimated that 10% to 44% of individuals will experience moderate to severe symptoms, even when withdrawal is carefully managed.[16,21,40] Severity may be assessed using any one of a number of scales that have been developed. Examples include the Benzodiazepine Withdrawal Symptom Questionnaire[41] and the Clinical Institute Withdrawal Assessment—Benzodiazepines.[42] In practice, however, these scales are not all that helpful, since tracking individual symptom severity is often more useful than global scores. A low numerical value may not reflect the intensity of one or two symptoms that need to be addressed.

Severity is dependent upon a number of factors. Most important is the manner of discontinuation, such as the speed of tapering. Mixed data suggest that being female or elderly is associated with greater difficulties during withdrawal.[43-51] Depression, alcohol overuse, passive-dependent personality traits, and lower educational achievement predict greater severity.[32-34,38,46,52,53] Most but not all evidence indicates higher dosage, shorter acting, and longer duration BzRA use correlates with increased symptom intensity.[21,30,32,33,38,40,47,48,54-63]

> "I felt like I was going to have a heart attack daily.
> [It felt like] toxins were seeping out of my pores."
> —Terri S.

Severe withdrawal can occur after only a few days of BzRA exposure but is more common with use of four weeks or more.[30,58,64] Onset of withdrawal may occur within one day of dose reduction for the shorter-acting agents and within several days of those that are longer acting.[65] The time to peak intensity is quite variable and may fluctuate dramatically thereafter. The potential for seizures during withdrawal is well recognized.[3,37,58,66-69] Other life-threatening outcomes include a delirium-catatonia spectrum, coma, and suicidality. Fatalities related to withdrawal do occur.[24,37,60,61,64,70-74]

No one symptom nor group of symptoms are pathognomonic for BzRA withdrawal. Some manifestations make physiologic sense, while others appear to be unrelated to currently understood neuropharmacology.[75] This can be challenging for medical providers and affected persons alike. Even so, there are certain features and patterns that are commonly seen.

BzRA withdrawal symptoms can be roughly divided into three categories: psychological, neurophysiologic, and somatic. Adverse psychological manifestations (Table 8.1) are very common but nonspecific. Correlation can be established if there is a temporal association between BzRA discontinuation and depression, mania, or psychosis.[30,56,62,76] If not evident before BzRA initiation, then depersonalization, derealization, and hallucinations during and/or after tapering are also likely to be the consequence of cessation as well.[16,21,30,77,78]

Determining the cause of emerging anxiety during BzRA withdrawal is a challenge. Since anxiety is the primary reason BZDs are prescribed, its return is typically interpreted as relapse (return to baseline intensity) or rebound (intensity rising above baseline).[17,21,32] Development of a new anxiety condition unmasked by BzRA discontinuation and fear

Table 8.1 PSYCHOLOGICAL WITHDRAWAL SYMPTOMS

Anxiety states

Agoraphobia

Aggressive behavior/homicidal ideation/rage/violence

Agitation/irritability/restlessness

Anhedonia/blunted emotions

Craving

Delusions/illusions/hallucinations

Depersonalization/derealization

Depression/sadness/suicidality

Excitability

Hallucinations

Hypochondriasis

Mania

Mood swings

Obsessions

Paranoia/feelings of persecutions

Posttraumatic stress disorder

Psychosis

about the withdrawal process itself are other considerations.[16,21,79] This puzzle can result in the misleading assumption BzRAs are beneficial long term.[17]

Although paradoxical, BzRA use itself can be a *source* of anxiety-related complaints. In a landmark paper in 1987, Ashton reported on 50 consecutive patients followed for 10 months to 3.5 years after BZD withdrawal had been concluded.[18] Most study participants reported that their anxiety actually increased during BZD therapy and improved after cessation. Even more striking, 20% developed agoraphobia after BZD initiation, and this too improved after discontinuation. These findings correspond to other observations,[16,33,34,80,81] suggesting that for a subset of the population using BZDs long term, not only do these medications become ineffective, but also can cause what might be termed *BZD-induced hyperanxiogenesis*, analogous to opioid-induced hyperalgesia. Surprisingly, Ashton's research has not since been adequately explored or extended.

Neurophysiologic symptoms (Table 8.2) in BzRA cessation are well documented. Seizures, dizziness, weakness, and cramps can be seen.[16,32,66,69] Dyscognition may encompass confusion and impairment of memory, as well as decrements in concentration and decision-making.[16,82] An altered level of consciousness can range from sedation to an organic brain syndrome.[16,71,72,83] Nightmares and hypnagogic hallucinations can be frightening. Insomnia usually worsens and includes rapid eye movement rebound that improves over time.[16,84–87] These do not surprise clinicians familiar with withdrawal from other addiction-prone substances.

Other symptoms, however, are not only unfamiliar but appear peculiar and even bizarre. These include alterations of any or all perceptual domains: visual, auditory, smell, taste, and tactile.[16,29,30,32,88] There may be marked and intolerable sensory hypersensitivity, tinnitus, photophobia, diplopia, and dysosmia.[16,32,88] Cutaneous reactions can be very disturbing: hot and cold sensations, numbness, paresthesia, pruritus, and formication.[16,32] Pain (allodynia, hyperesthesia, electric shock-like sensations) may be prominent and diffuse or present in various body regions.[16] Neuromuscular presentations include akathisia, dystonias, tics, tremor, tardive dyskinesia, and myoclonus.[16,88] Striking,

Table 8.2 NEUROPHYSIOLOGIC WITHDRAWAL SYMPTOMS

Altered level of consciousness

Auditory alterations/loss/hyperacusis/tinnitus

Alterations of taste/smell/vision/speech

Cutaneous sensory alterations

Dizziness/light-headedness

Dyscognition/amnestic states/dementia-like symptoms

Muscular/neuromuscular symptoms

Pain—ache/neuropathic/local or diffuse

Sense of motion

Sexual dysfunction

Sleep problems

unusual movement abnormalities may wrongly prompt the diagnosis of psychogenic nonepileptic seizures (pseudoseizures), especially if the electroencephalogram is found to be normal.[16,29,88]

Somatic adverse sequelae to BzRA cessation (Table 8.3) are also quite common and well documented.[8,16,17,21,29–32,66,73,78,79] Future research may determine a neurophysiologic basis for such manifestations, but here they are categorized separately. When temporally associated with BzRA withdrawal, both somatic and neurophysiologic symptoms are not likely to be psychiatric or psychosomatic in origin. Some point to activation of centralized mechanisms. Others suggest potential involvement of the mitochondrial-based peripheral BZD receptors (see Chapter 6 of this volume).[59,89,90] Whatever the explanation and however peculiar or dramatic, these symptoms should not be minimized nor patients discounted.

Although counterintuitive, all of these adverse consequences (psychological, neurophysiologic, somatic) can occur while patients are still taking BzRAs.[9,16,21,78,79,91] This interdose or tolerance withdrawal is seen more commonly with longer use and with shorter-acting BzRAs due to more rapidly falling drug concentrations, perhaps in part due to kindling mechanisms. Interdose withdrawal symptoms tend to worsen with dose decrements during discontinuation.[21,87] Obversely, they can improve temporarily if dosages are increased, followed by re-emergence as BzRAs are continued and worse yet again with subsequent dose reductions.[21]

The course of BzRA withdrawal symptom severity may differ from that of other drugs.[21,73,79,92,93] For withdrawal from most addiction-prone substances, an acute phase of greater intensity typically abates at a characteristic time. Linear in trajectory, symptoms become fewer and less bothersome. Some individuals may experience postacute withdrawal syndrome (PAWS) with effects that linger but steadily dissipate over weeks to months. A few will have permanent damage from the drugs themselves, although not due to the cessation process itself (*e.g.*, an organic brain syndrome). The course of BzRA withdrawal intensity, on the other hand, can be either linear or nonlinear. Several different patterns have been identified[21,73,79,88] as follows.

Table 8.3 SOMATIC WITHDRAWAL SYMPTOMS

Cardiovascular: flushing/palpitations/tachycardia/BP ↑ or ↓
Appetite increase/weight gain
Appetite decrease/weight loss
Breast engorgement
Dry mouth/thirst
Menstrual abnormalities
Fatigue/malaise
Food intolerance
GI: gas/constipation/diarrhea/dysphagia/nausea/vomiting
Hyperventilation/dyspnea
Urinary: frequency/incontinence/polyuria

1. No symptoms (rare)
2. A steady linear decline to resolution
3. An initial increase followed by decrease
4. An initial decline followed by resurgence
5. Sustained symptoms
6. Fluctuations in severity that cycle from hours to weeks in duration and overlie an otherwise static, declining, or worsening trajectory

When seen, nonlinear progressions are quite perplexing. Waves of increased intensity can alternate with windows of relative normality.[21,90] These vary not only in duration but also with respect to which symptoms increase or decrease at different times. For example, an individual might experience heightened sound sensitivity at one point and have markedly worsened depression or suicidality at another.

Indeed, withdrawal responses may present as a constantly changing mix of symptoms, severity, and time spans.[21] Clinically, this can be confusing. However, a number of indicators help differentiate BzRA withdrawal syndrome from alternative medical diagnoses[21,79] that might otherwise be considered.

1. Somatic symptoms, notably cardiovascular and gastrointestinal
2. Neurophysiologic symptoms, notably movement abnormalities, perceptual disturbances, and centralized pain
3. Psychological symptoms that are
   - Not present prior to BzRA initiation
   - Combined with neurophysiologic and/or somatic symptoms
4. Interdose symptoms while on BzRAs that worsen during discontinuation
5. Symptom decline followed by worsening
6. Waxing and waning symptom intensity
7. Sustained stereotypic symptom cluster

Although derived from the literature and consistent with extensive anecdotal reports, these are not researched criteria. When present, especially in combination, they highly suggest BzRA discontinuation as the source of symptoms. Even though there is nothing consistently characteristic about BzRA withdrawal, these features can guide diagnosis and subsequent treatment. More than that, clinician recognition validates patients who already feel unhinged by the symptoms themselves as well as dismissive responses by others, including many medical providers and loved ones who misinterpret them as having psychiatric or psychosomatic conditions.

When symptoms are sustained beyond six to eight weeks, the clinical picture is called prolonged, persistent, or protracted,[16,19,21,52,73,79] most often termed PAWS. While manifestations of BzRA cessation may be ongoing in an estimated 10% to 15%, ultimate resolution is expected and likely for most individuals.[16,79,94] Clinical management of discontinuation in this circumstance is challenging, but it is usually successful if tapering proceeds at a pace slow enough to be tolerable to the patient.

MANAGING BENZODIAZEPINE RECEPTOR AGONIST WITHDRAWAL

There are many reasons to consider and encourage BzRA discontinuation. Obvious and significant adverse reactions, diversion, and the absence or loss of efficacy are the most apparent. This is of particular importance when other sedating/depressant medications like opioids are used concurrently (see Chapter 9 of this volume). Postmortem detection of BzRAs in opioid-related unintentional deaths has increased from 13% in 1999 to 31% in 2011 to 52% in 2016–2017 and is even higher in some locales.[95-97] It is not unusual to see patients prescribed multiple BzRAs—even multiple BZD anxiolytics—without good rationale. Polypharmacy with the so-called Holy Trinity (BzRA, opioid, and carisoprodol taken together) is especially dangerous.[98] A careful review of all medications is indicated to determine which medication or combination of medications might be implicated in the presenting symptoms.

Overdose is addressed with the ABCs (airway, breathing, circulation) of basic life support, reversal agents (flumazenil, naloxone), avoidance of gastrointestinal decontamination (due to potential aspiration), urine alkalization (for barbiturates), and ventilator support as needed.[99] The potential risk for future respiratory depression can be identified with polysomnography, which can suggest the presence of central or peripheral sleep apnea. Although oxygen saturation per se is not a good measure of acutely impending respiratory depression, the risk of sleep apnea is a well-established harbinger of future risk. Close monitoring, sleep specialist referral, the use of continuous positive airway pressure or similar devices, and changes in dose of opioids and/or BZDs in such a patient would be warranted.[100-102]

Deprescribing is also recommended when BzRAs have been used long term: four weeks or more.[16,30,103-106] It is not at all unusual that benefit from BzRAs declines, although not always apparent to either prescribers or patients[107-110] These drugs may also inhibit the efficacy of psychotherapeutic modalities such as exposure therapy.[111,112] Symptoms might not be recognized as BzRA side effects, such as psychomotor decrements or dyscognition, as they may be incorrectly attributed to other causes.[99,113] Anxiety that increases during BZD therapy might be thought of as worsening of the underlying condition and lead to increased dosage, when, in fact, for some individuals, tapering results in improvement in anxiety.[16,18,33,34,77] Such a conclusion could be called into question due to the subjective nature of anxiety reports; however, loss of BZD efficacy has also been seen when used for seizures. In a clonazepam discontinuation study, 75% showed no worsening of this objective measure, and, in fact, 15% had fewer seizures after cessation.[114] Finally, worsening insomnia or anxiety during BzRA withdrawal can lead to the misperception that these agents continue to be effective.[16]

Prescribers first must discern the nature of these problems and then communicate their concerns about continued BzRA use to their patients. Patients may become willing to consider cessation once adequately informed of its importance. Initiating the offer with a simple, explanatory letter to the patient is effective.[115-118] A direct face-to-face consultation with a prescriber or pharmacist enhances patient engagement.[105-107]

In addition to such a discussion, the Ashton Manual (published in 1999 and 2002) and its supplement (published in 2011) are valuable, freely available resources to educate patients. These documents provide reliable information and guidance that is understandable and useful for patients and practitioners alike.[16,119] In clear, accessible language Ashton outlines the limited therapeutic utility of BzRAs, nonmedical use, and negative outcomes including withdrawal. With appropriate disclaimers (*i.e.*, insufficient researched evidence), she describes the often-baffling symptoms expressed during use and upon discontinuation. In a supportive manner, she walks through the cessation process, self-management strategies, best practice recommendations, and the challenges that may be encountered. It is considered essential reading for which this book is an update.

Although studies are unclear,[117] motivational interviewing delivered in a respectful, nonjudgmental manner facilitates patient recognition of BzRA-related difficulties and the desirability of deprescribing. The potential for loss of efficacy and nonobvious relationship to various symptoms should be conveyed and in a fair-balanced fashion— neither minimized nor exaggerated. It should be made clear that the extent of problems may not be fully evident until sometime after BzRA cessation has been completed. The goal is to encourage interest in making a change, share decision-making, manage expectations, and set the tone for the journey ahead.

If the patient declines to begin this process, ongoing monitoring for BzRA efficacy, risks, and adverse reactions is important. Mandated cessation without consent is inappropriate unless significant respiratory depression or other major side effects are identified.[16] Leveraged change, however, is recommended if serially measured functional screeners and sleep studies determine there are significant decrements in mood, cognition, psychomotor function, or oxygenation status.[95,96] It is important to keep in mind that, as Ashton points out, "in a small number of cases withdrawal may be inadvisable."[16] Consequently, close attention to patient reports, close monitoring, and good clinical judgment is warranted.

Preparation for deprescribing is critical. Frequently, insufficient or no informed consent had been provided[120]; therefore, education about risks, benefits, and alternatives needs to be provided. Ideally, patients have or can build a network of support from family, friends, and peer coaching.[16] Online communities can be helpful, but it is important to recognize that many peers do not have professional medical training.[16] Problematic co-prescribed medications like opioids and carisoprodol should be identified and addressed. Fluoroquinolones should be avoided, as they inhibit GABA interaction with receptors and can precipitate withdrawal.[16,121] If a written treatment agreement is used, it should support and not disrupt the therapeutic alliance: it should not instill fear.

If taken for more than a month, BzRAs should not be stopped abruptly (cold turkey), as this is dangerous.[57-63] Gradual tapering, even for those on low dosages, is safer and far more successful.[16,17,31,57,70,91,95] This may be accomplished using the agent the patient is already being prescribed.[16,29,38,49,54,68,69,79,99] Specific dose reduction schedules have been published[16,122,123]; however, utility is limited as suggested rates of reduction are too rapid for some patients. As emphasized by Ashton, there may be a need to go off-schedule with flexible dosing.[16]

Table 8.4 BENZODIAZEPINE RECEPTOR AGONIST DOSE CONVERSIONS BZRAS AVAILABLE IN THE UNITED STATES

BzRA	Ashton[16]	ClinCalc.com[125] Dose (range)
Diazepam (reference)	10 mg	10 mg
Alprazolam	0.5 mg	0.75 mg (0.5–2 mg)
Chlordiazepoxide	25 mg	33 mg (12–50 mg)
Clobazam	20 mg	—
Clonazepam	0.5 mg	0.75mg (0.5–4 mg)
Clorazepate	15 mg	13 mg (8–30 mg)
Estazolam	1–2 mg	—
Eszopiclone	3 mg	—
Flurazepam	15–30 mg	20 mg (8–30 mg)
Lorazepam	1 mg	1.3 mg (1–4 mg)
Midazolam po	—	7 mg (5–10 mg)
Oxazepam	20 mg	20 mg (5–40 mg)
Phenobarbital	20 mg	20 mg (15–60 mg)
Quazepam	20 mg	27 mg (15–40 mg)
Secobarbital	—	67 mg (50–100 mg)
Temazepam	20 mg	20 mg (5–40 mg)
Triazolam	0.5 mg	0.25 mg (0.25–1 mg)
Zaleplon	20 mg	—
Zolpidem	20 mg	—

Substitution with a longer half-life BzRA prior to tapering can minimize interdose withdrawal and facilitate better management.[16,25,49,54,60,69,80,99,124] Switching GABAergic agents is done through conversion tables (Tables 8.4 and 8.5), which are based on experience and expert opinion, not well-controlled studies.[16,125] The relative potencies listed are only rough estimates, as individual variation with respect to pharmacodynamics and pharmacokinetics can be significant. It is recommended that the transition proceed by cross tapering, a process that involves sequential reduction of the original BzRA paired with simultaneous incremental additions of the new longer-acting agent. After substitution, if needed, the dosage should be adjusted and stabilized for a period of time to ensure the effect is similar to the prior BzRA, with only minor new side effects before beginning the taper.[16] Patients are not always able to tolerate the selected substitute, and another switch may be necessary.

Diazepam (half-life 20–100 hours) is a good first choice as a long-acting agent for substitution.[16,68,79,126] Tablets in many strengths and a solution of low concentration (1mg/mL) allow for small incremental reductions.[16,108] Phenobarbital (half-life 50–120 hours), a non-BZD GABA$_A$ receptor agonist, is also reasonable because of minimal fluctuations of blood levels between doses.[19,113,126,127] The method of phenobarbital substitution of Smith and Wesson is well established and is recommended.[65,93,128] Clonazepam (half-life 20–50 hours) may be used, although it is more difficult to taper because of smaller

Table 8.5 ADJUNCTIVE MEDICATIONS
FOR BZRA WITHDRAWAL

Carbamazepine[32,55,106,109,110]

Flumazenil[16,30,109,122,123]

Pregabalin[43,121,124]

Gabapentin[124,125]

Imipramine[32,118,126]

Paroxetine[16,121,127]

Valproate[108,121,128]

available dosage sizes due to its greater potency.[16,87] Because duration of clinical effects does not always parallel elimination half-life, interdose withdrawal can still occur with these agents, which may, therefore, need to be divided throughout the day.[16]

Some sensitive individuals may find it quite difficult to make dose reductions small enough with available product sizes, even with scored tablets. Although challenging, compounding pharmacists can provide small dose decrements with improved accuracy.[129] Online lay communities have developed very sophisticated micro-tapering strategies, which have been successful anecdotally.[116,130] Dry-cutting is a technique that uses a razor blade and a jewel scale to make very small reductions. The amount ingested, however, may be inconsistent because of manufacturing variations, uneven distribution of the active agent within tablets, and technique.

Some patients report success with liquid titration methods, which allow for any rate of tapering.[16,116,118,120,130] A tablet can be pulverized and mixed in 100 mL of water, for example. While actively stirring the mixture, individuals can then remove and discard 1 mL of the mixture before ingesting the remaining amount. For the next reduction, 2 mL might be jettisoned and so forth over time. When BzRAs are mixed in this manner, however, even distribution of the suspension is not assured.

Caution is warranted for both dry-cutting and liquid titration techniques. Both are off-label and have not been formally researched. Inherent measurement inaccuracies can generate variations dose to dose, which can be very problematic for some patients. Still, many individuals report success and endorse these methods.[120,130] It is reasonable to support such strategies when other, more standard approaches have fallen short.

Although many patients tolerate dose reductions of greater than 10%, this is not recommended at the outset because for some individuals overwhelming symptoms may ensue.[16] Successful discontinuation can take anywhere from four weeks to several years, but as observed by Ashton, "the classic six weeks withdrawal period adopted by many clinics and doctors is much too fast for many long-term users."[16] To minimize the risk for a severe withdrawal response this author suggests calculating the initial dose decrement as if it will take 12 to 18 months to complete the taper. Beginning with a reduction of 1 mg of diazepam or diazepam equivalent may be reasonable, for instance, if this is less than 10% - better yet, less than 5% - of the original dose. Not only will this determine tolerability, but also it will help build trust of the prescriber by the patient who is worried about withdrawal that is too quick and could magnify the symptom burden.

Subsequent dose reductions can be increased or decreased depending on response. Patients generally experience an increase in symptoms after each dosage decrement, even with very small reductions. It is important to pause periodically to allow for a relative break in symptom intensity before making subsequent reductions, since continuous high-level severity is especially hard to tolerate. Formulaic, fixed amount, or percentage reduction plans are generally unsuccessful. A patient-led, flexible process is recommended.[16] Patients, after all, are the experts when it comes to their own experience.

In addition, the interval between reductions must be individualized.[16] Micro-tapering of very small amounts on a daily basis can be successful but requires very close attention to detail.[130] Alternatively, the cut-and-hold method involves a somewhat larger reduction that is sustained for a week, a month, or even longer.[130] Absent research to indicate otherwise, patient preference should be supported. Reduction intervals differ from person to person because of variation in neuro-readaptation. Again, a primarily patient-directed approach involving shared decision-making is most likely to result in favorable outcomes.[16]

Replicating an identical frequency and amount of dose decrements throughout the entire taper is unlikely to work. Similar to corticosteroid and buprenorphine tapers, at lower doses the amount reduced must be decreased and the interval between reductions increased in a hyperbolic fashion.[16] Setbacks are unfortunately frequent and, as mentioned, close monitoring is essential for these patients. Updosing or using as-needed BzRAs should be avoided,[16] as this risks kindling or priming the neurophysiologic pump, which can light the fire of withdrawal symptoms and make subsequent tapering much more difficult.[5,7]

Adding adjunctive approaches can be helpful. Cognitive behavioral therapy, relaxation, and peer support have demonstrated efficacy and can be initiated before tapering begins.[16,108,117,131–136] Adjunctive medications may be beneficial as well.[60,137,138] They, too, can be started prior to or during tapering and continued after complete BzRA cessation to address ongoing symptoms. All such adjunctive medications are off-label for this purpose, have potential side effects, and may themselves require tapering. In addition, it is important to note that data on these agents in BzRA withdrawal are limited and often mixed, and most studies are of low quality with a high risk of bias.

Some medications have been found to both increase the likelihood of complete BzRA cessation and reduce symptom intensity. Carbamazepine (200-400 mg po tid) has the best, although still relatively weak, researched support.[59,60,77,99,118,124,137–139] Less and somewhat mixed evidence also exists for the use of valproic acid (250 mg po bid-tid).[99,124,137,140,141] These agents do pose serious risks for hepatic decompensation, blood dyscrasias, and mood alterations including suicidality, and other side effects, for which surveillance is indicated. Other medications of potential value include oxcabazine,[142] pregabalin,[48,137,143–14] gabapentin,[143,147] paroxetine,[137,148,149] imipramine,[32,133,150] trazodone,[141,151,152] and magnesium.[137]

Flumazenil by intravenous or subcutaneous infusion may have a unique role, even though it is not an obvious therapeutic candidate. Widely referred to as a $GABA_A$ antagonist, it is used for reversal of BzRA overdose.[153] In fact, it is actually a very weak partial agonist[154] that may normalize $GABA_A$ receptor function[155] and thus explain its efficacy for both symptom suppression and completion of BzRA cessation.[16,124,137,155-160] Lader and Morton found it to be effective in a small pilot study of symptomatic patients who were already BzRA-free for one month to five years.[16] It is the only medication that has been studied in this specific population. On the other hand, durability of flumazenil benefit is unknown, and there are substantial risks such as precipitation of panic and seizures.[38,159,161] Use of this procedure, therefore, should be reserved to medical providers who are highly experienced.

Other agents have been found to reduce BzRA withdrawal sequelae but do not appear to improve the likelihood of complete cessation. These include propranolol (studies mixed),[34,60,162] buspirone (studies mixed),[60,150,163,164] and hydroxyzine.[165] On the other hand, clonidine,[166] progesterone,[60,167,168] melatonin,[169] and ondansetron[170] appear to be ineffective.

Individuals report employing other approaches to address discontinuation symptomatology—many that are nontraditional and have not been researched. Environmental stimuli can be overwhelming, and affected individuals find it worthwhile to calibrate their sensory exposure to keep their "net neural load" within tolerance. Activity and exercise can be useful but must be paced and advanced slowly to avoid doing too much.[16] Sleep hygiene measures are important.[117,171,172] Postural orthostatic tachycardia syndrome has been reported in BzRA withdrawal, so directed interventions could potentially help. Anecdotally, modalities that are self-directed after guidance (e.g., mindfulness, yoga) or professionally directed (e.g., acupuncture) may be valuable,[16] and, although not formally studied during BzRA discontinuation, these approaches have strong evidence for use to treat underlying conditions like anxiety and insomnia.

Because brains are biochemically active, it would be quite surprising if nutritional practices and deficiency states did not affect outcomes. Specific dietary approaches have not been researched in withdrawing populations. However, anecdotally some patients describe benefit from specific diets, yet others do not find those diets useful.[16] Reported successful dietary elements include an emphasis on complete proteins to support amino acid production and low glycemic-index carbohydrates. Various vitamins and supplements have been tried in BzRA discontinuation with inconsistent results—again without research.[16] L-methyl-folate use can benefit certain psychiatric conditions in those with genetically based reduced folate metabolism, but this is untested among those undergoing withdrawal.[173] Alcohol and tobacco should be avoided because both interact with the $GABA_A$ receptor and worsen both sleep and anxiety.[16,174-178]

Anecdotally, probiotics, niacin, oxaloacetate, N-acetylcystine, and nicotinamide adenine dinucleotide have had some success. GABA itself minimally crosses the blood–brain barrier and has no known utility.[179] Some products—valerian, cannabinoids, even phenibut—have proponents but are GABAergic and therefore cannot be recommended.[180-182] Lavender, on the other hand, might be a good option as it does not appear to work though the $GABA_A$ receptor and was compared favorably to lorazepam in a small anxiety trial.[183]

MANAGING BZRA NONMEDICAL USE AND BZRA USE DISORDER

Nonmedical use of a medication refers to use of a medication for other than its prescribed indication. BzRAs are used nonmedically to reduce alcohol withdrawal severity or ease the intensity of a stimulant high. This in and of itself is not BUD, although clearly problematic.[24-27] As mentioned previously, true BzRA addiction, although possible, is rare among users.[23,184] Flunitrazepam, a date-rape drug, may have the greatest addiction liability[185] and is now found in the United States only through illicit markets. Butalbital, a Food and Drug Administration–approved barbiturate that commonly causes medication overuse headache[186] and not necessarily addiction, presents unique challenges that are beyond the scope of this chapter.

SUD or addiction is driven by incentive salience or *wanting* a drug—more so than hedonic *liking* of the drug.[187] The disease of addiction is characterized neurophysiologically by a demand or perceived *needing* of a drug in the absence of a bona fide medical need along with loss of ability to choose to not use on a consistent basis. Despite major adverse consequences, affected individuals lose control over whether they use in the first place as well as the amounts consumed. This presents a real challenge for the few who are truly addicted to BzRAs.

BzRA tapering remains essential for safety reasons and to minimize withdrawal severity. Yet the person with BUD will experience the drive to overuse (craving) despite any professed, authentic commitment to a tapering regimen. Completing an entire taper in a restricted inpatient environment, however, is impractical because completion of the discontinuation process can take months or even years.[26,93,108] It is, therefore, recommended that when possible, outpatient tapering be done using BzRAs that are less euphorigenic (*i.e.*, less salient or less attractive). This means avoiding agents that have greater addiction liability, such as alprazolam, diazepam, and lorazepam (data are very limited).[65,188] Phenobarbital is a good choice, but selection must be determined on an individualized basis.[65,93,127,128]

The presence of a true BUD also means incorporating mutual help programs (12-step facilitation) and addiction therapy into the treatment plan. Although these modalities have not been specifically researched with respect to BUD, there is evidence that such integrated multidisciplinary treatment is beneficial for other SUDs and should be employed.[189]

While important in the context of serious co-occurring psychiatric or alcohol and other use disorders, traditional addiction-focused therapy, 12-step, detox centers, and inpatient care do not address the primary issues faced by those with BzRA physiologic dependence alone. In fact, such approaches anecdotally have not been helpful and even counterproductive when BUD is not present.[119,120] These individuals are caught in a cycle of continued use because of difficulties with discontinuation—not craving itself, which is the central focus of addiction treatment. This difference is evidenced, in part, by stable BzRA dosages in the vast majority of non-addicted users over time.[190]

Indeed, because of the absence of or pressured requests for escalating BzRA use by individual patients, addiction medicine providers as a whole have not fully recognized and addressed the challenges of BzRA physiologic dependence.

In simplest terms, nonaddicted BzRA users need effective withdrawal assistance, which they typically do not receive. Cognitive behavioral therapy and support are important but need to be focused on the challenges of withdrawal and not on the disease of addiction, which is generally irrelevant.[16,117,119,13] When the wrong diagnosis, addiction, is assigned, it should be no surprise that addiction-related interventions are ineffective. Favorable outcomes are far more likely when management is directed toward the actual medical challenges faced by those physiologically dependent with a fully engaged collaborative team: prescriber, pharmacist, behavioral health, peer coach, family, and patient.[118,135,136,191,192]

THE LEGACY PATIENT

Legacy patients are those who have been inherited from the care of other medical providers due to retirement, transfer of care, or by referral.[193] When the treatment approach varies significantly from that of the previous provider, this poses unique challenges. Establishing and maintaining an effective therapeutic alliance may be difficult when there are major differences in recognized efficacy and safety of therapeutic regimens.[192] The same can be said when prescribers themselves come to a new understanding that the medications they had been prescribing are no longer supportable for the medical conditions and/or duration for which they have been used.

Ethically, medical providers are obliged to implement best practices founded on researched evidence that is personalized to their patients. When consideration is given to current or potential therapies, the overriding principle is to "do *less* harm," not to "do *no* harm," since harm is possible along any therapeutic pathway. Balancing beneficence and nonmalfeasance is central to good medical decision-making.[194] However, simply being comfortable and/or maintaining inertia with respect to continued BzRA prescribing is unsustainable when the extent of actual risks become recognized.

Deprescribing in the legacy patient begins with a thorough review of the patient's current medications and medical conditions. Patient report should be verified through medical records, family/significant other corroboration, and online prescription databases. Urine drug screening by immunoassay (point of care or cup test) is unreliable for identifying BzRA exposure; therefore, testing by definitive technique (gas chromatography–mass spectrometry or liquid chromatography–mass spectrometry) is indicated.[195] Polypharmacy—variously defined as ≥2 to ≥11 medications (usually ≥5)[196]—may be identified, and while multiple medications may be rational and indicated for complex multimorbidities, this is not always the case. Frequently, drugs have been added in a prescribing cascade to improve efficacy, to address side effects, or because symptoms are (often erroneously) attributed to new medical conditions.[197]

There are a number of barriers to deprescribing. Medicine as practiced today sits within a culture that encourages adding—not subtracting—medications.[198] As Kafka states, "It is easy to write prescriptions, but difficult to come to an understanding with people.[199] Even though non-pharmacologic alternatives are first-line, access may be difficult. Patients may minimize BzRA side effects[113] or resist change because they believe their condition might get worse and withdrawal will be hard.[200] BzRAs inhibit cognitive processing,[111,112,201] which can interfere with thoughtful balancing of risks and benefits. Clinicians may be reluctant to change a plan in the absence of major overt problems or because significant covert negative consequences are not recognized as such. Prescriber deprescribing skills may be wanting as well.

In general, deprescribing proceeds along a series of steps. This is perhaps best described by the NO TEARS tool[202] as follows.

1. Need and indication
2. Open-ended questions
3. Tests and monitoring
4. Evidence and guidelines
5. Adverse events
6. Risk reduction or prevention
7. Simplification and switches

With what is known, BzRAs should rise to the top of list of medications to be discontinued. Indeed in the last 20 years the Food and Drug Administration's voluntary adverse event reporting system (MedWatch) received 300,000 complaints about BzRAs, including 66,000 associated deaths.[203] Too often, however, their cessation is neglected altogether when attention is directed solely towards other drugs like opioids, which, of course, also need to be addressed. Unilateral decision-making on the part of the prescriber is inappropriate unless severe negative outcomes from current use are identified.[16,193] Instead, it is the art of medicine centered on motivational interviewing, which best preserves the therapeutic relationship, promotes stages of change and encourages patient interest, willingness, and engagement.[117] To do otherwise may prompt dissatisfied patients to leave their practitioners for less scrupulous prescribers or street sources that will not serve them well.[193]

Patient education and informed consent is not only effective; they are ethical and legal obligations.[49,191,204] This is necessary not only in prescribing but also the discontinuation process and to manage expectations. Outright open critique of the patient's prior prescriber is not appropriate, as there may have been some, albeit limited and quite questionable, rationale for the previous prescribing[205] that is not appreciated at the time. For example, it can be explained that it is now known BZDs are ineffective and even contraindicated for anxiety at almost any time for posttraumatic stress syndrome and obsessive-compulsive disorder.[206-208] In the same way, patients can be advised that even when not obvious, benefits may have been lost and side effects may have mounted when BzRAs are used long term for medical conditions like anxiety,[107-110] insomnia,[209] and seizures.[114] BzRA discontinuation, then, should proceed upon the full understanding and acceptance by all involved.

Although many patients are able to complete BzRA cessation successfully, some will continue to be symptomatic for months and sometimes years beyond their last dose. This is poorly understood and unpredictable because no clinical study has not been of sufficient duration with large enough sample size to have identified the frequency, severity, and (often bizarre) nature of protracted problems. In addition, there is no proven explanatory neurophysiology for this phenomenon, even though LaCorte's hypothesis[12] of "overlapping vicious cycles" that perpetuate oxidative stress is of great interest.

A deficient scientific foundation should not negate the validity of observations made, however. The history of medicine, after all, is replete with syndromes described long before their pathophysiology is understood. In fact, there is a population of individuals about whom little is known through formal research, yet promises to be a rich source of information. Tens of thousands of BZD survivors have found their way into online communities, many reporting they did so because their conditions were unrecognized, discounted, or called out as psychosomatic by their medical providers. They often feel stigmatized, alienated, isolated, and inadequately treated.

Research about their medical circumstances, function, and psychosocial condition unfortunately is very limited. Pittman et al.[120] performed a survey of participants ($N =$ 493) on one online community, Benzo Buddies (2013 membership: 10,949). Half of them reported not being informed about potential adverse effects prior to or during prescribing. Of the 70% who completed BzRA cessation, withdrawal symptoms persisted in 96%. Almost half of these individuals did have resolution of their symptoms ultimately, but it took an average of 14 months. The majority, though, did not get assistance in this process from medical providers but rather from family, friends, and online communities.

Similar results were found in a survey of the Yahoo Benzo Group (2007 membership: 3,020) by Young[210] who examined the progression of symptoms and nine functional parameters through and beyond BzRA cessation where applicable. On the average, respondents ($N = 346$) had been taking BzRAs for average of eight years, and such use was associated with a greater than 50% decline in function. Those who discontinued BzRAs rated the water titration and diazepam substation plus tapering methods to be least difficult, although still challenging. Those with symptomatic resolution upon BzRA discontinuation reported that it took an average of 12.2 months (range 1–60 months) after their final BzRA exposure.

Using a qualitative methodology, Fixsen and Ridge researched withdrawal by narrative inquiry of internet postings on a range of internet platforms.[211] They found that these postings had millions of hits. Expressions of BzRA lived experiences were coded, and from that seven major themes were identified ranging from "hell and isolation" to "healing and renewal." Quite evident was the severity of distress as well as anger directed towards medical providers.

Limited as it is, this research shows that for a significant proportion of individuals, the process of withdrawal as well as symptoms and functional impairments after complete BzRA cessation can be far longer and more significant than generally recognized. It makes clear the need for informed consent, restrained prescribing, and competent discontinuation practices. It also makes clear that many clinicians are not sufficiently knowledgeable, engaged, and supportive—and they need to be.

CONCLUSIONS

Terri S. did not show evidence of SUD, but clearly had adverse reactions to medications. Because of this, she chose to taper off both opioids and BZDs. She resorted to her allergist who became her prescriber, medical advisor, and emergency contact. Tapering off BZDs over 10 weeks was "almost impossible, exponentially harder than opioids, and the most difficult thing I have ever done." It took 18 months after complete cessation to have a full day of feeling normal and 24 to 30 months before feeling better on a consistent basis.

> "It was as if a switch had been turned on again:
> my capacity to think, my energy, and my ability to laugh
> all returned."
> —Terri S.

More than three years after complete BZD cessation, her long-standing spine pain (unrelated to BZDs) accelerated. Procedures were considered. The pain, however, was so severe that on a single occasion she took 2.5 mg of cyclobenzaprine and 2.5 mg of hydrocodone, and upon doing so, she felt the familiar tightening of the neck and hypersensitivity to sound and touch—"just like withdrawing from BZDs."

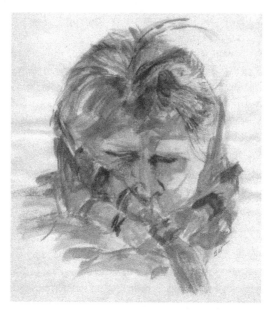

© Susan Wright

Medical decision-making is complicated. It goes beyond the essential calculus of balancing risks, benefits, and the availability of therapeutic options. Inertia and the challenges of change are significant barriers. Other priorities (*e.g.*, opioids) and perceived patient expectations are factored in. Prescribers conceptualize "deserving" patients and of what they might be deserving.[205] However, they may not be fully aware that these motivations are at play.

Pressured by time constraints, medical judgements are made heuristically: those efficient although imperfect mental strategies to address complex problems without the necessity of exhaustive information.[212] These short-cuts are not simple intuition, nor do they represent an abdication of responsibility, because at a minimum decision-making is uncertain whereby much is not known or unknowable. They are essential and valuable skills in clinical practice, but when BzRA prescribing is anchored narrowly in the erroneous assumption that short-term benefit will reliably translate into long-term gain, it can lead to harm. When such available "wisdom" is instead unexamined, BzRA-related fallacies inherited through generations of medical learners, patients on the whole will not do well.

Meant to improve on this, evidence-based medicine has become foundational for good reason: use of data is more reliable than that derived implicitly from clinical experience alone. But it is important to realize that evidence-based medicine deals with larger populations of patients, usually in a bell curve distribution. It does not deal with single individual patients. Although a major advance, research still describes a patient generically within the category studied, and when decision-making overrelies on similarity to a type (representativeness heuristics[205,212]) rather than as individualized (personalization), this, too, can cause harm. The view through cognitively biased glasses may cause well-meaning prescribers to tilt toward continuing BzRAs when more explicit considerations suggest otherwise.

Balancing BzRA benefit with problems based on available evidence today, certain recommendations can be made. Prescribing occurs in the context of uncertainty in which much is not known or unknowable and in which the principle "less is more"[213] is applicable. BzRA withdrawal is best avoided by limiting initiation and duration of use. As is true with the use of opioids in pain management, the goal is durable functional improvement and not simply symptomatic relief. When efficacy is lost, adverse reactions arise, and/or BzRAs are used for more than a month (*i.e.*, long-term), deprescribing is indicated. Best practices include a well-prepared integrated team with sufficient support, slow tapering, psychological therapies, and perhaps adjunctive medication. For the busy practitioner, these state-of-the-art heuristics will serve well.

It is recommended that an initial tapering rate be selected by anticipating 12 to 18 months to complete the cessation, *and only then* make adjustments up or down. The speed at which reductions take place should be based on the array and intensity of developing manifestations, anticipating wide variations over time. Fixed schedules are predictably problematic; the approach must be individualized. Symptoms and their patterns distinguish BzRA withdrawal from the re-emergence of conditions for which BzRAs were originally prescribed. The latter and other developing medical conditions require multidisciplinary management with evidence-based practices that should avoid an increase in BzRA dosage along the way.

Patients often arrive to their medical providers already traumatized by their experiences in the medical system and fear the whole catastrophe. Negative or harmful encounters with others (including prescribers) or the BzRA withdrawal itself may result in a picture "akin to post-traumatic stress disorder"[16] Many have been misdiagnosed as being psychosomatic or having addiction which prompts patient dismay and distress—and the use of ineffective, even harmful treatment strategies. Patients report it is not unusual for clinicians to discredit the validity of their lived experiences, discontinue prescriptions abruptly, or jump to alternative psychiatric diagnoses in error and with attendant inappropriate interventions. It is critical that prescribers respectfully and authentically listen to patients, who must be able to share their symptoms without fear. Actual individual responses to tapering determine ongoing decision-making—shared, to be sure—but primarily patient-directed.[16]

To help cope and manage expectations, patients, caregivers, and prescribers should be reminded that complete BzRA cessation may take longer than first expected. Prescribers and the involved collaborative team must remain engaged throughout tapering *and at least* until symptoms have abated, which may continue many months or years post-discontinuation. Several medications are known to be beneficial when symptoms are prominent during tapering but may have side effects. Flumazenil may be considered by those experienced in its use for patients with significant residual symptoms after BzRA cessation is fully concluded.[160]

This process can be very disruptive and in nightmare scenarios patients may be ostracized by family, friends, and even medical providers. Patient discomfort, withdrawal symptom severity, and alienation can largely be avoided by anticipation, planning, counseling, and support—and by becoming educated about BzRA withdrawal or "benzo-wise." While it is important to validate the frustrations experienced by families, it is critical also to validate the reality of patients' reports to their families and others no matter how severe or bizarre. Patients need direct reassurance. No one—certainly not the BZD survivor—signed on to this challenge by choice. Medical providers need to examine and adjust their own attitudes and biases to best serve their patients' need.

Hope must be nurtured throughout. Although benzodiazepine injury syndrome may be a more accurate description than prolonged withdrawal syndrome of an extended symptomatic course, it is not misleading to project optimism for a favorable outcome, which is true for most in due course. For most affected persons, healing proceeds and resolution is likely, although may take time and patience.

Sustained symptoms are to be met with sustained evidence-based practices individualized to the persons we serve. Medical care and caring are obligations that encompass prescribing, withdrawal, and for as long as symptoms and functional impairments persist beyond complete cessation—which may, in fact, be years. This journey, this enterprise, this gathering and unpredictable storm requires our full attention to the stories we hear and reasoned, empathetic responses to the hearts of those who are still struggling.

REFERENCES

1. Buire AC, Vitry F, Hoizey G, et al. Overdose of meprobamate: plasma concentration and Glasgow Coma Scale. *Br J Clin Pharmacol.* 2009;68(1):126–127.
2. Buckley NA, McManus PR. Changes in fatalities due to overdose of anxiolytic and sedative drugs in the UK (1983–1999). *Drug Saf.* 2004;27(2):135–141.
3. Hollister LE, Motzenbecker FP, Degan RO. Withdrawal reactions from chlordiazepoxide ("Librium"). *Psychopharmacologia.* 1961;2:63–68.
4. Barnes EM. Use-dependent regulation of $GABA_A$ receptors. *Int Rev Neurobiol.* 1996;39:53–76.
5. Allison C, Pratt JA. Neuroadaptive processes in GABAergic and glutamatergic systems in benzodiazepine dependence. *Pharm Ther.* 2003;98(3):171–195.
6. American Psychiatric Association. Substance-related and addictive disorders. In: *Diagnostic and Statistical Manual of Mental Disorders.* 5th ed. Arlington, VA, American Psychiatric Association; 2013:481–490, 550–560.
7. Stephens DN. A glutamatergic hypothesis of drug dependence: extrapolations from benzodiazepine receptor ligands. *Behav Pharmacol.* 1995;6(5–6):425–446.
8. Heberlein A, Bleich S, Kornhuber J, Hillemacher T. Neuroendocrine pathways in benzodiazepine dependence: new targets for research and therapy. *Hum Psychopharmacol.* 2008;23(3):171–181.
9. Vgontzas AN, Kales A, Bixler EO. Benzodiazepine side effects: role of pharmacokinetics and pharmacodynamics. *Pharmacology.* 1995;51(4):205–223.
10. Wichniak A, Brunner H, Ising M, et al. Impaired hypothalamic-pituitary-adrenocortical (HPA) system is related to severity of benzodiazepine withdrawal in patients with depression. *Psychoneuroendocrinology.* 2004;29(9):1101–1108.
11. Metten P, Crabbe JC. Genetic determinants of severity of acute withdrawal from diazepam in mice: commonality with ethanol and pentobarbital. *Pharmacol Biochem Behav.* 1999;63(3):473–479.
12. LaCorte S. How chronic administration of benzodiazepines leads to unexplained chronic illnesses: a hypothesis. *Medical Hypotheses.* 2018;118:59–67.
13. Mulkey SB, du Plessis AJ. Autonomic nervous system development and its impact on neuropsychiatric outcome. *Pediatr Res.* 2019;85(2):120–126.
14. Miller LG, Galpern WR, Byrnes JJ, et al. Chronic benzodiazepine administration. X. Concurrent administration of the peripheral-type benzodiazepine ligand PK11195 attenuates chronic effects of lorazepam. *J Pharmacol Exp Ther.* 1992;261(1):285–289.
15. Byrnes JJ, Miller LG, Perkins K, et al. Chronic benzodiazepine administration. XI. Concurrent administration of PK11195 attenuates lorazepam discontinuation effects. *Neuropsychopharmacology.* 1993;8(3):267–273.
16. Ashton H. *The Ashton Manual: Benzodiazepines: How They Work and How to Withdraw.* https://www.benzo.org.uk/manual/. Published 1999. Revised 2002. Supplement 2011.
17. Pecknold JC, Swinson RP, Kuch K, Lewis CP. Alprazolam in panic disorder and agoraphobia: results from a multicenter trial. III. Discontinuation effects. *Arch Gen Psychiatry.* 1988;45(5):429–436.
18. Ashton H. Benzodiazepine withdrawal: outcome in 50 patients. *Br J Addict.* 1987;82:655–671.
19. Landry MJ, Smith DE, McDuff DR, Baughman OL. Benzodiazepine dependence and withdrawal: identification and medical management. *J Am Board Fam Pract.* 1992;5(2):167–175.
20. World Health Organization. Dependence syndrome: definition. https://www.who.int/substance_abuse/terminology/definition1/en/. Accessed 8/5/20.

21. Ashton H. Protracted withdrawal syndromes from benzodiazepines. *J Subst Abuse Treat.* 1991;8(1–2):19–28.

22. Smith DE. Diagnostic, treatment and aftercare approaches to cocaine abuse. *J Subst Abuse Treat.* 1984;1(1):5–9.

23. Becker WC, Fiellin DA, Desai RA. Non-medical use, abuse and dependence on sedatives and tranquilizers among US adults: psychiatric and socio-demographic correlates. *Drug Alcohol Depend.* 2007;90(2-3):280–287.

24. Smith DE, Landry MJ. Benzodiazepine dependency discontinuation: focus on the chemical dependency detoxification setting and benzodiazepine-polydrug abuse. *J Psychiatr Res.* 1990;24 Suppl 2:145–156.

25. Laqueille X, Launay C, Dervaux A, Kanit M. Abuse of alcohol and benzodiazepine during substitution therapy in heroin addicts: a review of the literature. *Encephale.* 2009;35(3):220–225.

26. O'Brien CP. Benzodiazepine use, abuse, and dependence. *J Clin Psych.* 2005;66(Suppl 2):28–33.

27. Stein MD, Kanabar M, Anderson BJ, et al. Reasons for benzodiazepine use among persons seeking opioid detoxification. *J Subst Abuse Treat.* 2016;68:57–61.

28. Tyrer P. Benzodiazepine dependence: a shadowy diagnosis. *Biochem Soc Symp.* 1993;59:107–119.

29. Petursson H, Lader MH. Withdrawal from long-term benzodiazepine treatment. *Br Med J.* 1981;283:634–635.

30. Marriott S, Tyrer P. Benzodiazepine dependence: avoidance and withdrawal. *Drug Safety.* 1993;9(2):93–103.

31. Lader M, Kyriacou A. Withdrawing benzodiazepines in patients with anxiety disorders. *Curr Psychiatry Rep.* 2016;18(1):8.

32. Pelissolo A, Bisserbe JC. Dependence on benzodiazepines: clinical and biological aspects. *Encephale.* 1994;20(2):147–157.

33. Rickels K, Schweizer E, Case G, Greenblatt DJ. Long-term therapeutic use of benzodiazepines. I. Effects of abrupt discontinuation. *Arch Gen Psychiatry.* 1990;47(10):899–907.

34. Cantopher T, Olivieri S, Cleave N, et al. Chronic benzodiazepine dependence: a comparative study of abrupt withdrawal under propranolol cover versus gradual withdrawal. *Br J Psychiatry.* 1990;156:406–411.

35. Tyrer P, Owen R, Dawling S. Gradual withdrawal of diazepam after long-term therapy. *Lancet.* 1983;1(8339):1402–1406.

36. Lader M. Long-term anxiolytic therapy: the issue of drug withdrawal. *J Clin Psychiatry.* 1987;1(48 Suppl):12–16.

37. Hu X. Benzodiazepine withdrawal seizures and management. *J Okla State Med Assoc.* 2011;104(2):62–65.

38. Griffiths R, Evans S, Guarino J. Intravenous flumazenil following acute and repeated exposure to lorazepam in healthy volunteers: antagonism and precipitated withdrawal. *J Pharmacol Exp Ther.* 1993;265:1163–1174.

39. Kurko TAT, Saastamoinen LK, Tähkäpää S, et al. Long-term use of benzodiazepines: Definitions, prevalence and usage patterns - A systematic review of register-based studies. *Eur Psychiatry.* 2015;30:103–147.

40. Lugoboni F, Quaglio G. Exploring the dark side of the moon: the treatment of benzodiazepine tolerance. *Br J Clin Pharmacol.* 2014;77(2):239–241.

41. Couvée JE, Zitman FG. The Benzodiazepine Withdrawal Symptom Questionnaire: psychometric evaluation during a discontinuation program in depressed chronic benzodiazepine users in general practice. *Addiction.* 2002;97(3):337–345.

42. Busto UE, Sykora K, Sellers EM. A clinical scale to assess benzodiazepine withdrawal. *J Clin Psychopharmacol.* 1989;9(6):412–416.

43. Schweizer E, Rickels K, Case WG, Greenblatt DJ. Long-term therapeutic use of benzodiazepines. II. Effects of gradual taper. *Arch Gen Psychiatry*. 1990;47(10):908–915.
44. Kan CC, Mickers FC, Barnhoorn D. Short- and long-term results of a systematic benzodiazepine discontinuation program for psychiatric patients. *Tijdschr Psychiatr*. 2006;48(9):683–693.
45. Gorgels WJ, Oude Voshaar RC, Mol AJ, et al. Predictors of discontinuation of benzodiazepine prescription after sending a letter to long-term benzodiazepine users in family practice. *Fam Pract*. 2006;23(1):65–72.
46. Saxon L, Hiltunen AJ, Hjemdahl P, Borg S. Gender-related differences in response to placebo in benzodiazepine withdrawal: a single-blind pilot study. *Psychopharmacology (Berl)*. 2001;153(2):231–237.
47. Pomara N, Willoughby LM, Ritchie JC, et al. Sex-related elevation in cortisol during chronic treatment with alprazolam associated with enhanced cognitive performance. *Psychopharmacology (Berl)*. 2005;182(3):414–419.
48. Bobes J, Rubio G, Terán A, et al. Pregabalin for the discontinuation of long-term benzodiazepines use: an assessment of its effectiveness in daily clinical practice. *Eur Psychiatry*. 2012;27(4):301–307.
49. Tannenbaum C, Martin P, Tamblyn R, et al. Reduction of inappropriate benzodiazepine prescriptions among older adults through direct patient education: the EMPOWER cluster randomized trial. *JAMA Intern Med*. 2014;174(6):890–898.
50. Holton A, Riley P, Tyrer P. Factors predicting long-term outcome after chronic benzodiazepine therapy. *J Affect Disord*. 1992;24(4):245–252.
51. Schweizer E, Case WG, Rickels K. Benzodiazepine dependence and withdrawal in elderly patients. *Am J Psychiatry*. 1989;146(4):529–531.
52. Joughin N, Tata P, Collins M, et al. In-patient withdrawal from long-term benzodiazepine use. *Br J Addict*. 1991;86(4):449–455.
53. Pétursson H. The benzodiazepine withdrawal syndrome. *Addiction*. 1994;89(11):1455–1459.
54. MacKinnon GL, Parker WA. Benzodiazepine withdrawal syndrome: a literature review and evaluation. *Am J Drug Alcohol Abuse*. 1982;9(1):19–33.
55. Seivewright N, Dougal W. Withdrawal symptoms from high dose benzodiazepines in polydrug users. *Drug Alcohol Depend*. 1993;32(1):15–23.
56. O'Connor KP, Marchand A, Bélanger L, et al. Psychological distress and adaptational problems associated with benzodiazepine withdrawal and outcome: a replication. *Addict Behav*. 2004;29(3):583–593.
57. Schmauss C, Apelt S, Emrich HM. Characterization of benzodiazepine withdrawal in high- and low-dose dependent psychiatric inpatients. *Brain Res Bull*. 1987;19(3):393–400.
58. Ista E, van Dijk M, Gamel C, et al. Withdrawal symptoms in critically ill children after long-term administration of sedatives and/or analgesics: a first evaluation. *Crit Care Med*. 2008;36(8):2427–2432.
59. Paquin AM, Zimmerman K, Rudolph JL. Risk versus risk: a review of benzodiazepine reduction in older adults. *Expert Opin Drug Saf*. 2014;13(7):919–934.
60. Denis C, Fatséas M, Lavie E, Auriacombe M. Pharmacological interventions for benzodiazepine mono-dependence management in outpatient settings. *Cochrane Database Syst Rev*. 2006;(3):CD005194.
61. Lader M. Anxiety or depression during withdrawal of hypnotic treatments. *J Psychosom Res*. 1994;38 Suppl 1:113–123.
62. Ashton H. A problem with lorazepam? https://www.benzoinfo.com/. Published 1988.
63. Lapierre YD. Benzodiazepine withdrawal. *Can J Psychiatry*. 1981;26(2):93–95.
64. Ashton H. The diagnosis and management of benzodiazepine dependence. *Curr Opin Psychiatry*. 2005;18:249–255.

65. Haass-Koffler CL, McCance-Katz EF. The pharmacology of nonalcohol sedative hypnotics. In: Miller SC, Fiellin DA, Rosenthal RN, Saitz R, eds. *The ASAM Principles of Addiction Medicine*. 6th ed. New York, NY: Lippincott Williams & Wilkins, 2018: 125-135.

66. Fialip J, Aumaitre O, Eschalier A, et al. Benzodiazepine withdrawal seizures: analysis of 48 case reports. *Clin Neuropharmacol.* 1987;*10*(6):538–544.

67. Lann MA, Molina DK. A fatal case of benzodiazepine withdrawal. *Am J Forensic Med Pathol.* 2009;*30*(2):177–179.

68. Browne JL, Hauge KJ. A review of alprazolam withdrawal. *Drug Intell Clin Pharm.* 1986;*20*(11):837–841.

69. Martínez-Cano H, Vela-Bueno A, de Iceta M, et al. Benzodiazepine withdrawal syndrome seizures. *Pharmacopsychiatry.* 1995;*28*(6):257–262.

70. Rosebush PI, Mazurek MF. Catatonia after benzodiazepine withdrawal. *J Clin Psychopharmacol.* 1996;*16*(4):315–319.

71. Oldham MA, Desan PH. Alcohol and sedative-hypnotic withdrawal catatonia: two case reports, systematic literature review, and suggestion of a potential relationship with alcohol withdrawal delirium. *Psychosomatics.* 2016;*57*(3):246–255.

72. Hauser P, Devinsky O, De Bellis M, et al. Benzodiazepine withdrawal delirium with catatonic features. Occurrence in patients with partial seizure disorders. *Arch Neurol.* 1989;*46*(6):696–699.

73. Murphy SM, Tyrer P. A double-blind comparison of the effects of gradual withdrawal of lorazepam, diazepam and bromazepam in benzodiazepine dependence. *Br J Psychiatry.* 1991;*158*:511–516.

74. Martin-Kleisch A, Zulfiqar AA. Retrospective study of the assessment and management of benzodiazepine withdrawal syndrome in hospital between 2000 and 2015. *Ann Pharm Fr.* 2017;*75*(3):196–208.

75. Raffa R, Pergolizzi JV. Commentary: Benzodiazepine (BZD) and related BZD-receptor agonists: basic science reasons to limit to four weeks or less. *Pharmacol Pharm.* 2019;*10*(8):357–364.

76. Turkington D, Gill P. Mania induced by lorazepam withdrawal: a report of two cases. *J Affect Disord.* 1989;*17*(1):93–95.

77. Garcia-Borreguero D, Bronisch T, Apelt S, et al. Treatment of benzodiazepine withdrawal symptoms with carbamazepine. *Eur Arch Psychiatry Clin Neurosci.* 1991;*241*(3):145–150.

78. Mellor CS, Jain VK. Diazepam withdrawal syndrome: its prolonged and changing nature. *Can Med Assoc J.* 1982;*127*(11):1093–1096.

79. Bruce TJ, Spiegel DA, Gregg SF, Nuzzarello A. Predictors of alprazolam discontinuation with and without cognitive behavior therapy in panic disorder. *Am J Psychiatry.* 1995;*152*(8):1156–1160.

80. Ashton H. Benzodiazepine withdrawal: an unfinished story. *Br Med J.* 1984;*288*:1135–1140.

81. Cohen SI. Alcohol and benzodiazepines generate anxiety, panic and phobias. *J R Soc Med.* 1995;*88*(2):73–77.

82. Tata PR, Rollings J, Collins M, et al. Lack of cognitive recovery following withdrawal from long-term benzodiazepine use. *Psychol Med.* 1994;*24*(1):203–213.

83. Pecknold JC. Discontinuation reactions to alprazolam in panic disorder. *J Psychiatr Res.* 1993;*27* Suppl 1:155–170.

84. Ashton CH. Protracted withdrawal from benzodiazepines: the post-withdrawal syndrome. *Psychiatric Annals.* 1995;*25*(3):174–179.

85. Morin CM, Bastien C, Guay B, et al. Randomized clinical trial of supervised tapering and cognitive behavior therapy to facilitate benzodiazepine discontinuation in older adults with chronic insomnia. *Am J Psych.* 2004;*161*(2):332–342.

86. Belleville G, Morin CM. Hypnotic discontinuation in chronic insomnia: impact of psychological distress, readiness to change, and self-efficacy. *Health Psychol.* 2008;*27*(2):239–248.

87. Greenblatt DJ, Harmatz JS, Zinny MA, Shader RI. Effect of gradual withdrawal on the rebound sleep disorder after discontinuation of triazolam. *N Engl J Med.* 1987;*317*(12):722–728.

88. Busto U, Sellers EM, Naranjo CA, et al. Withdrawal reaction after long-term therapeutic use of benzodiazepines. *New Engl J Med.* 1986;*315*:654–659.

89. Yeliseev AA, Kaplan S. TspO of Rhodobacter sphaeroides. A structural and functional model for the mammalian peripheral benzodiazepine receptor. *J Biol Chem.* 2000;*275*(8):5657–5667.

90. Miller LG, Koff JM. Interaction of central and peripheral benzodiazepine sites in benzodiazepine tolerance and discontinuation. *Prog Neuropsychopharmacol Biol Psychiatry.* 1994;*18*(5):847–857.

91. Herman JB, Brotman AW, Rosenbaum JF. Rebound anxiety in panic disorder patients treated with shorter-acting benzodiazepines. *J Clin Psychiatry.* 1987;*48* Suppl:22–28.

92. Vikander B, Koechling UM, Borg S, et al. Benzodiazepine tapering: a prospective study. *Nord J Psychiatry.* 2010;*64*(4):273–282.

93. Smith DE, Wesson DR. Benzodiazepine dependency syndromes. *J Psychoactive Drugs.* 1983;*15*:85–95.

94. Tyrer P. The benzodiazepine post-withdrawal syndrome. *Stress Med.* 1991;*7*:1–2.

95. Chen LH, Hedegaard H, Warner M. Drug-poisoning deaths Involving opioid analgesics: United States, 1999-2011. *NCHS Data Brief.* 2014;(166):1–8.

96. Mattson CL, O'Donnell J, Kariisa M, et al. Opportunities to prevent overdose deaths involving prescription and illicit opioids, 11 states, July 2016–June 2017. *MMWR.* 2018;*67*(34):945–951.

97. Dasgupta N, Funk MJ, Proescholdbell S, et al. Cohort study of the impact of high-dose opioid analgesics on overdose mortality. *Pain Med.* 2016;*17*(1):85–98.

98. Horsfall JT, Sprague JE. The pharmacology and toxicology of the "Holy Trinity." *Basic Clin Pharmacol Toxicol.* 2017;*120*(2):115–119.

99. Eickelberg SJ, Dickinson WE. Attia RA. Management of sedative-hypnotic withhdrawal. In: Miller SC, Fiellin DA, Rosenthal RN, Saitz R, eds. *The ASAM Principles of Addiction Medicine.* 6th ed. New York, NY: Lippincott Williams & Wilkins; 2018:723–740.

100. Gonçalves M. Oliveira A, Leão A, Maia S, Brinca P. The impact of benzodiazepine use in nocturnal O2 saturation of OSAS patients. *Sleep Med.* 2013;*14*(1):e141–e142.

101. Wang S-H, Chen W-S, Tang S-E, et al. Benzodiazepines associated with acute respiratory failure in patients with obstructive sleep apnea. *Front Pharmacol.* 2019;*7*;9:1513.

102. Webster LR, Reisfield GM, Dasgupta N. Eight principles for safer opioid prescribing and cautions with benzodiazepines. *Postgrad Med.* 2015;*127*(1):27–32.

103. Lader M. Benzodiazepine harm: how can it be reduced? *Br J Clin Pharmacol.* 2014;*77*(2):295–301.

104. Pottie K, Thompson W, Davies S, et al. Deprescribing benzodiazepine receptor agonists: evidence-based clinical practice guideline. *Canadian Fam Phys.* 2018;*64*(5):339–351.

105. National Institute for Health and Clinical Excellence. Generalized anxiety disorder and panic disorder in adults. Clinical guideline CG113. https://www.nice.org.uk/guidance/cg113. Published January 2011. Updated July 26, 2019.

106. Ashton H. Guidelines for the rational use of benzodiazepines: when and what to use. *Drugs.* 1994;*48*(1):25–40.

107. van Balkom AJ, de Beurs E, Koele P, et al. Long-term benzodiazepine use is associated with smaller treatment gain in panic disorder with agoraphobia. *J Nerv Ment Dis.* 1996;*184*(2):133–135.

108. Curran HV, Collins R, Fletcher S, et al. Older adults and withdrawal from benzodiazepine hypnotics in general practice: effects on cognitive function, sleep, mood and quality of life. *Psychol Med.* 2003;*33*(7):1223–1237.

109. Fava GA. Fading of therapeutic effects of alprazolam in agoraphobia: case reports. *Prog Neuropsychopharmacol Biol Psychiatry.* 1988;*12*(1):109–112.
110. Pélissolo A, Maniere F, Boutges B, et al. Anxiety and depressive disorders in 4,425 long term benzodiazepine users in general practice. *Encephale.* 2007;*33*(1):32–38.
111. Marks IM, Swinson RP, Başoğlu M, et al. Alprazolam and exposure alone and combined in panic disorder with agoraphobia: a controlled study in London and Toronto. *Br J Psychiatry.* 1993;*162*:776–787.
112. Westra HA, Stewart SH, Conrad BE. Naturalistic manner of benzodiazepine use and cognitive behavioral therapy outcome in panic disorder with agoraphobia. *J Anxiety Disord.* 2002;*16*(3):233–246.
113. Cook JM, Biyanova T, Masci C, Coyne JC. Older patient perspectives on long-term anxiolytic benzodiazepine use and discontinuation: a qualitative study. *J Gen Intern Med.* 2007;*22*(8):1094–1100.
114. Specht U, Boenigk HE, Wolf P. Discontinuation of clonazepam after long-term treatment. *Epilepsia.* 1989;*30*(4):458–463.
115. Gorgels WJ, Oude Voshaar RC, Mol AJ, et al. Discontinuation of long-term benzodiazepine use by sending a letter to users in family practice: a prospective controlled intervention study. *Drug Alcohol Depend.* 2005;*78*(1):49–56.
116. Mugunthan K, McGuire T, Glasziou P. Minimal interventions to decrease long-term use of benzodiazepines in primary care: a systematic review and meta-analysis. *Br J Gen Pract.* 2011;*61*(590):e573–e578.
117. Darker CD, Sweeney BP, Barry JM, et al. Psychosocial interventions for benzodiazepine harmful use, abuse or dependence. *Cochrane Database Syst Rev.* 2015;(5):CD009652.
118. Lader M, Tylee A, Donoghue J. Withdrawing benzodiazepines in primary care. *CNS Drugs.* 2009;*23*(1):19–34.
119. Ashton H. The Ashton manual supplement. https://benzo.org.uk/ashsupp11.htm. Published 2011.
120. Pittman CM, Youngs W, Karle E. Social networking and benzodiazepine withdrawal: the realities of dependence and the necessity of support. Presented at the 33rd Annual National Conference of the Anxiety and Depression Association of America, La Jolla, California, April 2013.
121. Kamath A. Fluoroquinolone induced neurotoxicity: a review. *J Adv Pharmacy Ed Res.* 2013;*3*(1):16–19.
122. Ford C, Law F, Barjolin J, et al. Guidance for the use and reduction of misuse of benzodiazepines and other hypnotics and anxiolytics in general practice. 2014.
123. All Wales Medicines Strategy Group. Educational pack: Material to support appropriate prescribing of hypnotics and anxiolytics across Wales. http://www.awmsg.org/awmsgonline/rr_home.html. Published April 2011. Updated December 2016.
124. Janhsen K, Roser P, Hoffmann K. The problems of long-term treatment with benzodiazepines and related substances. *Dtsch Arztebl Int.* 2015;*112*(1-2):1–7.
125. ClinCalc. Equivalent benzodiazepine calculator. https://clincalc.com/Benzodiazepine/. Accessed 8/5/20.
126. Perry PJ, Alexander B. Sedative/hypnotic dependence: patient stabilization, tolerance testing, and withdrawal. *Drug Intell Clin Pharm.* 1986;*20*(7-8):532–537.
127. Kawasaki SS, Jacapraro JS, Rastegar DA. Safety and effectiveness of a fixed-dose phenobarbital protocol for inpatient benzodiazepine detoxification. *J Subst Abuse Treat.* 2012;*43*(3):331–334.
128. Landry MJ, Smith DE, McDuff DR, et al. Benzodiazepine dependence and withdrawal: identification and medical management. *J Am Board Fam Pract.* 1992;*5*:167–176.
129. Newton DW, Schulman SG, Becker CH. Limitations of compounding diazepam suspensions from tablets. *Am J Hosp Pharm.* 1976;*33*(5):450–452.

130. Inner Compass Initiative. The withdrawal project. https://withdrawal.theinnercompass. org/. Accessed 8/5/20.

131. Gould RL, Coulson MC, Patel N, et al. Interventions for reducing benzodiazepine use in elderly. *Br J Psychiatry.* 2014;*204*(2):98–107.

132. Parr JM, Kavanagh DJ, Cahill L, et al. Effectiveness of current treatment approaches for benzodiazepine discontinuation: a meta-analysis. *Addiction.* 2009;*104*(1):13–24.

133. Voshaar RC, Couvée JE, van Balkom AJ, et al. Strategies for discontinuing long-term benzodiazepine use: meta-analysis. *Br J Psychiatry.* 2006;*189*:213–20.

134. Lichstein KL, Peterson BA, Riedel BW, et al. Relaxation to assist sleep medication withdrawal. *Behav Modif.* 1999;*23*(3):379–402.

135. Tattersall ML, Hallstrom C. Self-help and benzodiazepine withdrawal. *J Affect Disord.* 1992;*24*(3):193–8.

136. Ng BJ, Le Couteur DG, Hilmer SN. Deprescribing benzodiazepines in older patients: impact of interventions targeting physicians, pharmacists, and patients. *Drugs Aging.* 2018;*35*(6):493–521.

137. Baandrup L, Ebdrup BH, Rasmussen JØ, et al. Pharmacological interventions for benzodiazepine discontinuation in chronic benzodiazepine users. *Cochrane Database Syst Rev.* 2018;*3*:CD011481.

138. Welsh JW, Tretyak V, McHugh RK, et al. Adjunctive pharmacologic approaches for benzodiazepine tapers. *Drug Alcohol Depend.* 2018;*189*:96–107.

139. Schweizer E, Rickels K, Case WG, Greenblatt DJ. Carbamazepine treatment in patients discontinuing long-term benzodiazepine therapy: effects on withdrawal severity and outcome. *Arch Gen Psychiatry.* 1991;*48*(5):448–452.

140. Harris JT, Roache JD, Thornton JE. A role for valproate in the treatment of sedative-hypnotic withdrawal and for relapse prevention. *Alcohol Alcohol.* 2000;*35*(4):319–323.

141. Bandrup, Rickels K, Schweizer E, Garcia España F, et al. Trazodone and valproate in patients discontinuing long-term benzodiazepine therapy: effects on withdrawal symptoms and taper outcome. *Psychopharmacology (Berl).* 1999;*141*(1):1–5.

142. Croissant B, Grosshans M, Diehl A, Mann K. Oxcarbazepine in rapid benzodiazepine detoxification. *Am J Drug Alcohol Abuse.* 2008;*34*(5):534–540.

143. Bramness JG, Sandvik P, Engeland A, Skurtveit S. Does pregabalin (Lyrica(*)) help patients reduce their use of benzodiazepines? A comparison with gabapentin using the Norwegian Prescription Database. *Basic Clin Pharmacol Toxicol.* 2010;*107*(5):883–886.

144. Hadley SJ, Mandel FS, Schweizer E. Switching from long-term benzodiazepine therapy to pregabalin in patients with generalized anxiety disorder: a double-blind, placebo-controlled trial. *J Psychopharmacol.* 2012;*26*(4):461–470.

145. Oulis P, Kalogerakou S, Anyfandi E, et al. Cognitive effects of pregabalin in the treatment of long-term benzodiazepine-use and dependence. *Hum Psychopharmacol.* 2014;*29*(3):224–229.

146. Oulis P, Konstantakopoulos G, Kouzoupis AV, et al. Pregabalin in the discontinuation of long-term benzodiazepines' use. *Hum Psychopharmacol.* 2008;*23*(4):337–340.

147. Mariani JJ, Malcolm RJ, Mamczur AK, et al. Pilot trial of gabapentin for the treatment of benzodiazepine abuse or dependence in methadone maintenance patients. *Am J Drug Alcohol Abuse.* 2016;*42*(3):333–340.

148. Bandrup, Nakao M, Takeuchi T, Nomura K, et al. Clinical application of paroxetine for tapering benzodiazepine use in non-major-depressive outpatients visiting an internal medicine clinic. *Psychiatry Clin Neurosci.* 2006;*60*(5):605–610.

149. Nakao M, Takeuchi T, Nomura K, et al. Clinical application of paroxetine for tapering benzodiazepine use in non-major-depressive outpatients visiting an internal medicine clinic. *Psychiatry Clin Neurosci.* 2006;*60*(5):605–610.

150. Rickels K, DeMartinis N, García-España F, et al. Imipramine and buspirone in treatment of patients with generalized anxiety disorder who are discontinuing long-term benzodiazepine therapy. *Am J Psychiatry.* 2000;*157*(12):1973–1979.

151. Ansseau M, De Roeck J. Trazodone in benzodiazepine dependence. *J Clin Psychiatry.* 1993;*54*(5):189–191.

152. Funk S. Pharmacological treatment in alcohol-, drug- and benzodiazepine-dependent patients - the significance of trazodone. *Neuropsychopharmacol Hung.* 2013;*15*(2):85–93.

153. Ngo AS, Anthony CR, Samuel M, et al. Should a benzodiazepine antagonist be used in unconscious patients presenting to the emergency department? *Resuscitation.* 2007;*74*(1):27–37.

154. Rusch D, Forman SA. Classic benzodiazepines modulate the open-close equilibrium in alpha1 beta2 gamma 2L gamma-aminobutyric acid type A receptors. *Anesthesiology.* 2005;*102*(4):783–792.

155. Gerra G, Zaimovic A, Giusti F, et al. Intravenous flumazenil versus oxazepam tapering in the treatment of benzodiazepine withdrawal: a randomized, placebo-controlled study. *Addict Biol.* 2002;*7*(4):385–395.

156. Faccini M, Leone R, Opri S, et al. Slow subcutaneous infusion of flumazenil for the treatment of long-term, high-dose benzodiazepine users: a review of 214 cases. *J Psychopharmacol.* 2016;*30*(10):1047–1053.

157. Penninga EI, Graudal N, Ladekarl MB, Jürgens G. Adverse events associated with flumazenil treatment for the management of suspected benzodiazepine intoxication: a systematic review with meta-analyses of randomized trials. *Basic Clin Pharmacol Toxicol.* 2016;*118*(1):37–44.

158. Hulse G, O'Neil G, Morris N, et al. Withdrawal and psychological sequelae, and patient satisfaction associated with subcutaneous flumazenil infusion for the management of benzodiazepine withdrawal: a case series. *J Psychopharmacol.* 2012;*27*(2):222–227.

159. Mintzer MZ, Stoller KB, Griffiths RR. A controlled study of flumazenil-precipitated withdrawal in chronic low-dose benzodiazepine users. *Psychopharmacology (Berl).* 1999;*147*(2):200–209.

160. Lader MH, Morton SV. A pilot study of the effects of flumazenil on symptoms persisting after benzodiazepine withdrawal. *J Psychopharmacol.* 1992;*6*(3):357–363.

161. Harrison-Read PE, Tyrer P, Lawson C, et al. Flumazenil-precipitated panic and dysphoria in patients dependent on benzodiazepines: a possible aid to abstinence. *J Psychopharmacol.* 1996;*10*(2):89–97.

162. Tyrer P, Rutherford D, Huggett T. Benzodiazepine withdrawal symptoms and propranolol. *Lancet.* 1981;7;*1*(8219):520–522.

163. Lader M, Olajide D. A comparison of buspirone and placebo in relieving benzodiazepine withdrawal symptoms. *J Clin Psychopharmacol.* 1987;*7*(1):11–15.

164. Rynn M, García-España F, Greenblatt DJ, et al. Imipramine and buspirone in patients with panic disorder who are discontinuing long-term benzodiazepine therapy. *J Clin Psychopharmacol.* 2003;*23*(5):505–508.

165. Lemoine P, Touchon J, Billardon M. Comparison of 6 different methods for lorazepam withdrawal. A controlled study, hydroxyzine versus placebo. *Encephale.* 1997;*23*(4):290–299.

166. Fyer AJ, Liebowitz MR, Gorman JM, et al. Effects of clonidine on alprazolam discontinuation in panic patients: a pilot study. *J Clin Psychopharmacol.* 1988;*8*(4):270–274.

167. Schweizer E, Case WG, Garcia-Espana F, et al. Progesterone co-administration in patients discontinuing long-term benzodiazepine therapy: effects on withdrawal severity and taper outcome. *Psychopharmacology (Berl).* 1995;*117*(4):424–429.

168. Schweizer E, Case WG, Garcia-Espana F, et al. Progesterone co-administration in patients discontinuing long-term benzodiazepine therapy: effects on withdrawal severity and taper outcome. *Psychopharmacology (Berl)*. 1995;117(4):424–429.

169. Wright A, Diebold J, Otal J, et al. The effect of melatonin on benzodiazepine discontinuation and sleep quality in adults attempting to discontinue benzodiazepines: a systematic review and meta-analysis. *Drugs Aging*. 2015;32(12):1009–1018.

170. Romach MK, Kaplan HL, Busto UE, et al. A controlled trial of ondansetron, a 5-HT3 antagonist, in benzodiazepine discontinuation. *J Clin Psychopharmacol*. 1998;18(2):121–131.

171. Lichstein KL, Peterson BA, Riedel BW, et al. Relaxation to assist sleep medication withdrawal. *Behav Modif*. 1999;23(3):379–402.

172. Morgan K, Dixon S, Mathers N, et al. Psychological treatment for insomnia in the regulation of long-term hypnotic drug use. *Health Technol Assess*. 2004;8(8):iii–iv, 1–68.

173. Gilbody S, Lewis S, Lightfoot T. Methylenetetrahydrofolate reductase (MTHFR) genetic polymorphisms and psychiatric disorders: a HuGE review. *Am J Epidemiol*. 2007;165(1):1–13.

174. Aguayo LG, Peoples RW, Yeh HH, Yevenes GE. GABA$_A$ receptors as molecular sites of ethanol action. Direct or indirect actions? *Curr Top Med Chem*. 2002;2(8):869–885.

175. Fluharty M, Taylor AE, Grabski M, Munafò MR. The association of cigarette Smoking with depression and anxiety: a systematic review. *Nicotine Tob Res*. 2017;19(1):3–13.

176. Boehm MA, Lei QM, Lloyd RM, Prichard JR. Depression, anxiety, and tobacco use: overlapping impediments to sleep in a national sample of college students. *J Am Coll Health*. 2016;64(7):565–574.

177. Tolu S, Eddine R, Marti F, et al. Co-activation of VTA DA and GABA neurons mediates nicotine reinforcement. *Mol Psychiatry*. 2013;18(3):382–393

178. Angarita GA, Emadi N, Hodges S, Morgan PT. Sleep abnormalities associated with alcohol, cannabis, cocaine, and opiate use: a comprehensive review. *Addict Sci Clin Pract*. 2016;11(1):9.

179. Kuriyama K, Sze PY. Blood-brain barrier to H3-gamma-aminobutyric acid in normal and amino oxyacetic acid-treated animals. *Neuropharmacol*. 1971;10(1):103–108.

180. Trauner G, Khom S, Baburin I, et al. Modulation of GABA$_A$ receptors by valerian extracts is related to the content of valerenic acid. *Planta Med*. 2008;74(1):19–24.

181. Pertwee RG. Diverse CB1 and CB2 receptor pharmacology of 3 plant cannabinoids: D9-THC, CBD, D9-tetrahydrocannabivarin. *Br J Pharmacol*. 2008;153(2):199–215.

182. Lapin I. Phenibut (beta-phenyl-GABA): a tranquilizer and nootropic drug. *CNS Drug Rev*. 2001;7(4):471–481.

183. Woelk H, Schläfke S. A multi-center, double-blind, randomised study of the lavender oil preparation silexan in comparison to lorazepam for generalized anxiety disorder. *Phytomedicine*. 2010;17(2):94–99.

184. Blanco C, Han B, Jones CM, et al. Prevalence and correlates of benzodiazepine use, misuse, and use disorders among adults in the United States. *J Clin Psychiatry*. 2018;79(6):18m12174.

185. Pauly V, Frauger E, Pradel V, et al. Monitoring of benzodiazepine diversion using a multi-indicator approach. *Int Clin Psychopharmacol*. 2011;26(5):268–277.

186. Feeney R. Medication overuse headache due to butalbital, acetaminophen, and caffeine tablets. *J Pain Palliat Care Pharmacother*. 2016;30(2):148–149.

187. Berridge KC. From prediction error to incentive salience: mesolimbic computation of reward motivation. *Eur J Neurosci*. 2012;35(7):1124–1143.

188. Griffiths RR, Wolf B. Relative abuse liability of different benzodiazepines in drug abusers. *J Clin Psychopharmacol*. 1990;10(4):237–243.

189. Watkins KE, Ober AJ, Lamp K, et al. Collaborative care for opioid and alcohol use disorders in primary care: the SUMMIT randomized clinical trial. *JAMA Intern Med.* 2017;*177*(10):1480–1488.

190. Soumerai SB, Simoni-Wastila L, Singer C, et al. Lack of relationship between long-term use of benzodiazepines and escalation to high dosages. *Psychiatr Serv.* 2003;*54*(7):1006–1011.

191. Martin P, Tannenbaum C. A realist evaluation of patients' decisions to deprescribe in the EMPOWER trial. *BMJ Open.* 2017;*7*(4):e015959.

192. DuPont RL, Swinson RP, Ballenger JC, et al. Discontinuation of alprazolam after long-term treatment of panic-related disorders. *J Clin Psychopharmacol.* 1992;*12*(5):352–354.

193. Guina J, Merrill B. Benzodiazepines II: waking up on sedatives: providing optimal care when inheriting benzodiazepine prescriptions in transfer patients. *J Clin Med.* 2018;*7*(2):E20.

194. Munyaradzi M. Critical reflections on the principle of beneficence in biomedicine. *Pan Afr Med J.* 2012;*11*:29.

195. Darragh A, Snyder ML, Ptolemy AS, Melanson S. KIMS, CEDIA, and HS-CEDIA immunoassays are inadequately sensitive for detection of benzodiazepines in urine from patients treated for chronic pain. *Pain Physician.* 2014;*17*:359–366.

196. Masnoon N, Shakib S, Kalisch-Ellett L, et al. What is polypharmacy? A systematic review of definitions. *BMC Geriatr.* 2017;*17*:230.

197. Mlodinow SG, Linn BS, Mahvan T, et al. Strategies to reduce and prevent polypharmacy in older patients. *J Fam Pract.* 2019;*68*(8):429–440.

198. Laursen J, Kornholt J, Better C, et al. General practitioners' barriers toward medication reviews in polymedicated multimorbid patients: how can a focus on the pharmacotherapy in an outpatient clinic support GPs? *Health Serv Res Manag Epidemiol.* 2018;*5*:1–7.

199. Kafka F. A country doctor. https://holybooks-lichtenbergpress.netdna-ssl.com/wp-content/uploads/A-country-doctor-by-Franz-Kafka.pdf. Accessed 8/5/20.

200. Liebrenz M, Gehring MT, Buadze A, Caflisch C. High-dose benzodiazepine dependence: a qualitative study of patients' perception on cessation and withdrawal. *BMC Psychiatry.* 2015;*15*:116.

201. Rosen CS, Greenbaum MA, Schnurr PP, et al. Do benzodiazepines reduce the effectiveness of exposure therapy for posttraumatic stress disorder? *J Clin Psychiatry.* 2013;*74*(12):1241–1248.

202. Lewis T. Using the NO TEARS tool for medication review. *BMJ.* 2004;*329*(7463):434.

203. US Food and Drug Administration. FDA Adverse Event Reporting System (FAERS) public dashboard. https://www.fda.gov/drugs/questions-and-answers-fdas-adverse-event-reporting-system-faers/fda-adverse-event-reporting-system-faers-public-dashboard. Accessed 8/5/20.

204. Hall DE, Prochazka AV, Fink AS. Informed consent for clinical treatment. *CMAJ.* 2012;*184*(5):533–540.

205. Sirdifield C, Anthierens S, Creupelandt H, et al. General practitioners' experiences and perceptions of benzodiazepine prescribing: systematic review and meta-synthesis. *BMC Fam Pract.* 2013;*14*:191.

206. Guina J, Rossetter SR, DeRhodes BJ, et al. Benzodiazepines for PTSD: a systematic review and meta-analysis. *J Psychiatr Pract.* 2015;*21*(4):281–303.

207. Jeffreys M, Capehart B, Friedman MJ. Pharmacotherapy for posttraumatic stress disorder: review with clinical applications. *J Rehabil Res Dev.* 2012;*49*(5):703–716.

208. Koran LM, Hanna GL, Hollander E, et al. American Psychiatric Association. Practice guideline for the treatment of patients with obsessive-compulsive disorder. *Am J Psychiatry.* 2007;*164*(Suppl 7):5–53.

209. Riemann D, Perlis ML. The treatments of chronic insomnia: a review of benzodiazepine receptor agonists and psychological and behavioral therapies. *Sleep Med Rev.* 2009;*13*(3):205–214.
210. Young A. Survey of benzodiazepine withdrawal outcomes of an Internet benzodiazepine group. 2007.
211. Fixsen AM, Ridge D. Stories of hell and healing: internet users' construction of benzodiazepine distress and withdrawal. *Qual Health Res.* 2017;*27*(13):2030–2041.
212. Tversky A, Kahneman D. Judgment under uncertainty: heuristics and biases. *Science.* 1974;*185*(4157):1124–1131.
213. Gigerenzer G. Why heuristics work. *Perspect Psychol Sci.* 2008;*3*(1):20–29.

CHAPTER 9

Benzodiazepines and Pain Management

JOHN F. PEPPIN AND STEVEN L. WRIGHT

Pain is a more terrible lord over mankind
than even death itself.
                    —Albert Schweitzer[1p652]

HIGHLIGHTS

- Chronic pain is common around the world as is the use of opioids in treating this aliment.
- Benzodiazepines are frequently co-prescribed with opioids in the setting of chronic pain.
- Increases of overdose death are correlated with the co prescribing of benzodiazepines and opioids. Benzodiazepines by themselves increase overall mortality.
- Few data exist for the long-term use of benzodiazepines in chronic pain for either sleep disorders, pain, or anxiety.
- A process of deprescribing of benzodiazepines should be implemented more frequently.

Pain is universal, and its management remains a monumental challenge for both patients and their caregivers. In the previous year, 40% of the world's population report having chronic pain.[2] In the United States, some 100 million have persistent pain, and 25 million have pain on a daily basis.[3] Pain is associated with major negative consequences both physiologic and psychologic, including suicidality and mortality.[4,5] Further, pain patients are frequently marginalized and their pain discounted.[6] As aptly expressed by

Naomi Wolf, "pain is real when you get other people to believe in it. If no one believes in it, pain is madness or hysteria." [7p254]

Although data on functional outcomes are scant, opioids provide analgesic benefit for both acute and chronic pain.[8–20] In fact, limited that they are, there are more data supporting long-term opioid use in carefully selected and managed patients than that for benzodiazepine receptor agonists (BzRAs).[14–17] However, opioids can cause serious adverse outcomes, including opioid use disorder and overdose death. In general, nonopioid approaches are considered first line, and nonpharmacologic approaches are strongly encouraged in guidelines. For example, the Center for Disease Control and Prevention is strongly cautionary and recommend limited opioid use, close monitoring, and careful risk management.[21–24]

The opioid crisis has brought renewed attention to other central nervous system depressants, especially BzRAs. BzRA use is prevalent in the general population: 5% in the United States, 4% in Canada, and 3% to 13% across Europe.[25–31] Their use has increased in the United States, Canada, and the European Union over the last few decades—in some cases, up to 16%.[32] In the United States, the number of prescriptions, strength, and quantity of BZRAs has increased dramatically between 1996 and 2013.[33] BzRA use increased significantly in the Veterans Administration between 2003 to 2011 in posttraumatic stress disorder patients.[34] In pain management, approximately 20% of those using opioids also use BzRAs, despite universal recommendations to avoid overlapping prescriptions. [24,33,35–37] Associated factors for co-prescribing include female gender, older age, disability, three or more types of musculoskeletal pain, current smoking, and residence in the southern United States.[36–40]

Concern over BzRA use is not new. In 1990, a review of BzRA use suggested caution and a weighing of benefit/risk in acute use, even more so with chronic use: "The question of benefit outweighing risks . . . becomes less clear when therapeutic doses are used over long periods of time."[41p59] With few exceptions, most research and published expert opinion supports the use of BzRAs for no longer than four weeks.[42–46] Consideration in their discontinuation is particularly important when opioids are co-prescribed due to unfavorable synergistic and cumulative effects, a recommendation that goes back as far as 1980 and has remained a concern.[24,47]

When co-prescribed with opioids, adverse outcomes can be accelerated and multiplied.[48] BzRAs blunt the respiratory drive in the medulla, but even in toxic amounts, by themselves they are unlikely to be lethal.[49–51] However, when taken in conjunction with other central nervous system depressants (e.g., alcohol or opioids), risk of death increases.[52–53] Combined opioids and BzRAs are associated with a 40% increase in overall mortality compared to opioids alone.[54]

Of greatest concern is mortality related to accidental overdose.[55] BzRAs appear to be "second only to opioids in their contribution to prescription-related deaths overall."[56,57] Drawing on 2016–2017 data of eleven states, Mattson et al. found that BzRAs were detected in 52% of opioid-related deaths, an increase from 31% in 2011 and 13% in 1999.[23,58] This appears to vary dramatically by state in the United States, the rationale for which is not clear.[36] Between 2009 and 2011 in North Carolina, 80% of opioid-related overdose deaths included BzRAs use.[59]

When BzRAs and opioids are co-prescribed, cognitive and psychomotor impairments are worse than when either drug is taken alone.[60–63] Falls are more frequent, especially in the elderly. Decreased driving ability and increased motor vehicle accidents are also seen.[58,59,64–66] Autopsy investigations of substance-related traffic fatalities frequently identify the presence of both classes of drugs in high concentrations.[64]

BzRAs do have a potential role in several clinical settings (e.g., alcohol withdrawal, spinal cord injury with spasticity) as a bridge for anxiety states or disorders and surgical anesthesia (analgoanesthesia).[67–69] However, these populations, although seen in a pain practice, do not constitute the majority of pain patients. Opioid use disorder is also associated with the nonmedical use of BzRAs, which can amplify euphoria or ameliorate opioid withdrawal intensity. Co-prescribing is associated with the presence of other substance use disorders (SUDs) as well.[68–72]

As expected, BzRAs are most often prescribed to pain patients to manage anxiety and insomnia. Persons with pain often experience fear, fear avoidance, kinesiophobia, and catastrophizing—all features of anxiety. Pain disrupts sleep, and disrupted sleep accelerates pain.[73–75] Fully 50% of patients with pain have sleep complaints or anxiety, and 50% of those who have insomnia or anxiety also have pain.[76,77,79] Generalized anxiety disorder is the condition most commonly associated with pain.[78]

The use of BzRAs for sleep, anxiety, and analgesia has a paucity of research support. This belies the common use of BzRAs in the setting of pain management and suggests that other issues support the continued prevalence of use. Attitudes about treating pain and use of certain medication classes are frequently imparted through mentors and attending physicians whose approaches were also formed by their attendings in training programs.[79] BzRAs have been part of this imparted, but not evidence-based mythology, for decades, including in pain management.

In large part, research does not support benzodiazepine use for the purpose of direct or indirect (muscle relaxation) analgesia. A large randomized double-blind design study compared naproxen, diazepam, and placebo, in an urban emergency department in 2016 in which BzRAs were used in over 300,000 visits for low back pain.[80] Naproxen and BzRAs did not improve functional outcomes or pain versus placebo. As the authors state, "benzodiazepines are often mentioned as useful for these patients . . . although scant evidence exists to determine the appropriateness of this approach."[85] There is no researched support for benzodiazepines where used historically in acute back pain with radiculopathy.[81] A Cochrane Review found that BzRA use for pain in rheumatoid arthritis was not beneficial.[82] In a separate Cochrane Review, there was no evidence BzRAs use was beneficial in fibromyalgia or neuropathic pain.[83] Indeed, among the various pain conditions, only burning mouth syndrome (using clonazepam) and perhaps pain associated with multiple sclerosis has any, although limited, research support for direct analgesia.[84,85]

Because of the range, severity, and hidden nature of adverse BzRA reactions, it is expected that most patients will experience significant improvements of multiple health parameters after cessation. Elimination of concurrent opioid-BzRAs co-prescribing is estimated to reduce opioid-related overdose by 15%.[36] In one study 75% of respondents agreed that eliminating BzRA–opioid co-prescribing would improve patient outcomes.[86]

However, there are multiple barriers to co-prescribing cessation. Recent focus has been on the risks and attendant risk management of opioids. Prescribers may be reluctant, because patients appear stable or discontinuation is believed to be too difficult. Further there is a medical culture in which deprescribing is not normative and a sense that BzRA-related problems are overly exaggerated. Poor patient or medical provider decision support, affordable health care, fear, risks, expense, time constraints, knowledge deficits, enabling, and even criminal intent can all impinge implementation of BzRA cessation.

BzRAs initiation should be limited by invoking alternative approaches. If necessary due to severe, function-limiting anxiety symptoms, BzRAs should be used only to bridge, for no more than four weeks, while awaiting the onset of efficacy of other treatments.[87]

Best practice risk management principles employed for opioids applies here as well. There is a stepwise process to address current and future problems: (i) risk screening, (ii) risk stratification, (iii) risk mitigation, (iv) risk monitoring, and (v) adverse outcome management.[88]

Risk screening begins by taking a complete history including a personal and family history of SUD and psychiatric problems or trauma. Drug testing and prescription drug monitoring programs can be helpful information, but do not diagnose SUD per se.[89] Those individuals at higher risk for SUD should be considered for closer monitoring, counseling, and referral to a specialty clinic.

A benzodiazepine use disorder is unlikely, but side effects and problems can be deceptive.[90,91] The presence of SUD, including benzodiazepine use disorder, require screening. Dyscognition can be determined through validated memory screens.[92] Risk for respiratory depression can be evaluated by overnight oxygenation studies (e.g., nocturnal oximetry, polysomnography).[72,73,93,98] Risk stratification, then, amounts to the adjudicating of these factors to rank the level of risk for continued BzRA (and opioid) use as low, intermediate, or high. Similar stratifications have been suggested for the evaluation of chronic pain patients.[94]

Motivational interviewing encourages patient expression of their hopes and goals followed by patient expression of their current medical circumstance.[95,96] Based on this, the medical provider facilitates the patient's recognition of the disconnect between goals and current BzRAs and/or opioid use. In large part, prescriber and patient share in decision-making about next steps—with one exception. Objectively defined high respiratory risk may require assertive intervention even in the face of patient resistance. Sufficient explanation by the prescriber of the need to taper BzRAs (and/or opioids) is to be provided along with the assurance of continued safety and management of the underlying conditions. The art of medicine involves the ability to retain the patient, remain engaged, and to do so without enabling bad outcomes.

Risk mitigation employs strategies to minimize future adverse outcomes.[66] Although some suggest that naloxone may help reverse BzRA respiratory depression, this claim is difficult to support based on opioid antagonist pharmacology.[97] It should be said the respiratory depression from solo BzRA overdose is a rare occurrence.[98] Current clinical recommendations suggest that the use of naloxone should be enough to reverse respiratory depression in the setting of opioids and BzRAs. In severe overdose cases where it is know that excessive BzRAs have been taken, both naloxone and flumazenil have been recommended.[99]

Risk monitoring thereafter improves the chance for early identification of BzRA- and opioid-related problems. This includes behavioral aberrancy surveillance, prescription drug monitoring programs review, and definitive quantitative urine drug testing.[98] Periodic nocturnal oxygenation studies and memory screening may be necessary as well. Adverse outcome management follows to address identified problems, ensure safety, and help leverage BzRA cessation.

For patients on BzRAs with no supportive diagnoses, use for longer than four weeks, or with respiratory compromise, these agents should be tapered to off and eliminated (*cf.*, Chapter 8). In a chronic pain management rational polypharmacy is the norm, but with respect to BzRAs, desprescribing is rational and ought to be done systematically. This should not be unduly delayed because of focused (although necessary) attention on opioids.[100] The addition of BzRAs with no clear beneficial diagnoses is not a rational approach to treating pain patients. As with any class of medications, the benefit risk profile must be taken into account. BzRAs risks in the setting of pain management, especially if opioids are part of the regimen, usually does not warrant their inclusion and does require their removal. Based on previous research, alprazolam should never be part of any pain management therapeutic regimen.[i]

CONCLUSION

Patients in pain bring complexity that belies any notion of easy treatment.[101] They require a full and thorough history, physical, and evaluation. This focuses the diagnoses, helps establish the therapeutic regimen, and reduces patient risk. Part of this evaluation is a review of the patients' medication list and a thoughtful consideration of additional or alternative medications and other therapies. For those patients without diagnoses that might benefit from BzRAs, the addition of this class of medication should be avoided or tapered off. Collaboration with other specialties (e.g., psychiatry, addiction, sleep specialists, etc.) is a critical part of any pain practice.

Anxiety, depression, sleep disorders, and SUD are just some of the issues that need to be screened for and addressed in the pain patient. As patients get older, chronic pain, depression, and anxiety increase, are underdiagnosed, and frequently ignored.[102] Jordan et al. suggests that due "to their negative outcomes" of long-term BzRAs use they be seriously evaluated in light of the Beers Criteria.[103] Other alternatives for treating sleep disorders, anxiety disorders, and analgesia are legion. Literature support for these options is much more robust than that for BzRAs. Limited space in this chapter does

---

i. Further, some BzRAs appear to be more toxic than others; for example, "alprazolam is significantly more toxic, has no additional therapeutic benefit, and is increasingly misused compared with other BzRAs" (Schaffer A, Buckley NA, Cairns R, Pearson SA, Interrupted time series analysis of the effect of rescheduling alprazolam in Australia: Taking control of prescription drug use. *JAMA Intern Med.* 2016;176:1223–1225).

not allow a full discussion of these alternatives in detail; however, muscle relaxants (*e.g.,* alpha 2 agonists) for muscle pain, nonpharmacologic approaches to sleep disorders and anxiety disorders, and pharmacologic and nonpharmalogic therapies for pain are all potentials that can replace BzRAs and their risks.[104–109]

Unfortunately, educational efforts to improve pain control, evaluate comorbidities, and use rational polypharmacy is wanting in medical schools and residencies training in pain management is poor to minimal at best.[110,111] This also impacts the treatment of pain patients and contributes to the continued myth and use of BzRAs in pain treatment regimens. The combination of opioids and BzRAs has caused authors to urgently call for increased education in these settings.[36]

Benzodiazepine receptor agonists should be rarely initiated in pain management and, if prescribed, used as a bridge and for no longer than four weeks. For those already on these agents (*i.e.,* legacy patients), tapering with the goal of discontinuation in a safe and person-centered process should be done (described elsewhere in this volume). With what we now know, it is no longer acceptable to allow "I'll get to it later" to morph into "It never got done." Further, educational efforts must be improved to deal with the overuse of this class of drug, similar to the efforts currently underway to curb the overuse of opioids in chronic pain.

REFERENCES

1. Schweitzer AS. *On the Edge of the Primeval Forest.* New York, NY: Macmillan; 1931.
2. Tsang A, Von Korff M, Lee S, et al. Common chronic pain conditions in developed and developing countries: gender and age differences and comorbidity with depression-anxiety disorders. *J Pain.* 2008;9(10):883–891.
3. Institute of Medicine. *Relieving Pain in America: A Blueprint for Transforming Prevention, Care, Education, and Research.* Washington, DC: National Academies Press; 2011.
4. Ilgen MA, Kleinberg F, Ignacio RV, et al. Noncancer pain conditions and risk of suicide. *JAMA Psychiatry.* 2013;70(7):692–697.
5. Smith D, Wilkie R, Uthman O, et al. Chronic pain and mortality: a systematic review. *PLoS One.* 2014;9(6):e99048.
6. Peppin JF. The marginalization of chronic pain patients on chronic opioid therapy. *Pain Physician.* 2009;12(3):493–498.
7. Wolf N. *The Beauty Myth: How Images of Beauty are used against Women.* New York, NY: Harper Perennial; 2015.
8. Practice guidelines for acute pain management in the perioperative setting: an updated report by the American Society of Anesthesiologists Task Force on Acute Pain Management. *Anesthesiology.* 2012;116:248–273.
9. Cantrill SV, Brown MD, Carlisle RJ, et al. Clinical policy: critical issues in the prescribing of opioids for adult patients in the emergency department. *Ann Emerg Med.* 2012;60:499–525.
10. Blondell RD, Azadfard M, Wisniewski AM. Pharmacologic therapy for acute pain. *Am Fam Physician.* 2013;87(11):766–772.
11. McNicol ED, Midbari A, Eisenberg E. Opioids for neuropathic pain. *Cochrane Database Syst Rev.* 2013 Aug 29;8:CD006146.

12. Chou R, Deyo R, Friedly J, et al. Systemic pharmacologic therapies for low back pain: a systematic review for an American College of Physicians Clinical Practice Guideline. *Ann Intern Med.* 2017;*166*(7):480–492.

13. Deyo RA, Von Korff M, Duhrkoop D. Opioids for low back pain. *BMJ.* 2015;*350*:g6380.

14. Trescot AM, Helm S, Hansen H, et al. Opioids in the management of chronic non-cancer pain. *Pain Physician.* 2008;*11*:S5–S62.

15. Kalso E, Edwards JE, Moore RA, McQuay HJ. Opioids in chronic non-cancer pain: systematic review of efficacy and safety. *Pain.* 2004;*112*(3):372–380.

16. Noble M, Treadwell JR, Tregear SJ, et al. Long term opioids for chronic noncancer pain. *Cochrane Database Syst Rev.* 2010;(1):CD006605.

17. da Costa BR, Nüesch E, Kasteler R, et al. Oral or transdermal opioids for osteoarthritis of the knee or hip. *Cochrane Database Syst Rev.* 2014;(9):CD003115.

18. Martell BA, O'Connor PG, Kerns RD. Systematic review: opioid treatment for chronic back pain: prevalence, efficacy, and association with addiction. *Ann Intern Med.* 2007;*146*(2):116–127.

19. Bicket MC, Long JJ, Pronovost PJ, et al. Prescription opioid analgesics commonly unused after surgery: a systematic review. *JAMA Surg.* 2017;*152*(11):1066–1071.

20. Chou R, Turner JA, Devine EB, et al. The effectiveness and risks of long-term opioid therapy for chronic pain: a systematic review for a National Institutes of Health Pathways to Prevention Workshop. *Ann Intern Med.* 2015;*162*(4):276–286.

21. Centers for Disease Control and Prevention. CDC guideline for prescribing opioids for chronic pain. https://www.cdc.gov/drugoverdose/prescribing/guideline.html. Page reviewed August 28, 2019.

22. Vowels KE, McEntee ML, Julnes PS, et al. Rates of opioid misuse, abuse, and addiction in chronic pain: a systematic review and data synthesis. *Pain.* 2015;*156*(4):569–576.

23. Mattson CL, O'Donnell J, Kariisa M, et al. Opportunities to prevent overdose deaths involving prescription and illicit opioids, 11 states, July 2016–June 2017. *MMWR.* 2018;*67*(34):945–951.

24. Dowell D, Haegerich TM, Chou R. CDC guideline for prescribing opioids for chronic pain - United States, 2016. *MMWR Recomm Rep.* 2016;*65*(RR-1):1–49.

25. Olfson M, King M, Schoenbaum M. Benzodiazepine use in the United States. *JAMA Psychiatry.* 2015;*72*(2):136–142.

26. Neutel CI. The epidemiology of long-term benzodiazepine use. *Int Rev Psychiatry.* 2005;*17*(3):189–197.

27. Kurko TA, Saastamoinen LK, Tähkäpää S, et al. Long-term use of benzodiazepines: definitions, prevalence and usage patterns—a systematic review of register-based studies. *Eur Psychiatry.* 2015;*30*(8):1037–1047.

28. Magrini N, Vaccheri A, Parma E, et al. Use of benzodiazepines in the Italian general population: prevalence, pattern of use and risk factors for use. *Eur J Clin Pharmacol.* 1996;*50*(1–2):19–25.

29. Petitjean S, Ladewig D, Meier CR, et al. Benzodiazepine prescribing to the Swiss adult population: results from a national survey of community pharmacies. *Int Clin Psychopharmacol.* 2007;*22*(5):292–298.

30. Rosman S, Le Vaillant M, Pelletier-Fleury N. Gaining insight into benzodiazepine prescribing in General Practice in France: a data-based study. *BMC Fam Pract.* 2011;*12*:28.

31. Sonnenberg CM, Bierman EJM, Deeg DJH, et al. Ten-year trends in benzodiazepine use in the Dutch population. *Soc Psychiatry Psychiatr Epidemiol.* 2012;*47*(2):293–301.

32. Patorno E, Glynn RJ, Levin R, Lee MP, Huybrechts KF. Benzodiazepines and risk of all cause mortality in adults: cohort study. *BMJ.* 2017;*358*:j2941.

33. Bachhuber MA, Hennessy S, Cunningham CO, Starrels JL. Increasing benzodiazepine prescriptions and overdose mortality in the United States, 1996–2013. *Am J Public Health.* 2016;*106*(4):686–688.

34. Hawkins EJ, Malte CA, Grossbard JR, Saxon AJ. Prevalence and trends of concurrent opioid analgesic and benzodiazepine use among veterans affairs patients with post-traumatic stress disorder, 2003–2011. *Pain Med.* 2015;*16*(10):1943–1954.

35. Bohnert ASB, Guy GP, Losby JL. Opioid prescribing in the United States before and after the Centers for Disease Control and Prevention's 2016 opioid guideline. *Ann Intern Med.* 2018;*169*(6):367–375.

36. Sun EC, Dixit A, Humphreys K, et al. Association between concurrent use of prescription opioids and benzodiazepines and overdose: retrospective analysis. *BMJ.* 2017;*356*:j760.

37. McClure FL, Niles JK, Kaufman HW, Gudin J. Concurrent use of opioids and benzodiazepines: evaluation of prescription drug monitoring by a United States laboratory. *J Addict Med.* 2017;*11*(6):420–426.

38. Evans TI, Liebling EJ, Green TC, et al. Associations between physical pain, pain management, and frequency of nonmedical prescription opioid use among young Adults: a sex-specific analysis. *J Addict Med.* 2017;*11*(4):266–272.

39. Skurveit S, Furu K, Bramness J, et al. Benzodiazepines predict use of opioids: a follow-up study of 17,074 men and women. *Pain Med.* 2010;*11*(6):805–814.

40. Paulozzi LJ, Mack KA, Hockenberry JM. Variation among states in prescribing of opioid pain relievers and benzodiazepines: United States, 2012. *J Safety Res.* 2014;*51*:125–129.

41. American Psychiatric Association. *Benzodiazepine Dependence, Toxicity, and Abuse: A Task Force Report of the American Psychiatric Association.* Washington, DC: American Psychiatric Publishing; 1990.

42. Uhlenhuth EH, Balter MB, Ban TA, Yang K. International study of expert judgment on therapeutic use of benzodiazepines and other psychotherapeutic medications: IV. Therapeutic dose dependence and abuse liability of benzodiazepines in the long-term treatment of anxiety disorders. *J Clin Psychopharmacol.* 1999;*19*(6 Suppl 2):23S–29S.

43. Perna G, Alciati A, Riva A, et al. Long-term pharmacological treatments of anxiety disorders: an updated systematic review. *Curr Psychiatry Rep.* 2016;*18*(3):23.

44. Pottie K, Thompson W, Davies S, et al. Deprescribing benzodiazepine receptor agonists: evidence-based clinical practice guideline. *Canadian Fam Phys.* 2018;*64*(5):339–351.

45. Ashton H. Guidelines for the rational use of benzodiazepines: when and what to use. *Drugs.*1994;*48*(1):25–40.

46. Ashton H. *The Ashton Manual: Benzodiazepines: How They Work and How to Withdraw.* https://www.benzoinfo.com/ashtonmanual/. Published 1999. Revised 2002. Supplement 2011.

47. Hendler N, Cimini C, Ma T, Long D. A comparison of cognitive impairment due to benzodiazepines and to narcotics. *Am J Psychiatry.* 1980;*137*(7):828–830.

48. Guimmarra MJ, Gibson SJ, Allen AR, et al. Polypharmacy and chronic pain: harm exposure is not all about the opioids. *Pain Med.* 2015;*16*(3):472–479.

49. Horsfall JT, Sprague JE. The pharmacology and toxicology of the "Holy Trinity." *Basic Clin Pharmacol Toxicol.* 2017;*120*(2):115–119.

50. Longo LP, Johnson B. Addiction: Part I. Benzodiazepines: side effects, abuse risk and alternatives. *Am Fam Physician.* 2000;*61*(7):2121–2128.

51. Schmitz A. Benzodiazepine use, misuse, and abuse: a review. *Ment Health Clin.* 2016;*6*(3):120–126.

52. Bair MJ, Bohnert AS. Overdoses in patients on opioids: risks associated with mental health conditions and their treatment. *J Gen Intern Med.* 2015;*30*(8):1051–1053.

53. Webster LR, Reisfield GM, Dasgupta N. Eight principles for safer opioid prescribing and cautions with benzodiazepines. *Postgrad Med.* 2015;*127*(1):27–32.

54. Gaither JR, Goulet JL, Becker WC, et al. The effect of substance use disorders on the association between guideline-concordant long-term opioid therapy and all-cause mortality. *J Addict Med.* 2016;*10*(6):418–428.

55. Bachhuber MA, Hennessy S, Cunningham CO, Starrels JL. Increasing benzodiazepine prescriptions and overdose mortality in the United States, 1996–2013. *Am J Pub Health.* 2016;*106*:686–688.

56. Webster LR, Reisfield GM, Dasgupta N. Eight principles for safer opioid prescribing and cautions with benzodiazepines. *Postgrad Med.* 2015;*127*(1):27–32.

57. Jones CM, Mack KA, Paulozzi LJ. Pharmaceutical overdose deaths, United States, 2010. *JAMA.* 213;*309*:657–659.

58. Chen LH, Hedegaard H, Warner M. Drug-poisoning deaths Involving opioid analgesics: United States, 1999–2011. *NCHS Data Brief.* 2014;*166*:1–8.

59. Dasgupta N, Funk MJ, Proescholdbell S, et al. Cohort study of the impact of high-dose opioid analgesics on overdose mortality. *Pain Med.* 2016;*17*(1):85–98.

60. Zacny JP, Paice JA, Coalson DW. Separate and combined psychopharmacological effects of alprazolam and oxycodone in healthy volunteers. *Drug Alcohol Depend.* 2012;*124*(3):274–282.

61. Brown TL, Milavetz G, Gaffney G, Spurgin A. Evaluating drugged driving: effects of exemplar pain and anxiety medications. *Traffic Inj Prev.* 2018;*19*(Suppl 1):S97–S103.

62. Gjerde H, Strand MC, Mørland J. Driving under the influence of non-alcohol drugs: an update. Part I: epidemiological studies. *Forensic Sci Rev.* 2015;*27*(2):89–113.

63. Edvardsen HE, Tverborgvik T, Frost J, et al. Differences in combinations and concentrations of drugs of abuse in fatal intoxication and driving under the influence cases. *Forensic Sci Int.* 2017;*281*:127–133.

64. French DD, Chirikos TN, Spehar A, et al. Effect of concomitant use of benzodiazepines and other drugs on the risk of injury in a veterans population. *Drug Saf.* 2005;*28*(12):1141–1150.

65. Gerlach LB, Olfson M, Kales HC, Maust DT. Opioids and other central nervous system-active polypharmacy in older adults in the United States. *J Am Geriatr Soc.* 2017;*65*(9):2052–2056.

66. Laqueille X, Launay C, Dervaux A, Kanit M. Abuse of alcohol and benzodiazepine during substitution therapy in heroin addicts: a review of the literature. *Encephale.* 2009;*35*(3):220–225.

67. Cheatle MD, Shmuts R. The risk and benefit of benzodiazepine use in patients with chronic pain. *Pain Med.* 2015;*16*(2):219–221.

68. Watanabe N, Churchill R, Furukawa TA. Combined psychotherapy plus benzodiazepines for panic disorder. *Cochrane Database Syst Rev.* 2009;*1*:CD005335.

69. Ciccozzi A, Marinangeli F, Colangeli A, et al. Anxiolysis and postoperative pain in patients undergoing spinal anesthesia for abdominal hysterectomy. *Minerva Anestesiologica.* 2007;*73*(7–8):387–394.

70. Chen KW, Berger CC, Forde DP, et al. Benzodiazepine use and misuse among patients in a methadone program. *BMC Psych.* 2011;*11*:90.

71. Jones JD, Mogali S, Comer SD. Polydrug abuse: a review of opioid and benzodiazepine combination use. *Drug Alcohol Depend.* 2012;*125*(1–2):8–18.

72. Hirschtritta ME, Delucchib KL, Olfson M. Outpatient, combined use of opioid and benzodiazepine medications in the United States, 1993–2014. *Prevent Med Rep.* 2018;*9*:49–54.

73. Beesdo K, Hoyer J, Jacobi F, et al. Association between generalized anxiety levels and pain in a community sample: evidence for diagnostic specificity. *J Anxiety Disord.* 2009;*23*(5):684–693.

74. Sivertsen B, Lallukka T, Petrie KJ, et al. Sleep and pain sensitivity in adults. *Pain.* 2015;*156*(8):1433–1439.

75. Finan PH, Goodin BR, Smith MT. The association of sleep and pain: an update and a path forward. *J Pain.* 2013;*14*(12):1539–1552.
76. Sagheer MA, Khan MF, Sharif S. Association between chronic low back pain, anxiety and depression in patients at a tertiary care centre. *J Pak Med Assoc.* 2013;*63*(6):688–690.
77. de Heer EW, Gerrits MM, Beekman AT, et al. The association of depression and anxiety with pain: a study from NESDA. *PLoS One.* 2014;*9*(10):e106907.
78. Stein MB, Sareen J. Generalized anxiety disorder. *New Engl J Med.* 2015;*373*: 2059–2068.
79. Sambunjak D, Straus SE, Marušić A. Mentoring in academic medicine: a systematic review. *JAMA.* 2006;*296*(9):1103–1115.
80. Friedman BW, Irizarry E, Solorzano C, et al. Diazepam is no better than placebo when added to naproxen for acute low back pain. *Anna Emergency Med.* 2017;*70*(2):169–176.
81. Chou R, Deyo R, Friedly J, et al. Systemic pharmacologic therapies for low back pain: a systematic review for an American College of Physicians Clinical Practice Guideline. *Ann Int Med.* 2017;*166*(7):480–492.
82. Richards BL, Whittle SL, Buchbinder R. Muscle relaxants for pain management in rheumatoid arthritis. *Cochrane Database Syst Rev.* 2012;*1*:CD008922.
83. Corrigan R, Derry S, Wiffen PJ, Moore R. Clonazepam for neuropathic pain and fibromyalgia in adults. *Cochrane Database Syst Rev.* 2012;*5*:CD009486.
84. Liu YF, Kim Y, Yoo T, et al. Burning mouth syndrome: a systematic review of treatments. *Oral Dis.* 2018;*24*(3):325–334.
85. Wright LJ. Identifying and treating pain caused by MS. *J Clin Psychiatry.* 2012;*73*(7):e23.
86. Wallis KA, Andrews A, Henderson M. Swimming against the tide: primary care physicians' views on deprescribing in everyday practice. *Ann Fam Med.* 2017;*15*(4):341–346.
87. Cheatle MD, Shmuts R. The risk and benefit of benzodiazepine use in patients with chronic pain. *Pain Med.* 2015;*16*(2):219–221.
88. Ozer S, Young J, Champ C, Burke M. A systematic review of the diagnostic test accuracy of brief cognitive tests to detect amnestic mild cognitive impairment. *Int J Geriatr Psychiatry.* 2016;*31*(11):1139–1150.
89. Heit HA, Gourlay DL. Using urine drug testing to support healthy boundaries in clinical care. *J Opioid Manage.* 2015;*11*(1):7–12.
90. Substance Abuse and Mental Health Services Administration. National survey of drug use and health: US behavioral health trends. https://www.samhsa.gov/data/sites/default/files/NSDUH-FRR1-2014/NSDUH-FRR1-2014.pdf. Published September 2015.
91. McCabe. BZ use in US high school seniors. *Addict Behav.* 2014;*39*(5):959–964
92. Cheatle MD, Webster LR. Opioid therapy and sleep disorders: risks and mitigation strategies. *Pain Med.* 2015;*16*(Suppl 1):S22–S26.
93. Hassamal S, Miotto K, Wang T, Saxon AJ. A narrative review: the effects of opioids on sleep disordered breathing in chronic pain patients and methadone maintained patients. *Am J Addict.* 2016;*25*(6):452–465.
94. Peppin JF, Cheatle MD, Kirsh KL, McCarberg BH. The complexity model: a novel approach to improve chronic pain care. *Pain Med.* 2015;*16*:653–666.
95. Aguerre C, Bridou M, Laroche F, et al. Specifications of motivational interviewing within a cognitive-behavioral therapy of chronic pain. *Encephale.* 2015;*41*(6):515–520.
96. Bohnert AS, Bonar EE, Cunningham R, et al. A pilot randomized clinical trial of an intervention to reduce overdose risk behaviors among emergency department patients at risk for prescription opioid overdose. *Drug Alcohol Depend.* 2016;*163*:40–47.
97. Solhi H, Mostafazadeh B, Khoddami Vishteh HR, Ghezavati RA, Shooshtarizadeh A. Benefit effect of naloxone in benzodiazepines intoxication: findings of a preliminary study. *Hum Exp Toxicol.* 2001;*30*(7):535–540.

98. Kaufmann CN, Spira AP, Alexander GC, Rutkow L, Mojtabai R. Emergency department visits involving benzodiazepines and non-benzodiazepine receptor agonists. *Am J Emerg Med.* 2017;35(10):1414–1419.

99. Sivilotti MLA. Flumazenil, naloxone and the "coma cocktail." *Brit J Clin Pharmacol.* 2016;81(3):428–436.

100. Backonja M-M, Irving G, Argoff C. Rational multidrug therapy in the treatment of neuropathic pain. *Curr Pain Headache Rep.* 2006;10(1):34–38.

101. Peppin JF, Cheatle MD, Kirsh KL, McCarberg BH. The complexity model: a novel approach to improve chronic pain care. *Pain Med.* 2015;16:653–666.

102. Karp JF, DiNapoli EA, Wetherell J, et al. Deconstructing chronic low back pain in the older adult—step by step evidence and expert-based recommendations for evaluation and treatment: Part IX: Anxiety. *Pain Med.* 2016;17(8):1423–1435.

103. Campanelli CM. American geriatrics society updated beers criteria for potentially inappropriate medication use in older adults: the American geriatrics society 2012 beers criteria update expert panel. *J Am Geriatr Soc.* 2012;60(4):616–631.

104. Abdel Shaheed C, Maher CG, Williams KA, McLachlan AJ. Efficacy and tolerability of muscle relaxants for low back pain: systematic review and meta-analysis. *Eur J Pain.* 2017;21(2):228–237.

105. Schroeck JL, Ford J, Conway EL, et al. Review of safety and efficacy of sleep medicines in older adults. *Clin Therapeutics.* 2016;38(11):2340–2372.

106. Newby JM, McKinnon A, Kuyken W, Gilbody S, Dalgleish T. Systematic review and meta-analysis of transdiagnostic psychological treatments for anxiety and depressive disorders in adulthood. *Clin Psychol Rev.* 2015;40:91–110.

107. Stein MB, Sareen J. Generalized anxiety disorder. *New Engl J Med.* 2015;373(21):2059–2068.

108. Chou R, Deyo R, Friedly J, et al. Nonpharmacologic therapies for low back pain: a systematic review for an American College of Physicians clinical practice guideline. *Anna Intern Med.* 2017;166(7):493–505.

109. Chou R, Deyo R, Friedly J, et al. Systemic pharmacologic therapies for low back pain: a systematic review for an American College of Physicians clinical practice guideline. *Anna Intern Med.* 2017;166(7):480–492.

110. Volkow ND, McLellan AT. Opioid abuse in chronic pain—misconceptions and mitigation strategies. *New Engl J Med.* 2016;374(13):1253–1263.

111. Webster F, Bremner S, Oosenbrug E, Durant S, McCartney CJ, Katz J. From opiophobia to overprescribing: a critical scoping review of medical education training for chronic pain. *Pain Med.* 2017;18(8):1467–1475.

CHAPTER 10

The Regulatory History of Benzodiazepines in the Age of the Dark Web and Other Threats

JOHN J. COLEMAN

HIGHLIGHTS

- Benzodiazepines (BZDs) and related drugs can be subject to nonmedical use (abuse).
- Regulatory agencies attempt to assess, inform, and limit such occurrence by a variety of control measures.
- One approach categorizes drugs in a paradigm of less to more likely to be problematic and assigns a level of concern according to schedules (low to high).
- The history of control efforts for the BZDs has been mixed, both in terms of consistency and effectiveness.
- Modern phenomena of counterfeit drugs and the Dark Web complicate the situation.

INTRODUCTION

In 1914, with the world on the brink of war, an international treaty to control the commerce in opium and cocaine—the first of its kind—risked being forgotten as the powers that signed it, including the United States, prepared for conflict. The Great War, also known as the First World War, broke out in July 1914 and consumed most of the world's attention and resources for the next four years until it came to an end on November 11, 1918.

At war's end, a peace treaty was drawn up by the victors who hoped it would serve not only to end all wars but also to establish a world order to forever preserve the peace. The formal surrender of the German Empire and its allies occurred with the signing of the Treaty of Versailles on June 28, 1919. At the request of American and British authorities, the nearly forgotten 1914 treaty to control opium and cocaine was included as a codicil to the agreement—locking in most of the world's nations, including Germany and others who in 1914 had refused to sign the drug treaty.

The Treaty of Versailles also included provisions creating a League of Nations whose primary task was to preserve world peace. The League also would oversee enforcement of the new drug treaty. Although the United States did not ratify the Treaty of Versailles, it had already and previously ratified the drug treaty and, as required, enacted domestic legislation to regulate the commerce in opium and coca.

With the invasion of Poland by Germany in 1939, the world once again was plunged into war. When the war ended in 1945, the League of Nations, having failed to preserve the peace, dissolved and was replaced by the United Nations (UN) that took over most of the global responsibilities of the League, including the management of the 1914 drug treaty.

In 1961, the UN proposed a Single Convention on Narcotic Drugs, a new treaty to consolidate agreements previously enacted or amended by the League into a single comprehensive treaty that added new substances and updated regulatory protocols. As a signatory to the Single Convention, the United States was obliged to enact domestic legislation to conform to its new and expanded provisions. To comply with this obligation and for other purposes, in 1970 the US Congress enacted the Comprehensive Drug Abuse Prevention and Control Act, Title II of which is called the Controlled Substances Act (CSA).

The CSA codified many of the control provisions set forth in the Single Convention, including a tiered structure for controlling drugs based on their potential abuse liability. The CSA contained five levels, or schedules, to identify drugs, ranging from those not approved for medical use (Schedule I) to those approved for medical use but having relative abuse liability ranging from high (Schedule II) to low (Schedule V).

TRANQUILIZERS AND BENZODIAZEPINES AND MODERN DRUG CONTROL

The CSA included a listing of specific drugs by schedule based on medical and scientific data available at the time. Meprobamate (Miltown®) was the only minor tranquilizer to make the list of controlled drugs (Schedule IV) when the CSA was enacted in 1970. Miltown® also was the first tranquilizer approved for marketing in the United States and made its debut in 1955. The media dubbed it "mother's little helper" and the "peace pill" because of its calming effect. Initially believed to be a nonaddicting substitute for barbiturates, it would take several years of clinical experience before experts would conclude that continued use had the potential to cause psychological and physical dependence.[1]

By the late 1960s, when the CSA was being drafted, prescription drug abuse was considered rare and mostly confined to the overprescribing of amphetamines ostensibly for weight control. High-dose extended release opioids like OxyContin® and MS Contin® were almost two decades away.[2] When Miltown® was introduced in 1955, followed several years later by Librium® (chlordiazepoxide; 1960) and Valium® (diazepam; 1963), there was little reason to suspect that these drugs would produce dependency even when taken over long periods or at excessive doses. "People weren't as cynical about new drugs as they are now," said historian Andrea Tone, author of *The Age of Anxiety*[1] during a 2009 interview by Newsweek Magazine. Some in the industry, Tone added, viewed the enormous success of Miltown® as "psychiatry's penicillin."[1,3]

It certainly was true that Miltown® was a financial success for Carter-Wallace, a successor to the modest family-owned laxative company that in 1859 introduced the world to "Carter's Little Liver Pills."[4] The success of Miltown® inspired the industry to pursue the development of new and improved tranquilizers. In 1960, Hoffman-La Roche introduced Librium®, followed three years later by Valium®.[3] To highlight their importance and boost sales, Hoffman-La Roche promoted them as a new class of drugs called *benzodiazepines*.[3]

By some accounts BZDs changed the way the industry did business. Until the postwar period, pharmaceutical companies seemed content to rely on products developed by independent research labs in academia or private settings. They bought or licensed promising formulations that fit within their portfolio of treatment specialties. The financial success of Miltown® changed this paradigm and inspired companies to move beyond their market segments. Companies began to rely more heavily on their in-house research and development for new formulations.

In the 1960s, with street drugs like heroin, cannabis, and cocaine vying with the new psychedelic drugs, BZDs remained under the radar of the regulatory agencies. For the most part, chronic use of these drugs by patients properly supervised by their physicians did not appear to produce tolerance or any of the other typical signs of physiologic dependence or addiction, as these terms were defined at the time. This, however, would change in time as studies of long-term BZD use by patients with sleep disorders showed evidence of withdrawal when they were taken off the medication.

HISTORY OF BZD CONTROL

When Congress passed the CSA, it included by chemical name all drugs and other substances known or believed at the time to have abuse potential. In addition, data from the UN's 1961 Single Convention, ratified by the US in 1967, were considered in categorizing drugs according to their known or presumed abuse liability. With the notable exception of meprobamate, sedative-hypnotic medications including benzodiazepines, were not included in either the 1961 Single Convention or the CSA.[5,6] Meprobamate, the active ingredient in Miltown®, was listed in Schedule IV of the CSA.[5] It was a peculiar situation that a drug could remain unscheduled while its active ingredient was in Schedule IV.

The omission of BZDs from the CSA did not mean that they escaped the scrutiny of the government's watchdog agencies. In 1965, Congress passed amendments to the Federal Food, Drug, and Cosmetic Act (FFDCA) that gave the Secretary of the Department of Health, Education, and Welfare (HEW) sweeping regulatory authority over depressant and stimulant drugs.[7]

In its preamble to the Drug Abuse Control Amendments Act of 1965, Congress called attention to the growing threat from the illicit traffic in pharmaceutical drugs:

> The Congress hereby finds and declares that there is a widespread illicit traffic in depressant and stimulant drugs moving in or otherwise affecting interstate commerce; that the use of such drugs, when not under the supervision of a licensed practitioner, often endangers safety on the highways (without distinction of interstate and intrastate traffic thereon) and otherwise has become a threat to the public health and safety, making additional regulation of such drugs necessary regardless of the intrastate or interstate origin of such drugs; that in order to make regulation and protection of interstate commerce in such drugs effective, regulation of intrastate commerce is also necessary because, among other things, such drugs, when held for illicit sale, often do not bear labeling showing their place of origin and because in the form in which they are so held or in which they are consumed a determination of their place of origin is often extremely difficult or impossible; and that regulation of interstate commerce without the regulation of intrastate commerce in such drugs, as provided in this Act, would discriminate against and adversely affect interstate commerce in such drugs.[7]

Besides authorizing the Secretary of HEW to regulate the commerce in depressant or stimulant drugs, the act allowed the regulation of "any drug which contains any quantity of a substance which the Secretary,[i] after investigation, has found to have, and by regulation designates as having, a potential for abuse because of its depressant or stimulant effect on the central nervous system or its hallucinogenic effect."[7]

Section 8 of the act gave the secretary authority to direct any officer or employee of the department to conduct examinations, investigations, or inspections under the act relating to depressant, stimulant, and/or counterfeit drugs.[7] Persons designated to perform these duties were authorized by the act to carry firearms, execute and serve search and arrest warrants, to make arrests, and obtain court authorizations for seizures and condemnations of certain drug-making equipment used in violation of the act.[7]

In November 1965, HEW Secretary John W. Gardner approved the establishment of the Bureau of Drug Abuse Control as the enforcement arm of the FDA that would carry out the provisions of the 1965 act.[8] Although the Bureau of Drug Abuse Control

---

i. Most of the regulatory and administrative law authorities granted to the Secretary of the HEW (renamed in 1979 the Department of Health and Human Services) and the attorney general in carrying out drug control provisions of the FFDCA; CSA and FFDCA were delegated to the Assistant Secretary for Health/Food and Drug Administration (FDA) and Administrator/Bureau of Narcotics and Dangerous Drugs (BNDD), respectively. In 1973, the BNDD was reorganized and renamed the Drug Enforcement Administration (DEA).

was a relatively small law enforcement agency (377 positions authorized in 1967), its accomplishments in its first year were noteworthy.

In August 1973, the DEA administrator requested the Assistant Secretary for Health to submit on behalf of the secretary a scientific and medical evaluation for chlordiazepoxide (Librium®) and diazepam (Valium®) and to concur in a recommendation to place these drugs in Schedule IV of the CSA.[9] This was in keeping with the newly enacted CSA requiring collaboration between the HEW secretary and the attorney general when scheduling drugs and other substances.[10]

By letter, dated November 25, 1974, Charles C. Edwards, MD, Assistant Secretary for Health, provided the DEA administrator with a recommendation to place chlordiazepoxide and diazepam in Schedule IV of the CSA.[9] Edwards informed the DEA administrator that these drugs and other members of the benzodiazepines class of drugs had been under scientific and medical review for several years by the FDA's Controlled Substance Advisory Committee pursuant to the secretary's authorities under the 1965 Drug Abuse Control Amendments Act.[9]

Edwards recommended on behalf of the secretary that the DEA also place flurazepam (Dalmane®), oxazepam (Serax®), and chlorazepate (Tranxene®) in Schedule IV because the department's scientific and medical evaluation of these BZDs determined that they possessed the same "potential for abuse and a dependence liability" as chlordiazepoxide and diazepam.[9] In addition, Edwards advised that the department was evaluating a New Drug Application (NDA) for clonazepam (Klonopin®), an unmarketed investigative drug. Edwards included a recommendation that, if approved, clonazepam should be placed in Schedule IV of the CSA because of its abuse and dependence liability that preliminary testing showed was similar to the other BZDs in its class.[9]

On January 27, 1975, DEA Administrator John R. Bartels, Jr., published a Notice of a Proposed Rulemaking in the Federal Register that would place chlordiazepoxide, diazepam, oxazepam, chlorazepate, flurazepam and clonazepam (when approved by FDA) in Schedule IV of the CSA.[11] Several months later, on June 4, 1975, DEA issued a Final Rule placing chlordiazepoxide, diazepam, oxazepam, clorazepate, flurazepam, and newly approved clonazepam in Schedule IV of the CSA.[11]

Of the public comments that DEA received to its proposed rule, only one, authored by William E. Langeland on behalf of Wyeth Laboratories, manufacturer of Serax® (oxazepam), received extensive analysis and discussion in the DEA's Final Rule.[11] Wyeth's position was that DEA didn't follow the procedures set forth in the CSA because it was improperly relying on an unsupported recommendation from HEW that it, the DEA, did not request (i.e., the assistant secretary's scheduling recommendation for BZDs that were not included in the DEA's original request).[11] It was, at best, a technical procedural challenge against the scheduling of Wyeth's Serax®.

DEA acknowledged that it had not formally requested a scientific and medical evaluation of oxazepam, as the law allows, but that this, alone, in no way invalidated the data furnished by the FDA that evaluated the drug and found its abuse liability to be similar to that of the BZDs for which DEA did ask for the secretary's evaluation and scheduling recommendation.[11] DEA conceded that it was scheduling a "class" of drugs and justified this by saying that each drug in the class known as benzodiazepines showed similar abuse and dependence liability in laboratory testing, as well as in actual drug abuse records compiled by state and local police and DEA's own forensic laboratories.[11] In rejecting Wyeth's challenge, DEA concluded that "it would be exalting form over substance to render the proceedings to control oxazepam moot under the guise of statutory non-compliance." DEA's Final Rule became effective on July 2, 1975.[11]

HOW DOES THE STATUTE DEFINE SCHEDULE IV?

Schedule IV of the CSA is reserved for drugs requiring minimal control. In placing a drug in this schedule, Congress required the scheduling authorities (delegated from the HEW Secretary to FDA and the attorney general to DEA) to find that

(A) The drug or other substance has a low potential for abuse relative to the drugs or other substances in Schedule III;

(B) The drug or other substance has a currently accepted medical use in treatment in the United States; and

(C) Abuse of the drug or other substance may lead to limited physical dependence or psychological dependence relative to the drugs or other substances in Schedule III.[12]

The relatively low schedule of the BZDs reflected the low actual abuse record for these drugs cited by DEA at the time. DEA's 1975 Final Rule placing chlordiazepoxide, diazepam, oxazepam, clorazepate, flurazepam and clonazepam in Schedule IV provides this interesting commentary on the difference between reports of adverse health effects considered relevant for NDA purposes and specific indicators of diversion and abuse considered relevant for scheduling purposes:

> It is fair to assume that where the primary object of a reporting system is to determine abuse instances for drug control purposes, rather than to determine adverse reactions for NDA purposes, larger and more meaningful actual abuse statistics could be expected. Even then, case and survey reports would not provide a true indication of actual abuse, overdose or dependence, as has been demonstrated in a study regarding amphetamine by Kalant. Evidence of this is in DEA's attempt to determine actual abuse of oxazepam for the period from July 1972 to December 1974. The published literature revealed seven cases. Unpublished reports, acquired by DEA through its own reporting network, have totaled 953 for the same period. Moreover, DEA laboratories have analyzed, from July 1970 through November 1974, 48 exhibits of oxazepam associated with 45 different law enforcement actions. A survey taken by DEA in August 1974, has revealed that samples of oxazepam were submitted to State and local police laboratories at least 101 times. In seven Federal cases, oxazepam was seized with such drugs as amphetamine, barbiturates, cocaine, heroin, LSD, marihuana, MDA and phencyclidine. Serax has been offered for sale, in large quantities, to an undercover Federal narcotics agent. New York, Ohio and Virginia have reported that Serax has achieved 'street status' and sold illicitly for as much as two dollars per capsule."[11] (Internal citations omitted.)

This excerpt reveals one of the early hurdles that DEA encountered when carrying out its new scheduling responsibilities under the CSA. Since 1914 and the passage of the Harrison Narcotic Tax Act, the federal government's role in regulating controlled substances was confined to opiates and cocaine.[13] The Marihuana Tax Act of 1937 added cannabis to this list.[14] These laws required handlers of these drugs, as well as those authorized to prescribe and dispense them for medical purposes, to be registered with the federal government, pay a modest tax, and prescribe and dispense them only upon issuance and presentation of a written prescription.[13,14]

Until 1930 and the creation of the Federal Bureau of Narcotics, enforcement of these laws was given first to the Internal Revenue Service and later to a branch of the Bureau of Prohibition. Other drugs, to the extent that they were regulated for safety and efficacy, were the responsibility initially of the Bureau of Chemistry and later, in 1927, the Food, Drug, and Insecticide Administration.[15] In 1930, Congress shortened the name of the agency to the Food and Drug Administration (FDA).[15]

In 1938, following a tragedy that killed 107 persons, mostly children, after they consumed tainted cough medicine, Congress enacted the Federal Food, Drug, and Cosmetic Act (FFDCA) that provided additional authority for the FDA to ensure the safety and efficacy of the nation's food and drug supply.[15] The Durham–Humphrey Amendment in 1951 defined drugs that cannot safely be used without medical supervision and restricted their sale to prescription by a licensed practitioner.[15] In 1965, the aforementioned Drug Abuse Control Amendments to the FFDCA gave the FDA regulatory control and law enforcement responsibility for depressants, stimulants, and hallucinogens.[15]

In 1970, when Congress was considering the CSA, the then-Nixon administration proposed that certain drug control responsibilities of the Secretary of HEW be transferred to the attorney general. Included was drug scheduling.[16] This, however, was vigorously opposed by HEW scientists and medical officers who had been performing these tasks for years. They objected to Department of Justice officials having sole responsibility for making scientific and medical decisions pertaining to medicinal controlled substances.[16] In May 1970, approximately 100 HEW physicians and scientists signed a letter opposing this provision in the legislation then being considered by Congress.[16]

The bill that was passed by Congress and signed into law by President Nixon split the responsibility for drug scheduling between the Secretary of HEW and the attorney general.[ii] Information about drugs whose NDA showed a stimulant, depressant, or hallucinogenic effect on the central nervous system henceforth would be required to be furnished to the attorney general.[17] The latter, upon receiving a scientific and medical evaluation and a recommendation for scheduling from the secretary, would be required to initiate rule-making proceedings to schedule the drug.[18] Without the secretary's recommendation, the attorney general would not be authorized to schedule the drug.[18] An exception to this was if the drug posed an imminent hazard to public safety, the

ii. As previously mentioned, these responsibilities were delegated by regulation from the secretary to the FDA and Assistant Secretary for Health and by the attorney general to the DEA administrator.

attorney general could place the drug in Schedule I on a temporary basis, not to exceed 18 months (later extended to two years), while conventional drug scheduling proceedings would be undertaken by the secretary and attorney general.[19]

Thus, in 1975, when DEA and FDA collaborated to place a group of BZDs in Schedule IV, the two agencies were still developing collaborative policies for carrying out their respective roles under the CSA. As the previous excerpt from the *Federal Register* indicates, determining the abuse potential of a class of drugs, in this case, BZDs, rested on performing an eight-factor analysis in accordance with criteria provided in the CSA. For the FDA, this meant reviewing the record of adverse events for the drugs reported to the FDA by drug sponsors. For the DEA, defining abuse potential for scheduling purposes included assessing actual records of abuse found in local police files, DEA laboratory reports, surveys, and other law enforcement-generated data.

NEW SOURCES OF DATA NEEDED TO EVALUATE ABUSE POTENTIAL OF MEDICINAL CONTROLLED SUBSTANCES

DEA recognized in the earliest days of its new drug scheduling authority that the dynamic process used to assess the abuse potential of street drugs (e.g., arrests, seizures, etc.) would not work as well or as reliably for medicinal controlled substances. The majority of adverse events reported to the FDA by drug sponsors involved specific reactions and responses (or lack thereof) observed in the clinical setting and experienced by patients lawfully prescribed or administered the drugs. Definitions of drug abuse differ considerably depending upon one's perspective, but all parties appear to agree that the concept centers on the taking of a drug, whether prescribed or not, for a nontherapeutic or nonmedical purpose.[iii]

Beginning in 1971, when BNDD (predecessor of the DEA) began to exercise its new authority to schedule medicinal drugs with abuse liability—a task previously and exclusively performed by the FDA—agency officials recognized the need for timely data that could be used to determine the actual abuse liability for all drugs, including

iii. It should be noted that these unique interpretations of abuse potential persisted in theory until the Food and Drug Administration Amendments Act of 2007. This act for the first time identified drug abuse as an adverse event, thus narrowing the difference between the FDA and the DEA's interpretations:

(b) Definitions.—For purposes of this section:
  (1) Adverse drug experience.—The term "adverse drug experience" means any adverse event associated with the use of a drug in humans, whether or not considered drug related, including—
    (A) an adverse event occurring in the course of the use of the drug in professional practice;
    (B) an adverse event occurring from an overdose of the drug, whether accidental or intentional;
    (C) an adverse event occurring from abuse of the drug;
    (D) an adverse event occurring from withdrawal of the drug; and
    (E) any failure of expected pharmacological action of the drug.[20]

medicinal agents. Agency officials understood that law enforcement arrest and seizure records alone would not satisfy the scheduling requirements of the CSA that also required assessing the public health consequences of abuse. Indeed, five of eight statutory factors that Congress included in the CSA for determining drug scheduling focus on health risks and pharmacological issues, while only three pertain specifically to abuse or nonmedical use.[iv]

In 1972, about a year after the CSA went into effect, BNDD awarded a contract for services to IMS America, Ltd. (Ambler, PA, US), a market research company serving the healthcare industry.[22,23] The contract called for IMS to manage Project DAWN,[v] a nationwide program co-sponsored by DEA and the National Institute on Drug Abuse (NIDA) and intended to gather, interpret, and disseminate data on drug abuse from selected sites within the continental United States.[23]

The purpose of Project DAWN, as stated in one of the initial reports by IMS, was to assist the DEA in its "enforcement, compliance, scheduling, and information and research programs" and to assist NIDA in gathering "information towards forecasting, education, prevention, treatment and rehabilitation programs."[23] The goal of the project, according to IMS, was to achieve the following:

1. Identification of drugs currently abused and/or associated with harm to the individual and society.
2. The determination of existing patterns of drug abuse in 24 standard metropolitan statistical areas and national monitoring of abuse trends, including detection of new abuse entities and new combinations.
3. Provision of current data for the assessment of the relative hazards to health, both physiological and psychological, and relative abuse potential for substances in human experience.
4. Provision of data needed for rational control and scheduling of drugs of abuse, both old and new.[23]

In March 1975, after completing a series of pilot studies, IMS Health was awarded a second contract for the continuation of the program. Specifically, the contract covered gathering drug abuse information on

---

iv. The eight factors in the CSA for determining drug scheduling are

(1) Its actual or relative potential for abuse.
(2) Scientific evidence of its pharmacological effect, if known.
(3) The state of current scientific knowledge regarding the drug or other substance.
(4) Its history and current pattern of abuse.
(5) The scope, duration, and significance of abuse.
(6) What, if any, risk there is to the public health.
(7) Its psychic or physiological dependence liability.
(8) Whether the substance is an immediate precursor of a substance already controlled under this subchapter [21]

v. The acronym DAWN referred to Drug Abuse Warning Network.

a. The use of prescription drugs in a manner inconsistent with accepted medical practice;
b. The use of over-the-counter drugs contrary to approved labeling;
c. The use of any other substance, heroin, marijuana, peyote, glue, aerosols, etc., for the previously cited reasons.[23] In addition, the IMS Health contract covered gathering data on drug-related deaths.[23]

After a series of meetings among officials from DEA, NIDA, and IMS Health, a methodology was agreed upon that would collect drug abuse-related data from a sampling of hospital emergency departments, county medical examiners/coroners, and crisis intervention centers.[vi][23]

In Project DAWN's first report, covering the 12-month period of May 1975 through April 1976, a total of 171,712 drug mentions were recorded by its sample of hospital emergency departments. This comprised 69% of the 246,524 drug mentions from all data collection points participating in the DAWN system.[23]

Remarkably, of all the drug mentions collected from more than 800 hospitals in the program, tranquilizer drugs topped the list in drug mentions with one-quarter of all drug mentions (42,968/171,712).[23] Diazepam accounted for more than half (52.3%) of all the tranquilizer mentions.[23] The closest class of drugs after the tranquilizers was narcotic analgesics with 11.4% of all drug mentions (19,659/171,712).[23] Heroin accounted for more than 70% of the narcotic analgesic mentions.[23]

In reviewing these data today, an obvious concern is the apparent incongruity between what these data showed at the time and the CSA's drug scheduling process, which was one of the primary reasons for creating the DAWN project in the first place. Diazepam, a Schedule IV drug, had 22,493 mentions; heroin, 13,803 mentions, LSD and PCP combined, 3,168 mentions; and marijuana/hashish, 3,020 mentions—all Schedule I drugs—had far fewer mentions. By definition, a Schedule IV drug "has a low potential for abuse relative to the drugs or other substances in schedule III." However, there is not a single Schedule I, II, or III drug on the initial DAWN list with more mentions than diazepam.

In fairness, the eight factors in the CSA that must be evaluated when scheduling a drug contain a number of criteria—besides potential or actual abuse—that must be considered in determining the appropriate level of control. As previously mentioned, most of the eight factors pertain to public health and pharmacological-related issues. The frequency of misuse or abuse is not synonymous with the severity of the public health consequences resulting from such use. Surely, it can be said that the public health risks and consequences associated with the nonmedical use of diazepam are qualitatively less severe than those associated with the nonmedical use of higher scheduled medicinal and nonmedicinal opioids, stimulants, hallucinogens, and cannabis.

In March of 1981, the DEA administrator received a letter from the acting Secretary for Health that recommended that triazolam (Halcion®) be placed in Schedule IV of the

vi. The inclusion of data from crisis intervention centers was later dropped from the data collection set.

CSA.[24] Shortly after this, the DEA administrator received a second letter from the acting assistant secretary recommending that alprazolam (Xanax®) be placed in Schedule IV of the CSA.[24] The following month, DEA published a Notice of Proposed Rulemaking in the *Federal Register* stating its intention to place halazepam (Paxipam®), alprazolam, and triazolam in Schedule IV of the CSA. Halazepam had been previously proposed for scheduling but its final approval by FDA had been delayed. In view of this, DEA used this opportunity to renew its proposed rulemaking to place it in Schedule IV of the CSA.[24]

On October 29, 1981, DEA published a Final Rule in the Federal Register placing Halazepam in Schedule IV of the CSA.[25] As in the two previously mentioned cases, only one comment in support of the scheduling was received and it came from the American Society for Hospital Pharmacists.[25] The Final Rule was effective on October 29, 1981, the date it was published.[25]

On November 12, 1981, DEA published a Final Rule in the Federal Register placing alprazolam in Schedule IV of the CSA.[26] One comment was received from the American Society for Hospital Pharmacists in support of the scheduling of alprazolam in Schedule IV of the CSA.[26] No other comments or objections were received. The Final Rule was effective on November 12, 1981, the date it was published.[26]

On December 28, 1982, DEA published a Final Rule in the Federal Register placing triazolam in Schedule IV of the CSA.[27] As in the case of alprazolam, there was one comment in support of the scheduling action and it came from the American Society for Hospital Pharmacists.[27] The Final Rule was effective on December 28, 1982, the date it was published.[27]

LONGITUDINAL ABUSE RECORD OF BZDS

In 1980, Project DAWN, by then renamed DAWN, became the sole responsibility of NIDA.[28] In 1988, DAWN was transferred within the Department of Health and Human Services (HHS) from NIDA to the Substance Abuse and Mental Health Services Administration (SAMHSA).[28]

In 1997, a new probability sample was constructed by SAMHSA along with an improved methodology that permitted a re-analysis of historic DAWN data collected since 1978.[28] In August 1996, SAMHSA published a detailed document titled, *Historic Estimates from the Drug Abuse Warning Network,* that presented estimates from 1978 to 1994 of drug-related emergency department episodes.[28]

The 1996 SAMHSA report presents the following qualitative assessment of BZD abuse for the period 1978 to 1994:

Tranquilizers

- Diazepam (Valium) is a benzodiazepam used in the treatment of anxiety disorders, seizures, and muscle spasms. Diazepam-related emergency department episodes decreased by 78% (from 60,400 to 13,600) from 1978 to 1994. In 1978, diazepam-related episodes composed 19% of all drug-related emergency department episodes compared with 3% in 1994.

- Alprazolam (Xanax), a benzodiazepine used in the treatment of anxiety disorders, was first reported to DAWN in 1982. Alprazolam-related emergency department episodes increased from 1,200 to 17,200 from 1982 to 1994. In 1982, alprazolam-related episodes composed 0.4% of all drug-related emergency department episodes compared with 3% in 1994.
- Lorazepam (Ativan) is a benzodiazepine used in the treatment of anxiety disorders. Lorazepam-related emergency department episodes increased from 1,600 to 12,200 from 1978 to 1994. In 1978, lorazepam-related episodes composed 0.5% of all drug-related emergency department episodes compared with 2% in 1994.[28]

LIMITATIONS IN THE DAWN PROGRAM

Although the DAWN program was innovative, unique, and forward-thinking for its time, it had limitations that were difficult to reconcile. Even in its best years, only about half of its emergency department drug episodes were confirmed by toxicology records. This means that the other half relied on the verbatim record contained in intake forms completed by hospital staff at the emergency department that handled the episode. In drug-related overdose emergencies, it is vital that attending clinicians know the identity of substance(s) consumed by the victim. This may come in the form of observations made at the scene by police or emergency medical technicians (EMTs), or from statements that the overdose victim may be able to communicate to the EMTs. Friends or witnesses may come forth to inform the EMTs or hospital staff of what the victim consumed.

Each of these methods for learning what the overdose victim consumed is fraught with potential error. Decades of DAWN data obtained both from emergency departments and medical examiners/coroners in drug-related cases show that most drug overdoses and almost all drug fatalities involve polypharmacy, that is, the co-ingestion of multiple drugs, including beverage alcohol. The toxic interaction of some drugs, for example, the co-ingestion of an opioid and a stimulant such as cocaine or methamphetamine—called a speedball—is known to greatly increase the risk of fatal overdose. Likewise, the co-ingestion of an opioid and a BZD, sometimes accompanied by a muscle relaxant—called the "Trinity" or "Holy Trinity"—has been known to greatly increase the risk of fatal overdose.

Evidence found at the scene of an overdose or the good-faith statements rendered by a friend or witness at the time of an emergency may not tell the full story but only the part observed or assumed by the witness or the responding authorities. Only a laboratory analysis of the patient/victim's urine or serum can determine the full story. In the absence of toxicology results in about half the DAWN emergency department cases, we are left with having to rely on the verbatim record prepared by first responders and/or hospital staff.

DAWN data were criticized by drug sponsors claiming that their branded drug products were unfairly maligned by being named without verification in official records. Users of generic forms of popular drugs of abuse often inaccurately refer to them by their brand names. After 1996, with the popularity of OxyContin® increasing among those with a substance use disorder, the brand name on the street for this extended-release form of oxycodone became synonymous with any form of oxycodone.

To illustrate this, Purdue Pharma L.P., the sponsor of OxyContin, commissioned a study of oxycodone-related overdose deaths in Florida and was able to show that only a small percentage of them unequivocally were caused by OxyContin.[29] The study found that routine toxicology screening, even in the postmortem setting, cannot distinguish between an immediate-release or an extended-release form of oxycodone. Forensic testing confirms only the presence and serum concentration of a drug's metabolite(s) identified from the sample(s) analyzed.

To placate drug sponsors, SAMHSA used special software to convert verbatim drug data in the DAWN field reports to the generic or chemical name of the drug(s) in question. Ironically, it was OxyContin that almost halted the DAWN program when SAMHSA was criticized for having missed the outbreak of OxyContin abuse that began in the late 1990s in rural regions of Appalachia, Maine, and parts of Ohio. Known as "hillbilly heroin" in these areas, OxyContin was blamed for numerous overdoses and deaths in places where such activity was not expected and, therefore, not tracked. At the time, the DAWN program was focused on major urban areas and did not sample rural hospitals in areas where OxyContin abuse was most prevalent. As a result, some policymakers questioned the warning ability of the Drug Abuse *Warning* Network.

By the time the OxyContin crisis occurred, DAWN already was in trouble. In 1995, the Rand Corporation published a report critical of DAWN, claiming that the quality of its data was subject to significant measurement errors.[30,31] Because DAWN monitored episodes, not individuals, the Rand report claimed that its data are often misinterpreted as prevalence measures.[30] Perhaps the most damaging criticism and a harbinger of what was to come was that delays in reporting DAWN data undermined its utility as an early warning mechanism for identifying emerging drug problems.[30]

In 1997, SAMHSA undertook to correct these deficiencies, but it was evident several years later, after missing the outbreak of OxyContin abuse, that the corrections failed to resolve them.[30] By 2002, pressure was mounting on SAMHSA to either correct DAWN's deficiencies or terminate the program. SAMHSA temporarily discontinued DAWN in 2003 while it assembled a blue-ribbon panel of experts to decide what to do. Ultimately, the decision was made to continue the program but with significant changes and modernization of collection instruments and protocols. The year 2003 was considered a year of transition for old and new DAWN.[32]

NEW DAWN REPLACES OLD DAWN

The New DAWN, as the revamped program was called, was relaunched by SAMHSA in 2004 with an interim report of drug-related emergency department visits.[32] The report explained in detail how the New DAWN differed from the old DAWN and why the two data sets were not comparable. Data collection methodology, the number and location of hospitals in the sampling, and case selection criteria were among differences noted between the old and new systems and accounted for why their data could not be compared.[32]

SAMHSA continued publishing annual DAWN reports from 2004 until 2011 when the program was abruptly terminated during the height of the opioid abuse crisis. The reason for its termination provided by letter to respondent hospitals and other participants at the time explained that the DAWN program was being ended because of budget constraints.[33] However, a budget document for FY2011[vii] shows that SAMHSA received an increase of $110 million for a total budget authority of $3.7 billion.[34] For FY 2012, the first year after DAWN was terminated, the SAMHSA budget was reduced 0.05%, from $3.651 billion to $3.650 billion.[34] Despite this modest decrease, SAMHSA's overall budget in FY2012 included $26 million in new funding for "health surveillance and program support . . . including increased costs associated with ongoing efforts as well as enhancing data collection on drug related emergency room visits and deaths."[34]

In 2002, the final year under the old DAWN system, the top four BZDs mentioned in emergency departments were (i) alprazolam (27,659 mentions), (ii) clonazepam (17,042 mentions), (iii) diazepam (11,193 mentions), and (iv) lorazepam (11,042 mentions).[35,36] In 2011, the final year under the New DAWN system, the same four BZDs led the list of BZDs although lorazepam exchanged places with diazepam: (i) alprazolam (154,016 mentions), (ii) clonazepam (76,557 mentions), (iii) lorazepam (50,399 mentions), and diazepam (29,804 mentions).[37] See Table 10.1.

In the original 2011 DAWN data, alprazolam accounted for 36.2% of all BZDs mentioned and 48.8% of all BZDs mentioned by name. In 2002, alprazolam accounted for 26.2% of all BZDs mentioned and 39.3% of all BZDs mentioned by name. Clonazepam ranked second in both years, in 2011 accounting for 18% of all BZDs mentioned and 24.3% of all BZDs mentioned by name. In 2002, clonazepam accounted for 16.1% of all BZDs mentioned and 24.2% of all BZDs mentioned by name. The percentages for alprazolam and clonazepam remain fairly consistent over time.

In 2014, SAMHSA published an abstract of DAWN data for the period of 2005 to 2011 in which it illustrated the relationships between BZDs used alone or in combination with alcohol and/or opioids.[38] In 2011, the final year of DAWN data, there were 175,552 estimated visits to hospital emergency departments in which BZDs were mentioned.[38] Of this figure, 89,310 visits (50.9%) involved BZDs alone, while 50,561 visits (28.8%) involved BZDs and opioids.[38] BZDs and alcohol accounted for 27,452 visits (15.6%), while BZDs, alcohol, and opioids accounted for 8,229 visits (4.7%).[38] See Figure 10.2.

Today's opioid abuse epidemic has caused government regulatory and health agencies to examine what some have called "our other prescription drug problem."[39] This other prescription drug problem involves the BZDs, particularly alprazolam, clonazepam,

vii. Fiscal years in the US Government begin October 1 and end on September 30. The DAWN program was terminated at the end of fiscal year 2011.

Table 10.1 DAWN EMERGENCY DEPARTMENT DRUG MENTIONS BY DECADE, 1981 TO 2011, FOR SELECTED BZDS AND OTHER DRUGS

Category (CSA Schedule)	1981	1991	2001	2011[a]
Cocaine (C-II)	9,750	101,189	193,034	173,799
Heroin (C-I)	17,112	35,898	93,064	258,482
Methamphetamine (C-II)	6,469	4,887	14,923	102,961
Oxycodone (C-II)	4,202	3,941	18,409	175,229
Hydrocodone (C-III)	314	5,012	21,567	97,183
Methadone (C-II)	4,436	2,632	10,725	75,693
Alprazolam (C-IV)	**NA**	**16,235**	**25,644**	**154,016**
Diazepam (C-IV)	**43,569**	**14,637**	**11,447**	**29,804**
Lorazepam (C-IV)	**4,573**	**6,910**	**11,902**	**50,399**
Clonazepam (C-IV)	**71**	**6,467**	**19,117**	**76,557**
Triazolam (C-IV)	**NA**	**3,363**	**235**	**NA**

Notes: BZDs are in bold. BZDs = benzodiazepines. NA = data unavailable.
[a]DAWN's data collection and methodology changed in 2002; comparisons between 2011 and years prior to 2002 are not considered reliable or accurate.
Source: SAMHSA.[28,35]

diazepam, and lorazepam. Between 1996, when OxyContin was introduced, and 2013, the number of adults filling a prescription for BZDs increased 67%, from 8.1 million to 13.5 million. Of additional concern is that the quantity of BZDs received increased more than threefold, from 1.1 kg lorazepam-equivalents per 100,000 adults to 3.6 kgs lorazepam-equivalents per 100,000 adults.[40]

Lembke and colleagues[39] reported that in 2012, prescribers wrote 37.6 BZD prescriptions per 100 population, placing alprazolam, clonazepam, and lorazepam among the 10 most commonly prescribed psychotropic medications in the United States. Despite the increased risk from taking BZDs and opioids, a study of insurance claims filed between 2001 and 2013 on behalf of 595,410 patients co-prescribed opioids and BZDs, showed that the rate of co-prescribing these drugs nearly doubled between 2001 and 2013, from 9% of patients to 17% of patients.[41]

COUNTERFEIT XANAX

The popularity of BZDs, particularly alprazolam, has attracted interest from criminal organizations specializing in manufacturing and distributing counterfeit drugs. The underground drug market involved in making and selling three types of products: drugs that are made using unapproved but pharmaceutical-grade API (active pharmaceutical ingredient) corresponding to their label; drugs that are labeled as branded or well-known medicines but contain no API of the branded or well-known drugs; and drugs that are look-alike products that resemble branded or well-known drugs but contain a psychoactive ingredient that is unapproved and toxic.

For simplicity, these categories can be described as (i) *counterfeit-real*, (ii) *counterfeit-unreal*, and (iii) *counterfeit-toxic*. Generally, all counterfeit drugs will have physical characteristics, packaging, and labeling that resemble the branded or well-known product(s) but will differ in their content.

Counterfeit-Real

This category consists of drugs that appear identical with the branded or licensed product they fraudulently claim to be—right down to perfectly reproduced brand labels, product logos, shapes, colors, and lot numbers—but they contain nonapproved API obtained from underground commercial suppliers in places like India and China where chemical and drug industries are poorly regulated. Counterfeit-real drugs, even those containing API as labeled, also may contain toxic contaminants. They are not manufactured to approved standards and may contain more or less of the labeled (and safe) dosage indicated on the bogus label. Counterfeit-real drugs often are sold online to patients and others seeking a bargain or wanting to buy controlled substances without a valid prescription. Fraudulent webpage descriptions are used to deceive buyers into thinking they are dealing with bona fide pharmacies in, for example, Canada or some other trustworthy nation.

Counterfeit-Unreal

This category of counterfeit drugs mostly involved expensive drugs in high demand, such as chemotherapy or lifestyle drugs. The drugs in this category, however, will contain none of the labeled ingredient(s). Instead, they may contain fillers, buffers, and other inactive excipients, some of which may be contaminated or toxic. Over the past decade, opioids and BZDs have entered the counterfeit-unreal (CU) drug trade. Suppliers of this category of counterfeit drugs do not expect to attract or maintain a customer base but, instead, seek to insert their bogus products into legitimate channels where they can generate enormous profits or, in the case of controlled substances, sell to drug abusers and other drug dealers via Dark Web or Internet advertising.

Traditionally, suppliers of CU drugs have specialized in high-end cancer drugs because the risk of detection of their bogus ingredients was low. Victimized cancer patients and their caregivers unlikely question the integrity of a drug when it does not work for them.

In 2002, counterfeiters expected to make an estimated $28 million in profit from a shipment of 11,000 boxes of counterfeit Epogen and Procrit—two very expensive drugs for treating cancer-related anemia.[viii] US Customs agents in Florida, however, inspected

---

viii. Testimony given by the U.S. Government Accountability Office before Congress in 2013 showed that Epogen/Procrit (same drug, different brand name) ranked number one in Medicare drug expenditures ($2 billion) in 2010. [42]

a shipment of these drugs being imported and found that the entire shipment was bogus and contained only tap water. The labeling and packaging resembled the real thing right down to the smudged lot numbers stamped on each container.[43]

Unlike the high-end CU cancer drugs whose reliability may not be questioned, when it comes to CU opioids and BZDs, users quickly can discern whether they are bogus by the absence of expected effects. This, in turn, may have given rise to the third category of bogus drugs— a very dangerous category that has caused many accidental drug overdose deaths.

Counterfeit-Toxic

This category of counterfeit drugs has emerged more recently and involves products manufactured to resemble branded and generic forms of legitimate controlled substances but, instead of the labeled API, they contain deadly fentanyl. In 2006, DEA reported one of the first cases involving counterfeit OxyContin tablets containing fentanyl. The tablets were round, colored green with a logo "OC" on one side and the number "80" on the other side—made to resemble a genuine OxyContin 80 mg tablet.[44]

DEA has reported numerous other seizures of counterfeit OxyContin tablets containing fentanyl in New York, New Mexico, Iowa, Ohio, and California.[45] In 2006, in a suburb of Los Angeles, authorities sized a commercial pill press and thousands of counterfeit OxyContin tablets—each found to contain 1.5 mg of fentanyl HCL, a potentially lethal dose.[ix] In addition to counterfeiting OxyContin tablets, the authorities reported the seizure of tablets containing MDA (ecstasy), fentanyl, and caffeine.[45,47]

Of considerable interest is the recent emergence of counterfeit alprazolam (Xanax) tablets, many of which have been found to contain fentanyl. This is particularly dangerous because, unlike those who may inadvertently consume a fentanyl-laced counterfeit OxyContin tablet, those expecting the effects of a BZD may be opioid-naïve, and the dose of fentanyl they ingest may prove lethal.

From October 15 to December 31, 2015, the California Poison Control System, San Francisco division, identified eight patients who experienced adverse events after ingesting what turned out to be counterfeit alprazolam tablets containing fentanyl and etizolam.[48] The latter is a BZD available for sale online but not approved in the United States.[48] In addition, a fatal case involving counterfeit fentanyl-laced Xanax was reported to the San Francisco medical examiner during this same time period.[48] Patients were treated for serious life-threatening effects that included one case of cardiac arrest.[48] An infant, eight months old, was among the patients who were successfully treated. The child had consumed a fentanyl-laced Xanax tablet that it found on the floor.[48]

---

ix. According to the Centers for Medicare and Medicaid Services, 1.5 mg of fentanyl taken parenterally is the equivalent of 150 mg of morphine.[46] A dose of this magnitude would likely be lethal if taken by an opioid-naïve person. Fentanyl's bioavailability when taken orally is much less than that of either morphine or oxycodone, but the risks, nonetheless, remain substantial.

In 2018, police in Santa Ana, California, arrested three suspects and seized a pill press and several kilograms of powder believed used to make counterfeit oxycodone and Xanax tablets.[49]

The largest seizure to date of counterfeit Xanax tablets occurred in Switzerland where, in October 2013, Swiss authorities seized 440 kilograms of fake Xanax tablets in a large shipment en route to Egypt from China. More than a million pills containing no active ingredients were seized.[50] It should be noted that counterfeit Xanax tablets are very popular in Europe, especially the United Kingdom, where genuine alprazolam cannot lawfully be obtained via the National Health Service but is available only through private physicians. This has inspired a robust black market in counterfeit tablets that, according to British media reports, have caused 204 deaths since 2015, including 126 deaths in Scotland.[51]

In September 2017, Interpol coordinated a worldwide operation called Pangea X in which 197 police, customs, and health authorities in 123 countries carried out a series of coordinated raids on counterfeit drug makers and websites offering online services to purchase illicit pharmaceuticals, including BZDs, dietary supplements, pain pills, epilepsy medications, erectile dysfunction pills, antipsychotic medications, and nutritional products.[52]

The Interpol operation was global and focused on a variety of drugs and medicines. In the Congo, for example, officials seized 650 kgs of counterfeit antimalaria pills, and in Vietnam, authorities seized 1.2 tons of erectile dysfunction pills. This was the 10th year that the Interpol operation has been in operation and each year the number of participating nations and the coordinated seizures of counterfeit drugs increase.[52] Important, too, is the annual crackdown on thousands of websites that openly advertise the illegal sale of controlled substances.

In November 2018, the leader of a team of counterfeit Xanax makers was sentenced in federal court, Baltimore, Maryland, to 57 months in prison following a guilty plea to charges that from 2013 to 2017, he and a partner illegally distributed 920,000 counterfeit Xanax pills on the Dark Web,[x] amassing more than $5 million in currency and bitcoin. In a press release, the US attorney for Maryland stated that the defendant

> purchased narcotics manufacturing equipment, including pill presses and counterfeit 'Xanax' pill molds, which he used to press loose alprazolam powder into tablet or pill form, to resemble genuine Xanax pills. [He] solicited orders for the alprazolam pills on Dark Web marketplaces and sold alprazolam pills directly to buyers in exchange for Bitcoin.[53]

---

x. The Dark Web (sometimes called *Deep Web*) is an encrypted segment of the Internet accessible by special software that anonymizes users and content and is not indexed or accessible through conventional search engines. The Dark Web is considered a hotbed of criminal activity providing opportunities not only for international drug dealers but also for commerce in other illicit commodities and activities. Although promising its users encrypted anonymity, recent well-publicized criminal cases, some described in this chapter, suggest that authorities have developed ways for monitoring Dark Web browser traffic.

The Baltimore case was similar in many respects to a case uncovered by authorities in Utah in May 2017. After a year-long investigation, federal and local authorities broke up a ring of college-aged persons operating a bogus pharmacy on the Dark Web. The group manufactured and sold counterfeit alprazolam tablets made to look like a popular generic form and containing pharmaceutical-grade alprazolam unlawfully imported from China. The group also manufactured and sold counterfeit 30 mg oxycodone tablets made to look like a popular generic form but containing, instead, fentanyl, also unlawfully imported from China. An indictment charged this ring with manufacturing and distributing more than 175,000 counterfeit alprazolam tablets and more than 66,000 counterfeit 30 mg oxycodone tablets containing fentanyl. Authorities seized more than $6 million in cash, gold, and Bitcoin from this group. The leader of this ring was convicted in August 2019 of charges that carry a mandatory life prison sentence. Testimony at trial suggested that more than a dozen overdose deaths may have been caused by fentanyl drugs sold by this group. (*USA v. Arron Michael Shamo, et al.*)

The appearance of counterfeit drugs in the United States is alarming, and while federal authorities are aware of the potential harm these drugs pose to the public health, thus far, there have been few technical strategies put forth to reduce or prevent these activities. In July 2009, the FDA issued a draft document titled, *Guidance for Industry: Incorporation of Physical-Chemical Identifiers Into Solid Oral Dosage Form Drug Products for Anticounterfeiting.*[54] The document received more than a dozen comments from industry, academia, and standard-setting organizations. The Pharmaceutical Research and Manufacturers of America, the lobbying arm of the pharmaceutical industry, submitted the following comment that succinctly describes just one of several potential obstacles to the proposed guidance:

> Without protection, counterfeiters are more likely to be able to circumvent the anticounterfeiting measure by reverse engineering the product. Hence, disclosure of the [physical-chemical identifiers] (e.g., on the drug product labeling and/or package insert) becomes counterproductive [although we do acknowledge the resulting complexity of not listing an additive that may cause adverse events (e.g., allergic reactions) in a small number of patients].[54]

Besides the possibility of physical-chemical identifiers (PCIDs) being reversed engineered or causing adverse events, the fact of their presence in a drug would not, by itself, enable a user to know if a drug was authentic. This determination would have to be made by a forensic analysis of the substance in question. Nonetheless, requiring PCIDs might reduce large scale commercial counterfeiting schemes involving international shipments of drugs when, for example, a customs examination of a sample of an inbound shipment might detect counterfeit forms. In 2011, the FDA issued its formal guidance document under the same name as the draft, stressing that the guidance was nonbinding and represented only the current thinking of the FDA.[55]

DISCUSSION

The primary theme of this chapter was to describe the regulatory history of BZDs, when they were introduced to the public and how they were initially and subsequently treated by government regulatory agencies like the DEA and FDA. To the extent possible, we tried to avoid discussing the clinical use of these drugs beyond mentioning their labeled indications as approved by the FDA or cited in scheduling documents. It is difficult to discuss scheduling issues without taking into consideration important public health risks posed by a drug with abuse potential. Indeed, as we mentioned in the text, five of the eight criteria established by Congress and which must be evaluated by FDA and DEA when considering the scheduling status of a drug pertain to the drug's pharmacology and the public health consequences of its misuse.

In this chapter we addressed important factors pertaining to the association between the use of opioids and BZDs and one's higher risk for fatal overdose when these drugs are co-ingested. There are questions that we could not address, nor offer further analysis because the available data for doing so are weak or inadequate; however, they are discussed elsewhere in this volume. The government's efforts to measure prescription drug abuse has been plagued since the 1970s—almost a half century ago—with flawed information systems that no doubt have wasted resources that might have been used to reduce drug-related morbidity and mortality.

A good deal of attention was paid in this chapter and elsewhere in this book to describing some of these flawed information systems, particularly the DAWN emergency department program and the Center for Disease Control and Prevention's (CDC) system for tracking drug overdose deaths. Whatever one may think of these programs, there can be little doubt that their data over the years have greatly influenced public policies in health and national drug control.

Even so, it must be asked rhetorically, why the FDA and DEA agreed in 1981 to place three BZDs (halazepam, alprazolam, and triazolam) in Schedule IV—despite several years of solid data collected from over 800 hospital emergency departments showing that diazepam, one of the first BZDs approved in 1975 and similar to several new BZDs under review, was mentioned more frequently in emergency department drug-abuse episodes than any other prescription drug? The criteria for Schedule IV includes finding that the drug in question "has a low potential for abuse relative to the drugs or other substances in schedule III."[56]

Taking into consideration the statutory criteria, the actual nonmedical use, according to DAWN, of diazepam when it was placed in Schedule IV was much higher than drugs in Schedule III, and even some drugs in Schedules I and II—including heroin (Schedule I), cocaine (Schedule II), and oxycodone (Schedule II).

Under DAWN's revised methodology introduced in 2003, BZDs continued to account each year for a sizable percentage of DAWN mentions. In 2011, the final year of DAWN's existence, the top four BZDs—alprazolam (154,016 mentions), diazepam (29,804 mentions), lorazepam (50,399 mentions), and clonazepam (76,577 mentions)—collectively accounted for 310,716 mentions.[57] See Table 10.2.

Table 10.2 EMERGENCY DEPARTMENT MENTIONS FOR BZDS REPORTED BY DAWN FOR 2004 TO 2011

Drug Name	Total 2004	Total 2005	Total 2006	Total 2007	Total 2008	Total 2009	Total 2010	Total 2011
Benzodiazepines	170,474	221,454	233,119	259,515	330,229	373,328	408,021	425,616
Alprazolam	56,658	70,023	78,130	97,546	132,462	140,657	152,168	154,016
Chlordiazepoxide	1,441	2,552	2,780	1,818	1,904	2,547	2,675	
Clonazepam	32,414	36,576	42,506	48,525	59,868	69,620	73,452	76,557
Clorazepate				180	233	308	288	
Diazepam	19,096	22,332	23,368	24,413	33,214	30,214	31,970	29,804
Flurazepam		805						
Lorazepam	20,849	25,535	27,972	32,462	44,465	42,602	44,407	50,399
Oxazepam	750	399	810	934		485		
Temazepam	6,339	5,205	4,983	5,156	5,741	4,954	5,380	4,686
Triazolam				643				
Benzodiazepines NOS	42,337	68,983	67,128	62,833	75,041	98,973	115,605	129,654

Notes: Reported data are national estimates for entire United States by year. An omitted result means that it does not meet the standards of precision and has been suppressed because the relative standard error exceeds 50% or the unweighted count is less than 30. NOS = not otherwise specified.
Source: SAMHSA.[57]

While one of the original designs and purposes of DAWN was to collect data for use in scheduling drugs, we must repeat here that abuse potential or actual abuse liability, as determined by DAWN data, satisfy only some of the criteria considered in the government's medical and scientific evaluation used to determine the schedule of a drug. As we mentioned in the text, five of the eight statutory criteria used for scheduling are related to its public health risks and pharmacology. Given the structure and language of the CSA, Congress clearly intended the secretary of HHS and the attorney general to parse these differences between concerns for public health and public safety.

With the previous discussion in mind, Schedule IV may have been an appropriate level of BZD control at a time when the nation's drug abuse problem involved primarily nonprescription drugs like cocaine, heroin, cannabis, and hallucinogens. Until the final years of the 20th century, prescription drug abuse was a minor aspect of the nation's drug problem, involving mostly the abuse of amphetamine drugs overprescribed for weight control. Until the mid- to late 1990s, the boundary line between abusers of street drugs and abusers of prescription drugs was clear and rarely crossed. The introduction of OxyContin in 1996, and its subsequent widespread misuse, brought prescription drug abuse to the fore while blurring the boundary line between abusers of street drugs and abusers of prescribed drugs. Today's opiate "addict" is very likely to alternate between street and pharmaceutical opioids, depending upon which is more available at any given time.

Realistically, we no longer have the conditions that existed in 1970 when the CSA was enacted or, for that matter, in the 1970s and 1980s, when the BZDs were scheduled. Today, the nation's drug problem is far more complex than it was a half century ago. It has progressed beyond the capabilities of information systems designed to address a 1970 problem that, in retrospect and by today's standards, was manageable and confined to a handful of street drugs and a relatively small population of users clustered in major urban areas.

By comparison, a typical chronic abuser of controlled substances today likely uses a greater variety of drugs, often in combination, to achieve a desired effect. The campaign to emphasize opioids in the treatment of chronic pain that began in the mid-1990s with the introduction of OxyContin had the unfortunate side effect of causing pain patients and opioid "addicts" to share common health risks. Polypharmacy, the simultaneous co-ingestion of drugs that may produce adverse drug interactions, no longer is associated only with users of street drugs.

The number of patients prescribed both an opioid analgesic prescription and a BZD prescription increased 41% between 2002 and 2014.[58] Nearly 30% of opioid overdose deaths in 2015 involved BZDs.[59] The CDC reports that in 2016, synthetic opioids (primarily illicitly manufactured fentanyl) were involved in 23.7% of deaths involving prescription opioids, 37.4% of deaths involving heroin, and 40.3% of deaths involving cocaine.[60] Using a revised methodology, the CDC reports that more than two-thirds (67.8%) of the 70,237 drug overdose deaths reported in 2017 involved opioids.[61]

These data illustrate just how different today's drug abuser is from those of previous generations. This also may explain why systems like DAWN and the CDC's National Vital Statistics System—designed decades ago—are unable to capture important changes that have occurred over time, not only in the variety of abusable substances, but also in the demographics and drug-taking behavior of drug abusers.

In an effort to clarify how the CDC reconciles cause-of-death classification and definition of drug overdose deaths, in September 2019, the CDC reported:

> Drug overdose deaths may involve multiple drugs; therefore, a single death might be included in more than one category when describing the number of drug overdose deaths involving specific drugs. For example, a death that involved both heroin and fentanyl would be included in both the number of drug overdose deaths involving heroin and the number of drug overdose deaths involving synthetic opioids other than methadone.[62]

While categorizing drug-related deaths in this manner may have statistical value, it is almost devoid of value for understanding and preventing future drug overdose deaths. The tendency to view frequency of drug mentions as a risk metric obscures the important role of polypharmacy as a principal cause of accidental drug overdose deaths.

Besides designing better information systems to track drug overdose deaths, it may be time to revisit the scheduling status of BZDs, either by administrative rule-making or by legislation. The key players in this global market, according to industry sources, are AstraZeneca plc, Eli Lilly and Company, Forest Laboratories, Inc., GlaxoSmithKline plc, H. Lundbeck A/S, Johnson & Johnson, Merck & Co., Inc., Pfizer, Inc., and Sanofi S.A.[63]

These sponsors of BZDs likely would oppose any agency rule-making proceedings to reschedule this class of popular drugs. North America is the largest market for BZDs, followed by Europe and Asia. Industry sources forecast that the North American market alone will reach $2.4 billion in BZD sales by 2022.[63] Currently, 26 companies, large and small, have active NDAs in the United States and are authorized to manufacture and distribute alprazolam, the sales leader in the BZD market.[64] The potential loss of market share that would likely follow a rescheduling of BZDs no doubt would force the industry to oppose any administrative rescheduling proceeding initiated by the agencies.

In 2012, two years before all hydrocodone products were rescheduled from Schedule III to Schedule II, DEA data from the Automation of Records and Consolidated Orders (ARCOS) program showed that 39,786,938.75 grams of hydrocodone were distributed by pharmacies in the United States In 2017, three years after all hydrocodone products were rescheduled, this figure had dropped 35.5%, to 25,666,888.29 grams.[65] It should be noted that studies conducted since the rescheduling action show that the decline in the prescribing of hydrocodone products was offset to some degree by increases in the prescribing of other, often lower scheduled, analgesic drugs.[66,67]

The legislative route for rescheduling BZDs would be fast and final and unencumbered by years by costly legal challenges, assuming, that is, that Congress would agree to reschedule BZDs in the face of what expectedly would be fierce industry opposition to such a move. In 2018, according to the Center for Responsive Politics, the pharmaceutical industry led all sectors of the economy in lobbying expenditures ($280.3 million), followed in a far-distant second place by the insurance industry ($156.9 million).[68]

Although a reasonable case can be made that alprazolam poses the most likely BZD candidate for rescheduling because it figures so prominently and consistently in drug-related morbidity and mortality, if singled out in this way, rescheduling alprazolam, alone, likely would drive abusers to diazepam and the other remaining Schedule IV BZDs.

Thus, despite evidence of differential abuse liability among the BZDs, it is almost certain that the entire class would have to be rescheduled if the choice were to be made that alprazolam must be rescheduled. There is legislative precedence for scheduling an entire class of drugs to prevent misuse of substitute varieties having less abuse liability. In 1990 and 2004, Congress amended to CSA to place an entire class of anabolic steroids in Schedule III.[69,70]

Similar precedence exists for administratively scheduling an entire class of drugs. The first (and, possibly, only) example of this was when the Bureau of Narcotics and Dangerous Drugs in 1971 rescheduled amphetamine, methamphetamine and their optical isomers in Schedule II.[71] The original CSA listed injectable (liquid) forms of methamphetamine in Schedule II but left other forms of amphetamine and methamphetamine in Schedule III.[71] The BNDD rule-making closed this gap by placing the entire class of amphetamines, including all forms of methamphetamine, in Schedule II.[xi][71]

As we describe in the text, the drug scheduling schema devised by the UN relies on ill-defined criteria that may or may not be relevant to all member states. While many of the agreed upon obligations, such as licensing manufacturers and regulating import and export of controlled drugs, requiring dispensing by prescription, etc., are indeed commendable on a global basis, they alone are insufficient to address many of the problems identified in this chapter.

As we note in the text, the US Congress adopted the UN's drug scheduling process, in effect assigning the Secretary of HHS the role of the World Health Organization (WHO) and the attorney general the role of the UN's Commission on Narcotic Drugs. For a variety of reasons, it may be time for Congress to revisit this process and to consider additional scheduling levels to categorize drugs with added risks when co-ingested with other controlled drugs. Additional levels or sublevels of existing schedules could be used to require the kind of additional surveillance presently required by the CSA for Schedule I and II drugs and selected other controlled substances. Presently, BZDs, as Schedule IV controlled substances, are not tracked by ARCOS or subject to procurement or manufacturing quotas.

To be sure, there may be pharmacological explanations beyond the scope of this chapter for why alprazolam commands such a large segment of the BZD market. Over several decades, alprazolam has remained the most frequently prescribed BZD for the treatment of generalized anxiety disorder and panic attack.[72] According to DEA, in 2011

---

xi. The BNDD's Proposed Rule placing the entire class of amphetamines in Schedule II was objected to by four makers of amphetamine products who requested administrative hearings. The National Wholesale Druggists Association, the Minnesota State Board of Pharmacy, the U.S. Pharmacopeial Convention, Inc., the Manufacturers Educational Drug Information Association, and the National Association of Chain Drug Stores, Inc. raised concerns about the added security requirements for Schedule II amphetamines. The Proposed Rule was supported by the Christian Life Commission, the City of New York, Abbott Laboratories, and the American Medical Association.[71]

there were 49 million prescriptions for alprazolam dispensed in the United States., 27.6 million for lorazepam, 26.9 million for clonazepam, 15 million for diazepam, and 8.5 million for temazepam.[73]

Industry sources report that in 2017 more than 5.8 billion prescriptions for various medicines were dispensed, with generics accounting for about 5.2 billion or 90% of them.[74] Alprazolam was the only BZD to make the top 20 list of prescribed medicines, with 45 million dispensed prescriptions in 2017.[74]

The US market for alprazolam appears to be stable and, based on the DEA and industry estimates as previously noted, the market for alprazolam appears to have declined 8.2% between 2011 and 2017. Assuming for the sake of discussion the aforementioned association between the use of alprazolam and the use of opioids, prescribed or otherwise, a decrease in the prescribing of one should be matched by a corresponding decrease in the prescribing of the other. Data from independent sources suggest that this, in fact, can be shown. During the peak year of 2011, according to industry sources, prescription opioid volume reached 240 billion mgs of morphine equivalents, but by 2017, this figure had declined 29% to 171 billion mgs.[74]

Thus, we have reductions of 8.2% and 29% in the prescribing of alprazolam and opioids, respectively, in the years between 2011 and 2017. This, in turn, should have produced a corresponding drop in mortality associated with the concomitant ingestion of these drugs. This, however, did not occur.

According to the CDC, in 2016, the most frequent concomitant drugs for drug overdose deaths involving alprazolam were fentanyl (28.3%), heroin (26.9%), hydrocodone (26%), oxycodone (25.3%), and methadone (22%).[75] The most frequent concomitant drugs for drug overdose deaths involving diazepam were oxycodone (28.5%), fentanyl (24.8%), and heroin (20.0%).[75] The linear relationship between opioids and BZDs in national drug overdose deaths between 1999 and 2017, as measured by the CDC, is striking.[76] See Figure 10.1.

Unfortunately, we do not have CDC mortality data like this for years prior to 2016 so we are unable to test the hypothesis that declining prescriptions for alprazolam and opioids should produce a corresponding decline in their combined presence in drug-related overdose deaths. As we discuss in another chapter, the CDC's methodology tracking drug-related mortality was found unreliable when agency scientists acknowledged that the coding system used to categorize drug-related overdose deaths did not distinguish between licit and illicitly manufactured fentanyl, and, as a result, the CDC's report of prescription opioid-related deaths for 2016 was overstated, possibly by as much as 47.3%.[77]

Relying solely on published market data to detect drug abuse trends is risky for a number of reasons, not the least of which is the sizable increase of counterfeit pharmaceuticals, especially alprazolam and fentanyl. Drug abuse databases that depend on collecting information from hospital emergency departments and medical examiners by default attribute drug-related morbidity and mortality to lawfully manufactured drugs even when counterfeit drugs are involved. Identifying a counterfeit or illicitly manufactured drug after it has been consumed is generally not possible when the drug in question also is available as a lawful product. As we mention in the text, a typical

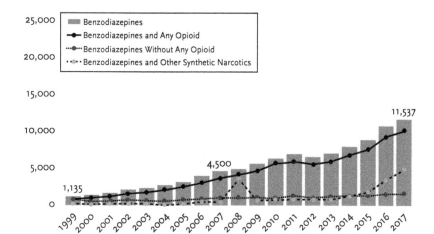

Source: Centers for Disease Control and Prevention, National Center for Health Statistics, Multiple Cause of Death 1999–2017 on CDC WONDER Online Database, released December, 2018

Figure 10.1 National overdose deaths involving BZDs, by opioid involvement, 1999–2017. From National Institute on Drug Abuse.[76]

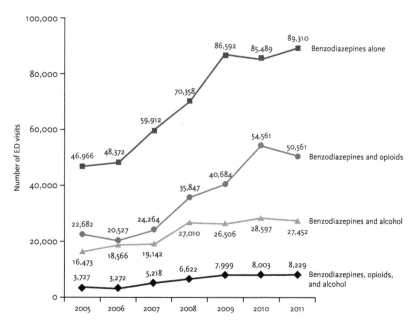

Figure 10.2 Estimated number of DAWN ED visits involving BZDs alone or in combination with opioids or alcohol, by year, 2005–2011. *Source:* SAMHSA.

toxicology screen cannot distinguish between licit and illicitly manufactured drugs if they both have APIs that produce identical metabolites.

In 2018, the US Congress recognized the shortcomings in the CDC's system for tracking drug overdose deaths and enacted legislation authorizing the CDC to modernize its systems to overcome this deficiency.[78] At the same time, recognizing that HHS and CDC are no longer tracking drug-related morbidity via the nation's hospital emergency departments, Congress directed and authorized the reinstitution of DAWN.[78] As mentioned in the text, the DAWN program was halted in 2011 by HHS at the height of what the White House at the time was describing as an epidemic of prescription drug abuse.[79] SAMHSA has awarded a contract to the company formerly responsible for DAWN to reinstitute the program.[80]

While Congress deserves credit for trying to address inaccurate reporting of drug-related overdose deaths by the CDC and requiring SAMHSA to reinstitute the DAWN program, there remains much more that Congress and HHS could do to address the nation's drug problems. In another chapter where we discuss in detail the CDC's use of the WHO's *International Classification of Diseases* (ICD) taxonomy for categorizing drug-related mortality, we note how deficient this system is for differentiating individual drugs within their classes. This problem is even more pronounced with the BZDs—all of which are identified by single code (T42.4) in the ICD. Because of this, when used for reporting BZD-related mortality, the result will show no difference between, say, alprazolam and triazolam.[xii]

As we also note in another chapter, it would take very little to correct this serious flaw, and the WHO permits member states to make clinical modifications to ICD codes when needed to distinguish specific characteristics of interest (such as the chemical name of a drug and whether it is licitly or illicitly manufactured). Each five-digit ICD code may be modified up to a total of seven alpha digits. If the CDC and HHS had adopted clinical modifications to distinguish licit from illicit fentanyl when street fentanyl emerged in 2005 and then again in 2013, the integrity of the data reporting prescription opioid overdose deaths in 2016 (and earlier years) would have been preserved. Clinical modifications to the ICD codes need to be made for all medicinal controlled substances, notably opioids and BZDs, if this system is to be maintained.

Finally, FDA's frequent issuance of guidance documents has come under fire in recent years for being a backdoor way of creating administrative rules without going through the administrative rule-making procedures of the FFDCA and the Administrative Procedure Act.[81] Although the FDA, like other regulatory agencies of the federal government, is quick to note that a guidance document, per se, is nonbinding on the regulated entity, critics nonetheless sometimes view these documents as covert threats that skirt executive regulatory review and public accountability.[82,83]

How a guidance document is viewed by the industry is secondary to the fact that they are nonbinding and, therefore, often ignored by those for whom the guidance is intended.

---

xii. Just for reference, in a five-year period between 2007 and 2011, the DAWN program reported 676,849 visits involving alprazolam to hospital emergency departments. In the same five-year period, the DAWN program reported only 643 visits involving triazolam.[37]

Consequently, we believe that the FDA should seek legislative authority to impose as a requirement on manufacturers of all solid dosage drugs the recommended guidance it provided in its 2011 document titled, *Guidance for Industry: Incorporation of Physical-Chemical Identifiers Into Solid Oral Dosage Form Drug Products for Anticounterfeiting.*[55]

There is no public information to show that any drug maker thus far has responded to this guidance. Moreover, given the anticipated costs of reformulating drug products with a special chemical identifier, it is unlikely any drug maker would comply unless required by law to do so and immunized against adverse events caused by FDA-approved PCIDs. The technology for doing this exists and would be useful in detecting counterfeit drugs, especially those containing the labeled API in unapproved products and formulations. Hopefully, the PCID tracing materials added to solid dosage units for this purpose would be designed to survive hepatic metabolism and be detectible in post-mortem toxicology examinations.

We believe that the most significant issue uncovered in this chapter about the history of BZD regulation is how it led us to the ongoing presence of a Dark Web pharmaceutical industry that is mostly immune from sovereign control. The accounts of counterfeit Xanax tablets and how and where they enter the channels of the drug supply chain should concern us all, including healthcare providers, patients, and regulators alike, as there is no logical reason why an international criminal infrastructure created to make and sell counterfeit Xanax should confine itself to making and marketing a single type of BZD.

Today's counterfeit drug makers import their API from commercial sources in China or India where controls are lax, and they use improvised manufacturing processes and pill presses to replicate designs and logos of popular drugs. International criminal organizations may soon discover—if they have not already—the enormous profit potential in mass producing counterfeit drugs and getting them to market, whether that market is the retail pharmacy in New York, London, or Tokyo or a virtual pharmacy on the Internet or Dark Web. We note that as part of the current administration's trade talks with China, tighter control over the manufacture and export of drugs and chemicals from sources in China has been a key topic of discussion. Thus far, as a result, China has agreed to place greater control on fentanyl and other harmful substances being manufactured in China and sold to customers in the United States. Some policy analysts, however, believe that these controls will have minimal effect and, if enforced, will drive the highly profitable illicit chemical and drug industry underground where it will continue providing the world with unapproved and potentially deadly drugs.

REFERENCES

1. Dokoupil T. America's long love affair with anti-anxiety drugs. *Newsweek Magazine.* https://www.newsweek.com/americas-long-love-affair-anti-anxiety-drugs-77967. Published January 21, 2019. Accessed February 21, 2019.
2. US Food and Drug Administration. Orange book: Approved drug products with therapeutic equivalence evaluations. https://www.accessdata.fda.gov/scripts/cder/ob/search_product.cfm. Published 2017. Accessed September 6, 2017.

3. Tone A. *The Age of Anxiety: A History of America's Turbulent Affair With Tranquilizers*. New York, NY: Basic Books; 2009.

4. History of Carter-Wallace, Inc. *Referenceforbusiness.com*. https://www.referenceforbusiness. com/history2/86/Carter-Wallace-Inc.html. Accessed March 5, 2019.

5. Controlled Substances Act, Title II, 21 USC 812; Pub.L. 91-513, 84 Stat. 1242 (1970). http://uscode.house.gov/. Accessed February 24, 2019.

6. United Nations. Single Convention on Narcotic Drugs of 1961. https://www.unodc. org/pdf/convention_1961_en.pdf. Published 1961. Amended 1972. Accessed January 14, 2015.

7. Drug Abuse Control Amendments of 1965: An act to protect the public health and safety by amending the Federal Food, Drug, and Cosmetic Act to establish special controls for depressant and stimulant drugs and counterfeit drugs, and for other purposes; P.L 89-75, 79 Stat. 236 (1965). http://law2.house.gov/statutes/pl/89/74.pdf. Accessed February 25, 2019.

8. US Bureau of Drug Abuse Control. BDAC: a review, Mar. 1966, Through Apr. 1967. https://catalog.hathitrust.org/Record/100673304. Published 1967, Accessed February 25, 2019.

9. Proposed placement of chlordiazepoxide, diazepam, oxazepam, clorazepate, flurazepam, and clonazepam in Schedule IV. *Fed Regist*. 197540(18):40FR4016. https://www. federalregister.gov/

10. Controlled Substances Act, Title II, 21 USC 811(a); Pub.L. 91-513, 84 Stat. 1242 (1970). http://uscode.house.gov/. Accessed January 14, 2019.

11. Final rule: placement of chlordiazepoxide, diazepam, oxazepam, clorazepate, flurazepam, and clonazepam in Schedule IV. *Fed Regist*. 1975;40(108):40FR23998. https://www. federalregister.gov/

12. Controlled Substances Act, Title II, 21 USC 812; Pub.L. 91-513, 84 Stat. 1242, Sect. 812(b)(4)(A-C) (1970). http://uscode.house.gov/. Accessed February 25, 2019.

13. Harrison Narcotic Tax Act; P.L. 63-223, 38 Stat. 785 (1914). http://www.druglibrary.org/ schaffer/history/e1910/harrisonact.htm. Accessed December 23, 2017.

14. Marihuana Tax Act of 1937, 75th Cong., 1st sess; P.L. 75-238; 50 Stat. 551 (1937).

15. US Food and Drug Administration. About FDA: milestones in U.S. food and drug law history. https://www.fda.gov/aboutfda/history/forgshistory/evolvingpowers/ ucm2007256.htm. Published January 31, 2018. Accessed February 28, 2019.

16. Schmeck HM. H.E.W. Scientists score drug bill: 100 sign a letter criticizing administration proposal. *The New York Times*. May 2, 1970.

17. Comprehensive Drug Abuse Prevention and Control Act, Title II: Controlled Substances Act; Pub. L. No. 91-513, 84 Stat. 1236, Title 21 US Code, Sect 811(f) (1970). http:// uscode.house.gov/. Accessed February 22, 2013.

18. Controlled Substances Act. Title 21, USC, Sect. 811(b); Evaluation of drugs and other substances (1970). http://uscode.house.gov/. Accessed August 29, 2016.

19. Controlled Substances Act. Title 21, USC, Sect. 811(h); Temporary scheduling to avoid imminent hazards to public safety (1970). http://uscode.house.gov/. Accessed August 29, 2016.

20. Food and Drug Administration Amendments Act of 2007; Pub. L. 110-85, Page 121 STAT. 823. (2007). https://www.gpo.gov/fdsys/pkg/PLAW-110publ85/html/PLAW-110publ85.htm. Accessed February 28, 2019.

21. Comprehensive Drug Abuse Prevention and Control Act, Title II: Controlled Substances Act. Pub. L. No. 91-513, 84 Stat. 1236; Title 21, USC, Sect 811(c) Factors determinative of control or removal from schedules (1970). http://uscode.house.gov/. Accessed March 1, 2019.

22. IMS Health, Inc. *Company-Histories.com*. http://www.company-histories.com/IMS-Health-Inc-Company-History.html. Accessed March 1, 2019.

23. IMS America Ltd. Drug Abuse Warning Network: phase IV report, May 1975–April 1976. Washington, DC: The Administration; 1977.

24. Schedules of controlled substances; proposed placement of halazepam, alprazolam and triazolam into Schedule IV. *Fed Regist.* 1981;46(82):46FR23953. https://www.federalregister.gov/

25. Schedules of controlled substances; placement of halazepam in Schedule IV. *Fed Regist.* 1981;46(209):46FR53407. https://www.federalregister.gov/.

26. Schedules of controlled substances; placement of alprazolam in Schedule IV. *Fed Regist.* 1981;46(218):46FR23998. https://www.federalregister.gov/.

27. Schedules of controlled substances; placement of trazolam in Schedule IV. *Fed Regist.* 1982;47(249):47FR57693. https://www.federalregister.gov/.

28. McCaig L. *Historical Estimates from the Drug Abuse Warning Network; 1978–1994: Estimates of Drug-Related Emergency Department Episodes.* DHHS Publication No. (SMA) 96-3105. Washington, DC: SAMHSA; 1996.

29. Cone EJ, Fant RV, Rohay JM, et al. Oxycodone involvement in drug abuse deaths: a DAWN-based classification scheme applied to an oxycodone postmortem database containing over 1000 cases. *J Anal Toxicol.* 2003;27(2):57–67; discussion 67.

30. Substance Abuse and Mental Health Services Administration. *Drug Abuse Warning Network: Development of a New Design (Methodology Report).* DAWN Series M-4, DHHS Publication No. (SMA) 02-3754. Rockville, MD: Department of Health and Human Services; 2002.

31. Caulkins JP, Ebener PA, McCaffrey DF. Describing DAWN's dominion. *Contemp Drug Prob.* 1995;22:547–567.

32. Substance Abuse and Mental Health Services Administration. *Drug Abuse Warning Network, 2003: Interim National Estimates of Drug-Related Emergency Department Visits.* Rockville, MD: Department of Health and Human Services; 2004.

33. Delany PD. Draft of letter from Director Delany to DAWN-participating hospitals announcing the termination of DAWN. 2011 [Obtained by John J. Coleman via Freedom of Information Act, December 27, 2011, from SAMHSA (unpublished document)].

34. Department of Health and Human Services. Budgets in Brief and Performance Reports: HHS Budgets in Brief (2011 and 2012). https://www.hhs.gov/about/agencies/asfr/budget/budgets-in-brief-performance-reports/index.html. Accessed March 5, 2019.

35. Substance Abuse and Mental Health Services Administration. *Emergency Department Trends From the Drug Abuse Warning Network, Final Estimates 1994–2001.* DAWN Series: D-21, DHHS Publication No. (SMA) 02-3635. Rockville, MD: US Department of Health and Human Services; 2002.

36. Substance Abuse and Mental Health Services Administration. *Emergency Department Trends From the Drug Abuse Warning Network, Final Estimates 1995–2002,* DAWN Series: D-24, DHHS Publication No. (SMA) 03-3780. Rockville, MD: US Department of Health and Human Services; 2003.

37. Substance Abuse and Mental Health Services Administration. Drug Abuse Warning Network (DAWN) national & metro tables, 2004–2011 ("All misuse and abuse"). https://www.datafiles.samhsa.gov/study-series/drug-abuse-warning-network-dawn-nid13516. Accessed March 4, 2019.

38. Substance Abuse and Mental Health Services Administration. The DAWN report: benzodiazepines in combination with opioid pain relievers or alcohol: greater risk of more serious ED visit outcomes. https://www.samhsa.gov/data/sites/default/files/DAWN-SR192-BenzoCombos-2014/DAWN-SR192-BenzoCombos-2014.pdf. Published 2014. Accessed March 4, 2019.

39. Lembke A, Papac J, Humphreys K. Our other prescription drug problem. *New Engl J Med.* 2018;378(8):693–695.

40. Bachhuber MA, Hennessy S, Cunningham CO, Starrels JL. Increasing benzodiazepine prescriptions and overdose mortality in the United States, 1996–2013. *Am J Public Health.* 2016;*106*(4):686–688.

41. Sun EC, Dixit A, Humphreys K, Darnall BD, Baker LC, Mackey S. Association between concurrent use of prescription opioids and benzodiazepines and overdose: retrospective analysis. *BMJ (Clin Res Ed).* 2017;356:j760–j760.

42. Testimony Before the Subcommittee on Health, Committee on Energy and Commerce, House of Representatives, Friday, June 28, 2013; Medicare: information on highest-expenditure Part B drugs; Statement of James Cosgrove, Director, Health Care. Report# GAO-13-739T. https://www.gao.gov/assets/660/655608.pdf. Published 2013. Accessed October 8, 2019.

43. Hoilmberg M. Counterfeit drugs: a real cause for alarm. *Pharmacy Times.* https://www.pharmacytimes.com/publications/issue/2004/2004-12/2004-12-9093. Published December 1, 2004. Accessed March 8, 2019.

44. Drug Enforcement Administration, Office of Forensic Sciences. Intelligence alert: OxyContin mimic tablets (containing fentanyl) near Atlantic, Iowa. *Microgram Bull,* 2006;39(1):2.

45. Coleman JJ. Special report: fentanyl analogs in street drugs (unpublished; prepared for Center for Substance Abuse Treatment, Department of Health and Human Services). 2007. Accessed March 12, 2019.

46. Centers for Medicare and Medicaid Services. Opioid oral morphine milligram equivalent (MME) conversion factors. https://www.cms.gov/Medicare/Prescription-Drug-Coverage/PrescriptionDrugCovContra/Downloads/Opioid-Morphine-EQ-Conversion-Factors-Aug-2017.pdf. Published August 2017. Accessed March 9, 2019.

47. Drug Enforcement Administration, Office of Forensic Sciences. Intelligence alert: large fentanyl/MDA/TMA laboratory in Azuza (sic), California—possibly the "OC-80" tablet source. *Microgram Bull.* 2006;39(4):45.

48. Arens AM, van Wijk XMR, Vo KT, Lynch KL, Wu AHB, Smollin CG. Adverse effects from counterfeit alprazolam tablets: letters. *JAMA Intern Med.* 2016;*176*(10):1554–1555.

49. Three O.C. men face federal narcotics charges that allege distribution of counterfeit opioid pills containing fentanyl. US Attorney's Office, Central Office of California. https://www.justice.gov/usao-cdca/pr/three-oc-men-face-federal-narcotics-charges-allege-distribution-counterfeit-opioid. Published April 15, 2018. Accessed March 9, 2019.

50. Torsoli A. Switzerland seizes bogus Pfizer pills in Zurich Airport. *Bloomberg Business Report.* https://www.bloomberg.com/news/articles/2013-10-18/swiss-authorities-seize-bogus-pfizer-pills-in-zurich-airport. Published October 18, 2013. Accessed March 9, 2019.

51. Devereux-Taylor R. Grieving Edinburgh mum warns of counterfeit pill dangers after son dies from Xanax overdose. *Edinburgh Evening News.* https://www.edinburghnews.scotsman.com/news/crime/grieving-edinburgh-mum-warns-of-counterfeit-pill-dangers-after-son-dies-from-xanax-overdose-1-4868483. Published February 6, 2019. Accessed March 9, 2019.

52. Millions of medicines seized in largest INTERPOL operation against illicit online pharmacies. Interpol. https://www.interpol.int/News-and-Events/News/2017/Millions-of-medicines-seized-in-largest-INTERPOL-operation-against-illicit-online-pharmacies. Published 2017. Accessed March 9, 2019.

53. US Attorney's Office, District of Maryland. Maryland man sentenced to 57 months in federal prison and ordered to forfeit at least $5.665 million as a result of his conviction on charges relating to Dark Web drug distribution and money laundering. https://www.justice.gov/usao-md/pr/maryland-man-sentenced-57-months-federal-prison-and-ordered-forfeit-least-5665-million-s. Published November 30, 2018. Accessed March 9, 2019.

54. Wertheimer AI, Wang PG. *Counterfeit Medicines: Policy, Economics and Countermeasures*. 1 ed. Glendale, AZ: ILM; 2012.

55. US Food and Drug Administration. Guidance for industry: incorporation of physical-chemical identifiers into solid oral dosage form drug products for anticounterfeiting. https://www.fda.gov/downloads/drugs/guidances/ucm171575.pdf. Published October 2011. Accessed March 9, 2019.

56. Controlled Substances Act, Title II, 21 USC 812(b)(4)(A); Pub.L. 91-513, 84 Stat. 1242 (1970). http://uscode.house.gov/.

57. Substance Abuse and Mental Health Services Administration. *Drug Abuse Warning Network*, 2011: *selected tables of national estimates of drug-related emergency department visits*. https://www.samhsa.gov/data/sites/default/files/DAWN2k11ED/DAWN2k11ED/DAWN2k11ED.pdf. Published 2013.

58. Hwang CS, Kang EM, Kornegay CJ, Staffa JA, Jones CM, McAninch JK. Trends in the concomitant prescribing of opioids and benzodiazepines, 2002–2014. *Am J Prev Med*. 2016;51(2):151–160.

59. National Institute on Drug Abuse. Benzodiazepines and opioids. https://www.drugabuse.gov/drugs-abuse/opioids/benzodiazepines-opioids. Revised March 2018. Accessed January 12, 2019.

60. Scholl L, Seth P, Kariisa M, Wilson N, Baldwin G. Drug and opioid-involved overdose deaths: United States, 2013–2017. *MMWR*. 2018;67(5152):1419–1427.

61. Centers for Disease Control and Prevention, National Center for Injury Prevention and Control. Drug overdose deaths. https://www.cdc.gov/drugoverdose/data/statedeaths.html. Accessed October 15, 2019.

62. Centers for Disease Control and Prevention, National Center for Health Statistics. NVSS vital statistics rapid release: provisional drug overdose death counts. 2019; https://www.cdc.gov/nchs/nvss/vsrr/drug-overdose-data.htm. Accessed October 14, 2019.

63. Benzodiazepine market research report: forecast to 2022. MRFR/Pharma/1674-HCR. *Marketresearchfuture.com*. https://www.marketresearchfuture.com/reports/benzodiazepine-market-2281. Updated June 2020.

64. US Food and Drug Administration. Orange book: approved drug products with therapeutic equivalence evaluations. 2019; http://www.accessdata.fda.gov/scripts/cder/ob/docs/obdetail.cfm?Appl_No=019516&TABLE1=OB_Rx. Accessed March 13, 2019.

65. Drug Enforcement Administration, Office of Diversion Control. ARCOS retail drug summary reports. https://www.deadiversion.usdoj.gov/arcos/retail_drug_summary/index.html. Accessed September 30, 2019.

66. Seago S, Hayek A, Pruszynski J, Newman MG. Change in prescription habits after federal rescheduling of hydrocodone combination products. *Proceedings (Bayl Univ Med Cent)*. 2016;29(3):268–270.

67. Bernhardt MB, Taylor RS, Hagan JL, et al. Evaluation of opioid prescribing after rescheduling of hydrocodone-containing products. *Am J Health Syst Pharm*. 2017;74(24):2046–2053.

68. Center for Responsive Politics. Lobbying expenditures for 2018 by amount and industry sector. *OpenSecrets.org*. https://www.opensecrets.org/lobby/top.php?showYear=2018&indexType=i. Accessed March 13, 2019.

69. Anabolic Steroid Control Act; Pub. L. 101-647, Title XIX (1990). https://www.govinfo.gov/content/pkg/STATUTE-104/pdf/STATUTE-104-Pg4789.pdf. Accessed January 3, 2012.

70. Anabolic Steroid Control Act of 2004, Publ. L. 108-358 (118 Stat. 1661) (2004). https://www.congress.gov/108/plaws/publ358/PLAW-108publ358.pdf. Accessed December 29, 2011.

71. Bureau of Narcotics and Dangerous Drugs, Department of Justice. Final rule: amphetamine, methamphetamine, and optical isomers. *Fed Regist*. 1971;36:12734. https://www.federalregister.gov/.

72. Ait-Daoud N, Hamby AS, Sharma S, Blevins D. A review of alprazolam use, misuse, and withdrawal. *J Addict Med.* 2018;*12*(1):4–10.

73. Drug Enforcement Administration. Benzodiazepines (street names: benzos, downers, nerve pills, tranks). https://www.deadiversion.usdoj.gov/drug_chem_info/benzo. pdf#search=benzodiazepine%20. Published December 2019.

74. Medicine use and spending in the U.S.: a review of 2017 and outlook to 2022. *Iqvia Institute.* https://www.iqvia.com/insights/the-iqvia-institute/reports/medicine-use-and-spending-in-the-us-review-of-2017-outlook-to-2022. Published April 19, 2018.

75. Hedegaard H, Bastian BA, Trinidad JP, et al. Drugs most frequently involved in drug overdose deaths: United States, 2011–2016. *CDC Nat Vital Stat Rep.* 2018;*67*(9):14.

76. National Institute on Drug Abuse. Overdose death rate. https://www.drugabuse.gov/related-topics/trends-statistics/overdose-death-rates. Revised January 2019. Accessed February 26, 2019.

77. Seth P, Rudd RA, Noonan RK, Haegerich TM. Quantifying the epidemic of prescription opioid overdose deaths. *Am J Public Health.* 2018;*108*(4):500–502.

78. Support for Patients and Communities Act, H.R. 6, 115th Congress; Pub. L. 115-271 (October 24, 2018). 2018; https://www.govinfo.gov/content/pkg/PLAW-115publ271/html/PLAW-115publ271.htm.

79. Executive Office of the President, Office of National Drug Control Policy. Epidemic: responding to America's prescription drug abuse crisis. https://www.hsdl.org/?abstract&did=4609. Published 2011. Accessed October 14, 2017.

80. Westat wins Drug Abuse Warning Network (DAWN) contract. *Westat.com* https://www.westat.com/articles/westat-wins-drug-abuse-warning-network-dawn-contract. Published November 12, 2018. Accessed January 22, 2019.

81. Administrative Procedure Act; Pub. L. 79–404, 60 Stat. 237 (1946). https://www.law.cornell.edu/uscode/text/5/part-I/chapter-5. Accessed March 11, 2019.

82. Cortez N. Regulating disruptive innovation. *Berk Technol Law J.* 2014;*29*(1).

83. Brito J. "Agency threats" and the rule of law: an offer you can't refuse. *Harv J L Pub Policy.* 2014;*37*(2):553–577.

CHAPTER 11

Benzodiazepines Today and Tomorrow

What We Know and Don't Know About Them

JOHN J. COLEMAN

HIGHLIGHTS

- Benzodiazepines (BZDs) and related drugs were originally promoted as being virtually free of the problems associated with barbiturates, including nonmedical use (abuse).
- Experience has taught that the unconcern was unjustified.
- The combination of BZDs with opioids is a particularly lethal mix.
- Efforts at regulatory control have been varied and generally inadequate.
- This chapter discusses specific aspects of the problem, plus the broader societal issues.
- New challenges include counterfeit drugs, the existence of a Dark Web, and others.

INTRODUCTION

Benzodiazepines comprise a class of drugs prescribed extensively to treat anxiety and sleep disorders and are used as adjuvant therapy for depression and pain management and as muscle relaxants.[1] Today, they are among the world's most widely used drugs.[2] Diazepam (Valium™), one of the first BZD drugs and one of the more popular members of this growing class of drugs, is on the World Health Organization's (WHO) list of essential medicines.[3] Since the introduction of chlordiazepoxide (Librium®) in 1960, several thousand BZD compounds have been developed from the core molecule of which about a dozen are approved for marketing in the United States by the Food and Drug Administration (FDA).[4]

As beneficial as BZD drugs are for treating certain conditions, their long-term use can be problematic. Introduced as nonaddictive substitutes for barbiturates, it since has become clear that BZD drugs, indeed, do have addictive potential. In addition, they are often used nonmedically alone or, more likely, in combination with other drugs.[4] We discuss this and other factors in this chapter.

In 1984, the United Nations (UN) placed 36 BZDs, including some that are not approved in the United States under international control pursuant to the 1971 UN Convention on Psychotropic Substances.[5] The BZDs were placed in Schedule IV of the Convention, the lowest category requiring control by member states.[6]

In 1990, the UN added midazolam (Versed® in the United States) to its Schedule IV, followed by brotizolam (not approved in the United States) in 1995, and phenazepam (not approved in the United States) in 2016.[5] In 1995, the UN placed flunitrazepam (Rohypnol®, in United States) in Schedule III of the Convention.[5] Schedule III generally is reserved for drugs having a higher likelihood of misuse than Schedule IV drugs. As of October 16, 2019, a total of 181 nations, including the United States, have ratified the UN Convention.[6]

In 1970, the US Congress enacted the Comprehensive Drug Abuse Prevention and Control Act, Title II of which contained the Controlled Substances Act (CSA).[7] The CSA had at least two major purposes, the first of which was to update and consolidate federal drug laws, including those enacted since the 1914 Harrison Narcotic Tax Act, the Marihuana Tax Act of 1937, and the 1965 Drug Abuse Control Amendments to the Federal Food, Drug, and Cosmetic Act. The second major purpose was to bring US domestic law in conformance with obligations occasioned by the Senate's 84–0 vote on May 8, 1967 ratifying the UN's 1961 Single Convention on Narcotic Drugs.

In drafting the CSA, Congress adopted the scheduling schema of the 1961 Single Convention. Instead of four schedules, the CSA contained five, including a schedule (Schedule I) to categorize prohibited drugs and other substances for which there is no acceptable medicinal use. The US Congress also included specific criteria for categorizing drugs and other substances according to each of five schedules.

It should be noted that the UN process and the US process for scheduling drugs differ in substantive ways in deference to the respective jurisdictional interests of both parties. In the case of UN drug scheduling, a medical and scientific evaluation and recommendation is made by the WHO to place a drug is a particular schedule and this recommendation is then voted upon by members of the UN's Commission on Narcotic Drugs (CND).[8] A two-thirds majority of the members of the CND is required for scheduling a drug. Not all member states agree on the legal status, threat of abuse, or medical usefulness of psychotropic drugs, which explains why CND member states vote on scheduling matters to reach consensus.[8]

By comparison, drug scheduling pursuant to the CSA is determined by statutory or administrative rule-making based on medical and scientific evaluations by the FDA and Drug Enforcement Administration (DEA) and a scheduling recommendation from the Assistant Secretary for Health. Collaborative decisions on scheduling are made principally on evaluating a drug or other substance's abuse potential and health consequences. Unlike the UN's drug scheduling process that relies for enforcement on the cooperation of member states, the US drug scheduling process, when completed by legislation or administrative rulemaking has the force of law.

In the United States, BZD drugs have been designated by the CSA as Schedule IV controlled substances.[9,10] This is the next-to-last level in a five-tiered matrix in which level 1 (Schedule I) drugs are prohibited substances because of their high abuse potential and perceived lack of medical utility. Level 5 (Schedule V) drugs are estimated to have the lowest abuse potential needing control. Drugs in Schedules II through V are approved for medical use. Schedule I drugs are available for research only and in accordance with protocols specified in the CSA and requiring the approval of the DEA and the FDA.[i,12] Flunitrazepam, also known as Rohypnol or the "date-rape drug," is unique among the BZD drugs. Although listed as a Schedule IV drug in the CSA, Rohypnol is not approved for medical use in the United States and because of its statutory definition as a date-rape drug, it carries harsher Schedule I penalties for unlawful distribution/possession.[13]

The CSA identifies Schedule IV controlled substances as having "a low potential for abuse relative to the drugs or other substances in schedule III . . . a currently accepted medical use in treatment . . . [and] abuse of the drug or other substance may lead to limited physical dependence or psychological dependence relative to the drugs or other substances in schedule III."[14] Whether and to what extent these criteria may be affected by a drug's interaction with another drug—as in the case of co-ingesting a BZD with an opioid—is not part of the decision-making process for scheduling under the CSA.

The FDA requires a boxed warning on nearly 400 product labels for BZDs, opioids, and opioid-containing cough products to warn prescribers and patients of potentially toxic interactions.[15] The boxed warning advises that the concomitant use of opioids and BZDs may result in profound sedation, respiratory depression, coma, and death.[15]

The FDA took this action in response to a petition from state health officials asking that warnings be included in the prescribing information (labels) of BZDs and opioids.[15] In its evaluation of the petition, the FDA considered data from the Drug Abuse Warning Network (DAWN) showing that hospital emergency department visits between 2004 and 2011 involving the nonmedical use of both classes of drugs increased significantly while overdose deaths involving them nearly tripled.[15] Additional review showed that between 2002 and 2014 there had been an increase of 41% in the number of patients prescribed both BZDs and opioids at the same time.[16] The FDA's review also noted that more than 2.5 million chronic pain patients on opioid medications in 2016 also had been prescribed BZDs.[15]

i. The levels of UN schedules and US schedules are not comparable. Schedule I under the UN's definition are "substances with addictive properties, presenting a serious risk of abuse," while Schedule II includes "substances normally used for medical purposes and given the lowest risk of abuse."[11] Schedule III under the UN's definitions, include "preparations of substances listed in Schedule II, as well as preparations of cocaine," and substances in Schedule IV are "the most dangerous substances, already listed in Schedule I, which are particularly harmful and extremely limited medical or therapeutic value."[11]

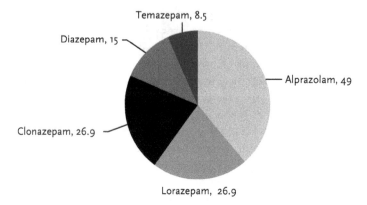

Figure 11.1 Top five BZD by total prescriptions (in millions), 2011.

The DEA reports that in 2011 almost 127 million prescriptions were dispensed for the top five BZD drugs: alprazolam (Xanax®): 49 million (38.6%); lorazepam (Ativan®): 26.9 million (21.2%); clonazepam (Klonopin®): 26.9 million (21.2%); diazepam (Valium®): 15 million (11.8%); and temazepam (Restoril®): 8.5 million (6.7%).[10] See Figure 11.1.

FEDERAL AUTHORITIES REACH OUT TO PRIVATE SECTOR AND STATES FOR BZD DATA

In 2013, to identify the volume of prescribed BZD drugs and opioids, Centers for Disease Control and Prevention (CDC) researchers obtained access to a commercial database (National Prescription Audit) owned and managed by IMS Health, an industry information and intelligence source.[17] Data in this system are collected from approximately 57,000 pharmacies representing about 80% of the retail pharmacies in the United States.[17] The CDC researchers found that in 2012, prescribers wrote 82.5 opioid prescriptions per 100 persons and 37.6 BZD prescriptions per 100 persons in the United States.[17]

Observing that prescribed opioids were involved in 16,917 overdose deaths in 2011, the CDC researchers noted that 31% of these deaths (~5,244) involved BZDs.[17] Persons in the United States, according to the researchers, consumed opioids at a rate greater than any other nation and at twice that of Canada, the second-ranked nation. Opioids and BZDs, they found, often are prescribed for the same patient—a practice, they noted, that increases the risk of overdose.[17]

In 2011, the CDC and FDA established the Prescription Behavior Surveillance System to study data obtained from prescription drug monitoring programs in eight participating states.[ii] Initial findings showed that opioid analgesics were prescribed

---

ii. California, Delaware, Florida, Idaho, Louisiana, Maine, Ohio, and West Virginia.[18]

approximately twice as often as stimulants or BZDs.[18] In addition, prescribing rates were substantially higher for females than for males, and prescribing rates for BZDs for both males and females increased with age.[18]

As expected, alprazolam (Xanax®) was the most frequently prescribed BZD in the eight states, with lorazepam (Ativan®) and clonazepam (Klonopin®) coming in second and third, respectively.[18] See Table 11.1. Researchers noted that the prescription drug monitoring programs data confirmed that persons who are prescribed opioids also are often prescribed BZDs despite the known risks of their additive depressive effects.[18]

Further evidence showing the role of BZDs in opioid-related overdose deaths was cited in a 2018 report by the CDC that began by acknowledging limitations in using a taxonomy promulgated by the *International Classification of Diseases* (ICD) program managed by the WHO.[iii][21] The failure of this system to distinguish between illicitly manufactured fentanyl and prescription fentanyl resulted in the CDC's overstating the number of prescription opioid-related overdose deaths in 2016. Without specifically mentioning this, the CDC's report explained the limitation as follows:

> One limitation of this classification system is that, with few exceptions, ICD-10 codes reflect broad categories of drugs rather than unique specific drugs. For example, oxycodone and hydrocodone are both classified in the same category of natural and semisynthetic opioid analgesics (ICD-10 code T40.2). The broad drug categorizations used in ICD-10 make it difficult to use ICD-10-coded data to monitor trends in deaths involving specific drugs (e.g., deaths involving oxycodone specifically).[21]

What the CDC's report failed to note is that this limitation is not isolated to opioids but affects several other classes of controlled substances, including BZDs that are represented by a single ICD-10 code. Additionally, the ICD coding system does not distinguish between counterfeit and authentic versions of drugs if both contain the same active pharmaceutical ingredient (API).

To address some of these limitations, CDC analysts re-examined original source data—state-furnished death certificates—and tabulated the top 15 drugs involved in causing or contributing to drug-related overdose deaths between 2011 and 2016.[21] Alprazolam was ranked among the top six drugs for each of the years reviewed by the CDC analysts. Diazepam was ranked 9th, 10th, or 11th and clonazepam was ranked 12th or 13th in years 2013 to 2016.[21] Overall, for the six-year period, a total of 42,368 overdose deaths involved one of these three BZDs. This was 14.6% of all drug overdose deaths recorded for this period ($N= 289,915$).[21] See Table 11.2; Figure 11.2.

---

iii. By international convention, the United States and most other nations of the world use a coding taxonomy published by WHO's ICD. As we explain in detail in another chapter, the ICD is limited in the number of T-codes it assigns for tracking opioids and benzodiazepines. Virtually all prescribed opioid drugs are aggregated in just two T-codes (T40.2 and T40.4). All BZD drugs are aggregated in just one T-code (T42.4). Similarly, cocaine and methamphetamine, both available either as prescribed pharmaceutical products or illicitly manufactured versions are identified by the same ICD-10 code (T40.5).[19,20]

Table 11.1 PRESCRIBING RATES FOR BZDS, EIGHT STATES, 2013 (FROM PRESCRIPTION DRUG MONITORING PROGRAMS DATA)

Benzodiazepine	State							
	California	Delaware	Florida	Idaho	Louisiana	Maine	Ohio	West Virginia
Alprazolam	92.1	207.9	220.9	99.2	240.2	103.8	159.2	226.0
Chlordiazepoxide	1.5	1.5	3.7	1.4	3.0	2.4	1.9	2.5
Clonazepam	54.1	79.4	99.2	73.0	129.4	139.6	89.6	114.1
Clorazepate	0.7	1.2	4.4	1.6	8.7	1.7	2.9	2.6
Diazepam	34.3	43.2	50.9	39.3	67.0	61.2	53.9	72.0
Estazolam	0.4	0.3	1.0	0.4	0.6	0.3	0.4	0.4
Flurazepam	1.7	0.6	1.2	0.6	1.6	0.6	0.7	0.5
Lorazepam	90.1	69.5	87.3	83.3	77.2	160.5	115.2	119.5
Oxazepam	1.3	1.2	0.9	0.3	1.1	2.0	1.6	3.0
Temazepam	29.9	20.7	74.1	18.3	43.5	12.6	21.4	29.3
Triazolam	4.1	2.0	4.7	5.8	7.7	2.5	2.9	1.8
Other	0.6	0.9	0.5	1.2	0.7	1.1	1.0	0.5
Total	**310.7**	**428.2**	**548.8**	**324.3**	**580.8**	**488.3**	**450.7**	**572.1**

Note: Results are given per LOCO state residents.

Table 11.2 TOP 15 DRUGS IDENTIFIED IN DRUG OVERDOSE DEATHS IN UNITED STATES, 2011–2016

Rank[a]	2011 (n = 41,340)			2012 (n = 41,502)			2013 (n = 43,9621)		
	Referent Drug	Number of Deaths[b]	Percentage of Deaths[c]	Referent Drug	Number of Deaths[b]	Percentage of Deaths[c]	Referent Drug	Number of Deaths[b]	Percentage of Deaths[c]
1	Oxycodone	5,587	13.5	Heroin	6,155	14.8	Heroin	8,418	19.1
2	Cocaine	5,070	12.3	Oxycodone	5,178	12.5	Cocaine	5,319	12.1
3	Heroin	4,571	11.1	Cocaine	4,780	11.5	Oxycodone	4,967	11.3
4	Methadone	4,545	11.0	Methadone	4,087	9.8	Morphine	3,772	8.6
5	Alprazolam	4,066	9.8	Alprazolam	3,803	9.2	Alprazolam	3,724	8.5
6	Morphine	3,290	8.0	Morphine	3,513	8.5	Methadone	3,700	8.4
7	Hydrocodone	3,206	7.8	Hydrocodone	3,037	7.3	Methamphetamine	3,194	7.3
8	Methamphetamine	1,887	4.6	Methamphetamine	2,267	5.5	Hydrocodone	3,113	7.1
9	Diazepam	1,698	4.1	Fentanyl	1,615	3.9	Fentanyl	1,919	4.4
10	Fentanyl	1,662	4.0	Diazepam	1,577	3.8	Diazepam	1,618	3.7
11	Diphenhydramine	1,226	3.0	Diphenhydramine	1,300	3.1	Diphenhydramine	1,360	3.1
12	Oxymorphone	1,190	2.9	Citalopram	1,042	2.5	Tramadol	1,009	2.3
13	Citalopram	1,043	2.5	Tramadol	935	2.3	Clonazepam	946	2.2
14	Acetaminophen	879	2.1	Oxymorphone	866	2.1	Citalopram	914	2.1
15	Tramadol	849	2.1	Amitriptyline	835	2.0	Amitriptyline	815	1.9

(continued)

Table 11.2 CONTINUED

Rank[a]	2014 (n = 47,055) Referent Drug	Number of Deaths[b]	Percentage of Deaths[c]	2015 (n = 52,404) Referent Drug	Number of Deaths[b]	Percentage of Deaths[c]	2016 (n = 63,632) Referent Drug	Number of Deaths[b]	Percentage of Deaths[c]
1	Heroin	10,882	23.1	Heroin	13,318	25.4	Fentanyl	18,335	28.8
2	Cocaine	5,892	12.5	Fentanyl	8,251	15.7	Heroin	15,961	25.1
3	Oxycodone	5,431	11.5	Cocaine	7,324	14.0	Cocaine	11,316	17.8
4	**Alprazolem**	4,237	9.0	Oxycodone	5,792	11.1	Methamphetamine	6,762	10.6
5	Fentanyl	4,223	9.0	Methamphetamine	5,092	9.7	**Alprazolam**	6,209	9.8
6	Morphine	4,024	8.6	**Alprazolem**	4,801	9.2	Oxycodone	6,199	9.7
7	Methamphetamine	3,747	8.0	Morphine	4,226	8.1	Morphine	5,014	7.9
8	Methadone	3,498	7.4	Methadone	3,376	6.4	Methadone	3,493	5.5
9	Hydrocodone	3,299	7.0	Hydrocodone	3,051	5.8	Hydrocodone	3,199	5.0
10	**Diazepam**	1,748	3.7	Diphenhydramine	1,798	3.4	**Diazepam**	2,022	3.2
11	Diphenhydramine	1,614	3.4	**Diazepam**	1,796	3.4	Diphenhydramine	2,008	3.2
12	Tramadol	1,175	2.5	**Clonazepam**	1,328	2.5	**Clonazepam**	1,656	2.6
13	**Clonazepam**	1,139	2.4	Gabapentin	1,222	2.3	Gabapentin	1,546	2.4
14	Citalopram	1,014	2.2	Tramadol	1,177	2.2	Tramadol	1,250	2.0
15	Oxymorphone	909	1.9	Oxymorphone	1,006	1.9	Amphetamine	1,193	1.9

Notes: BZDs are in bold. Drug overdose deaths are identified using *International Classification of Diseases, Tenth revision* (ICD-10) underlying cause-of-death codes X40-X44, X60-X64, X85, and Y10-Y14. Deaths may involve other drugs in addition to the referent drug (i.e., the one listed). Deaths involving more than one drug (e.g., a death involving both heroin and cocaine) are counted in bath totals. Caution should be used when comparing numbers across years. The reporting of at least once specific drug or drug class in the literal text, as identified using ICD-10 multiple cause-of-death codes T36-T50.8, improved from 75% of drug overdose deaths in 2011 to 85% at drug overdose deaths in 2016.

[a]Ranks were rot tested for statistical significance.
[b]Number of drug overdose deaths involving the referent drug.
[c]Percentage of drug overdose deaths invoking the referent drug.
Source: NCHS, National Vital Statistic System, Mortality files linked with death certificate literal text, 2011–2016.

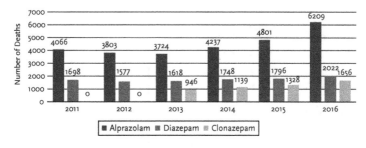

Figure 11.2 Overdose deaths involving BZDs, 2011–2016.
Source: NVSS/FDA data.

In 2012, the Substance Abuse and Mental Health Services Administration (SAMHSA) terminated the DAWN program that for several decades had tracked drug-related hospital emergency department episodes and drug-related overdose deaths.[22] As a result, states increased their tracking of drug-related mortality and morbidity. Currently, more than 30 states have funding agreements with the CDC to provide drug-related mortality information that identifies opioids involved in overdose deaths by specific chemical names.[23] This arrangement is somewhat peculiar, inasmuch as the states collect information from the very same source data (death certificates) furnished by them to the CDC for the very same purpose. Unlike the CDC, however, the states use the literal language of the certificates to classify drug overdose deaths rather than ICD coding algorithms.[24]

Florida has established a model for tracking drug-related mortality. For several decades, the Medical Examiners Commission (MEC), a division of the Florida Department of Law Enforcement, has published detailed data on drug-related overdose deaths investigated by the state's medical examiners.[25] In 2017, for example, the MEC reported that drugs were identified in 12,439 deaths in the state.[26] Each year, the MEC issues a report that presents toxicology data from the autopsies of drug overdose victims. When describing BZD-related deaths, the MEC's annual report identifies each of 13 specific BZD drugs by the number of drug overdose deaths in which they were found to be present.[iv] See Figures 11.3 and 11.4.

As expected, alprazolam figured prominently in the MEC 2017 report for drug-related deaths in Florida. The MEC report showed that alprazolam was identified in 37.4% of postmortem toxicology screens in which a BZD was present.[26] See Figures 11.3 and 11.4. This is remarkably consistent with findings that showed alprazolam accounted for approximately one-third of all the BZD drugs mentioned by name in DAWN hospital emergency department visits from 2004 to 2011. See Table 11.3.

---

iv. By comparison, the CDC's National Vital Statistics System transforms the literal language of the cause of death statements in drug overdose-related death certificates into aggregated categories by drug classes. This means that any mention of a BZD by specific chemical or brand name in a death certificate is recorded in the CDC's mortality database as a benzodiazepine as required by the ICD's coding (T42.4) for this entire class of drugs.[20]

DRUG PRESENT IN BODY		CAUSE	PRESENT	TOTAL OCCURRENCES
Amphetamine	Amphetamine	256	598	854
	Methamphetamine	464	394	858
Benzodiazepines	Alprazolam	791	394	858
	Chlordiazepoxide	18	79	97
	Clonazepam	106	437	543
	Diazepam	178	429	607
	Estazolam	2	2	4
	Flunitrazepam	1	0	1
	Flurazepam	1	5	6
	Lorazepam	40	262	302
	Midazolam	4	177	181
	Nordiazepam	109	529	638
	Oxazepam	39	296	335
	Temazepam	83	374	457
	Trizolam	2	2	4
	Ethanol	975	4,283	5,258
Hallucinogenics	Phencyclidine (PCP)	2	1	3
	PCP Analogs	2	0	2
	Phenethylamines/Piperazines	18	18	36
	Tryptamines	1	3	4

Figure 11.3 Summary of drug occurrences in decedents, 2017.

Note: Benzodiazepines not included individually constituted less than one percent of occurrences. Percentages may not sum to 100 percent because of rounding. Several benzodiazepines (for example, diazepam) are metabolized to other benzodiazepines in the body (for examble, nordiazepam, oxazepam, and temazepam). Thus, occurrences of nordiazepan, oxazepam, and temazepam may be due to the ingestion of diazepam, chlordiazepoxide, and/or temazepam.

Source: Florida Medical Examiners Commission Drug Report 2017.

Like all FDA-approved medications, BZDs provide therapeutic benefits that a vast majority of patients consider essential. These benefits are fully detailed elsewhere in this book by medical practitioners. What we wish to convey in this chapter first and foremost is that despite their beneficial uses for those who take them as prescribed, these drugs, when taken for nonmedical purposes (and even when taken appropriately), can pose serious health risks. These risks are significantly increased when BZDs are taken with other drugs, particularly opioids, and/or with beverage alcohol. These risks may carry over to legitimate patients requiring both opioids and BZDs to deal with common co-morbidities of depression/anxiety and pain.

The evidence discussed in this chapter shows more often than not that when BZDs are used nonmedically with other drugs, notably opioids, they can be deadly. The CDC acknowledged this formally in 2016 when it issued detailed guidance for primary care clinicians prescribing opioids for chronic pain.[27] The CDC's guidance recommended that clinicians discuss with patients receiving chronic opioid therapy the "increased risks for respiratory depression when opioids are taken with benzodiazepines, other sedatives, alcohol, illicit drugs such as heroin, or other opioids."[27]

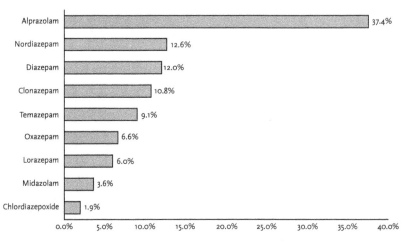

Figure 11.4 Frequency of occurrence of benzodiazepines, January–December 2017.
Source: Florida Medical Examiners Commission Drug Report 2017.

CDC's guidance did not recommend against prescribing BZDs and opioids together when therapeutically indicated but, instead, stressed the need for close medical supervision in such cases.[27] Chronic pain patients with mental health conditions, the CDC noted, often require BZDs to address depression, anxiety disorders, and posttraumatic stress disorder.[27]

Although drug scheduling has not been discussed thus far, it is worth taking a moment to review the relevant provisions of the Controlled Substances Act (CSA) that pertain to medicinal controlled substances. Pharmaceutical drugs determined by FDA and DEA to have abuse potential requiring control must be placed in tiered categories, or schedules, according to their relative abuse liability.[28]

Both Schedule I and II drugs have the same high abuse potential and differ only in that the therapeutic benefits of Schedule II drugs outweigh their abuse risks and, as a result, are approved by FDA for medical use under close supervision. Schedule I drugs are not approved for medical use and, therefore, cannot be prescribed or dispensed in the United States.[v] A Schedule III drug has less abuse potential than a Schedule II drug but greater abuse potential than a Schedule IV drug. A Schedule IV drug, in turn, has less abuse potential than a Schedule III drug, and a Schedule V drug has minimal abuse potential.[29]

In 1975, using its administrative law authority, DEA placed six BZD drugs[vi] in Schedule IV of the CSA (see also Chapter 12 of this volume).[30] In 1981, alprazolam was added to Schedule IV.[31] In 1984, estazolam and 20 other BZD drugs were placed in Schedule IV pursuant to a provision in the CSA requiring the United States to conform

v. The Code of Federal Regulations permits the use of Schedule I controlled substances under certain conditions and with the concurrence of the FDA for research.[12]
vi. Chlordiazepoxide, diazepam, oxazepam, clorazepate, flurazepam, and clonazepam.[30]

Table 11.3 DAWN DATA, 2004–2011, FOR BZD DRUG ED VISITS

National Estimates of Drug-Related Visits 2004-2011 by BZD Drug

	2004	2005	2006	2007	2008	2009	2010	2011
Benzodiazepines	58,601	81,686	86,948	85,879	109,824	131,869	146,983	152,179
Alprazolam	19,027	22,414	25,259	29,928	39,081	42,304	48,620	50,591
Chlordiazepoxide								
Clonazepam	7,082	7,794	9,054	10,593	14,270	14,437	14,639	16,252
Clorazepate								
Diazpem	5,739	5,930	5,544	7,082	8,577	6,472	6,250	8,158
Flurazepam								
Lorazepam	2,382	3,221	3,679	3,918	6,040	4,895	6,369	5,087
Oxazepam								
Temazepam	920	533	751	663	755	321	602	
Triazolam								
Benzodiazepines-NOS	28,028	45,721	46,274	38,575	48,866	68,618	75,259	81,514

Notes: An omitted result means that it does not meet the standards of precision and has been suppressed because the relative standard error exceeds 50% or the unweighted count is less than 30. NOS = not otherwise specified.

Source: Drug Abuse Warning Network, 2011: Selected tables of national estimates of drug-related emergency department visits. Rockville, MD: Center for Behavioral Health Statistics and Quality: SAMHSA, 2013.

its domestic drug controls to international treaties to which the United States is a party.[32,33]

The CSA provides for changing the schedule of a drug or other substance when warranted. After consulting with and receiving a medical and scientific evaluation from the Department of Health and Human Services (HHS), along with a scheduling recommendation, the DEA may initiate rule-making proceedings to schedule a drug or change the schedule of a drug—or, for that matter, remove a drug entirely from the schedules.[34] Besides the designated offices of the attorney general and Secretary of the Department of Health and Human Services, this action may be initiated by a petition by "any interested party."[35]

Thus far, there has been no expressed interest by the FDA or the DEA (or "any interested party) to move BZD drugs from Schedule IV to a higher schedule. Based on the information discussed in this chapter, one might argue that alprazolam warrants placement in a higher schedule, perhaps even Schedule II, because the frequency of its nonmedical use is similar to that of drugs in Schedule II. While true, we believe there are practical and legal considerations that argue against rescheduling alprazolam.

Given the variety of BZD drugs currently available, focusing increased control solely on one—alprazolam—likely would drive BZD abusers to other BZDs in Schedule IV. To be effective, a rescheduling action would have to include placing all BZD drugs in a higher schedule. The practical differences in regulatory control between Schedule III and Schedule IV drugs are minimal, so moving BZDs to Schedule III would have little or no effect on consumer access. Moving all BZDs to Schedule II, a category dominated by opioids and amphetamines would be unrealistic and difficult, if not impossible, to justify on legal grounds. Besides meeting the statutory criterion for having a high abuse potential, a Schedule II drug also must satisfy the criterion that "the drug or other substances may lead to severe psychological or physical dependence."[36]

While BZD drugs taken chronically are known to produce tolerance in some patients, this response is not uniform in all patients or with all BZD drugs, nor is it considered to have clinical significance when specific BZD drugs are used to treat certain conditions (elsewhere in this volume the issues of tolerance is dealt with in more detail).[2] These variables, it seems, would complicate the rescheduling of an entire class of drugs simply because of the abuse level of one member of the class—although, in truth, this has been done in the past by administrative rule-making for amphetamines and by statute for anabolic steroids.[37,38]

These rare administrative and statutory actions notwithstanding, it appears that reducing the misuse of BZDs will depend not on changing their schedule but, instead, on improved education for patients, prescribers, and the public. First and foremost, however, the government needs to improve its drug abuse data collection, specifically how it monitors drug-related morbidity and mortality. Understanding these dynamics in a timely and comprehensive manner is essential for designing public health strategies that reduce drug abuse and drug-related overdose deaths.

The popularity of alprazolam among BZD abusers has generated a secondary market for counterfeit Xanax tablets manufactured abroad and smuggled into the United States, or, as we discuss later in this chapter, manufactured in the United States by traffickers. Although beyond the scope of this chapter to go into great detail regarding the role of counterfeit drugs, it may be useful to cite briefly a few timely examples involving counterfeit BZDs (i.e., alprazolam) to illustrate the future threat this poses.

In 2018, a criminal complaint was filed in the US District Court for the District of Vermont charging Yazid Al Fayyad Finn with conspiracy to violate the CSA, "by attempting to possess with intent to distribute Alprazolam, which is a Schedule IV controlled substance under federal law."[39] Finn was linked to a Canadian accomplice named Cedrik Bougault-Morin, arrested in North Troy, Vermont, after crossing into the United States from Canada in possession "of approximately 90 kilograms of counterfeit Xanax tablets."[39] A footnote in the agent's affidavit explained: "Xanax© is a trade name pharmaceutical tablet manufactured by Pfizer Incorporated. The counterfeit Xanax tablets seized were later tested and confirmed to contain Alprazolam, a Schedule IV controlled substance."[39] In February 2018, DEA reported the arrest of an individual in San Diego, California, in possession of a pill press machine capable of manufacturing 10,000 counterfeit pills at a time. A search resulted in the seizure of a pistol with a silencer, approximately 8,000 counterfeit Xanax pills, and a quarter-pound of cocaine.[40]

In May 2017, DEA offices in Texas executed a search warrant and seized 35 pounds of fraudulent oxycodone tablets containing fentanyl. The search also uncovered four pill presses, 1 pound of fentanyl powder, 13 pounds of counterfeit Adderall and Xanax tablets containing methamphetamine, 1 pound of crystal methamphetamine, and multiple weapons.[40]

On May 31, 2017, an indictment was filed in the US District Court in Salt Lake City, Utah, charging six young adults with unlawfully importing fentanyl and alprazolam from China.[41] Charges included sales of thousands of counterfeit alprazolam tablets manufactured to resemble an approved form of this drug. Authorities seized a commercial pill press and die punches containing logos for a popular Xanax tablet (GG249) and for a well-known generic 30 mg oxycodone tablet. The indictment revealed that fentanyl, not oxycodone, was contained in the pills resembling the oxycodone tablets. [41]

On October 18, 2018, a superseding indictment in the Salt Lake City case charged the head of the organization with aiding and abetting the distribution of a controlled substance resulting in the death of at least one victim. The indictment added distribution charges totaling more than 66,000 fentanyl tablets counterfeited to resemble 30 mg oxycodone tablets and more than 175,000 alprazolam tablets counterfeited to resemble a well-known form of Xanax. More than $6 million in US currency, bitcoin, and silver bars were seized and held for criminal forfeiture.[42] On August 30, 2019, a jury convicted Aaron Michael Shamo, the ringleader of this group, of 12 felony counts, including one that carries a mandatory prison sentence of life without parole.[43]

In October 2015, a 29-year old resident of Aptos, California, took a Xanax tablet and a Benadryl tablet to help him sleep through a bout of hives that was causing him to itch relentlessly. Sometime during the night, he died. An autopsy revealed that the Xanax tablet he consumed contained fentanyl instead of alprazolam. Police later arrested a suspect in possession of a quantity of deadly counterfeit Xanax tablets.[44] A subsequent investigation linked a second death to this batch of counterfeit Xanax pills containing fentanyl.[45]

These stories highlight the rising threat from counterfeit versions of popular drugs like Xanax. As a drug gains market demand, the global underworld quickly moves to replicate its design and introduce it into the international drug commerce. This may happen as a result of Internet direct-to-consumer advertising or by clandestinely introducing bulk shipments into commercial drug supplies. The case previously described in Utah used the Dark Web, a compartmentalized and restricted segment of the Internet accessible by special software that purportedly enables users and operators to remain anonymous.

The authorities have managed to penetrate the Dark Web's technological veil of secrecy on several occasions. The latest example of this was reported on May 3, 2019 when a two-year international investigation was culminated by DEA, the German Federal Criminal Police (the Bundeskriminalamt), the German Public Prosecutor's Office in Frankfurt, the Dutch National Police (Politie), the Netherlands National Prosecutor's Office, Federal Police of Brazil (Policia Federal), Europol and Eurojust, the latter two organizations representing the consolidated law enforcement and liaison resources of the 28-nation European Union.[46-48]

Four defendants arrested in the United States and Germany operated a business on the Dark Web called "Wall Street Marketplace" (WSM), a Web hosting service that allowed approximately 5,400 vendors to sell illegal goods, including controlled substances, to about 1.15 million customers around the world.[48] Three defendants who were arrested in Germany supervised WSM and managed a sophisticated website accessible in six languages to accommodate WSM's vast global vendor network and customer base. One vendor connected to this operation is currently serving a 12-year prison sentence in the United States for selling a fentanyl nasal spray to a customer in Florida who suffered a fatal drug overdose.[48]

While this case shows that global law enforcement authorities can penetrate and immobilize Dark Web operations, there is no certainty that this will be the case in the future as criminals and the technicians that aid them develop more sophisticated ways to evade detection.

The emergence of large-scale criminal enterprises making and distributing counterfeit controlled substances greatly complicates the task of addressing the abuse of lawful drugs. Conventional control strategies, for example, that focus on DEA-registered commercial supply chain operations are completely irrelevant when it comes to stopping the flow of counterfeit drugs manufactured by criminals. It is clear just from the handful of examples that we cite in this chapter that the line between the illicit and licit drug trade has been blurred with the emergence of counterfeit BZDs containing alprazolam, the labeled API.

Dealing with this phenomenon will require new and improved technology, close cooperation between the regulatory community and lawful drug manufacturers, implementation of FDA's long-overdue "pedigree" requirements for prescription drugs, and, possibly, amendments to the CSA specifically to address the counterfeiting of controlled substances.[vii] In 2011, the FDA published guidance on the incorporation of physical-chemical identifiers (PCID) in solid oral dosage forms of drugs to identify and, possibly deter, counterfeit versions.[50] There is no public record indicating that any drug sponsor followed the FDA's guidance. It is time for this guidance to be mandated by agency rule-making or congressional legislation.

Presently, there is no way for any of the data systems we discussed in this chapter to distinguish illicitly manufactured Xanax from the real product if both contain alprazolam. Forensic testing may be able to make such a distinction, assuming, that is, that the chemistry and manufacturing processes for the authentic and counterfeit samples differ in some measurable way. Whether such a distinction can be made in a routine postmortem toxicology screening of bodily fluids is uncertain because the analytes of the counterfeit and the authentic drug—if both contain the same API—will be indistinguishable.

While some may view differences between counterfeit and authentic drugs containing the same API as unimportant, they have significant meaning for government authorities tasked with protecting the nation's public health and its drug supply. As we mentioned earlier, a strategy designed to address practices by DEA-registered manufacturers and distributors of controlled substances, by necessity, will be markedly different from a strategy intended to address criminal organizations manufacturing and distributing counterfeit drugs.

The successful government crackdown on pill mills, rogue Internet pharmacies, and corrupt practitioners that reduced the volume of prescription drug sales in the past several years created a vacuum in the illicit (i.e., diverted) supply of these drugs that, in turn, may have given rise to the deadly commerce in counterfeit versions of them. To be sure, the counterfeit drug phenomenon has been around for many years, but until recently, it focused mostly on counterfeiting chemotherapy drugs, lifestyle drugs, and expensive biologicals. An increased demand for prescription drugs, principally opioids and BZDs, has moved controlled substances into the counterfeiting arena.[viii]

Until recently, rogue Internet pharmacies offering to sell controlled substances without a prescription were largely considered fraudulent operations, often located in foreign areas where law enforcement and drug control were lax or nonexistent. For the most part, if these Web-based enterprises delivered drugs to their customers, there was a better-than-even chance that the drugs were bogus or contained little of the labeled and expected ingredients.

vii. The CSA already addresses counterfeit substances: "Unlawful acts . . . to create, distribute, or dispense, or possess with intent to distribute or dispense, a counterfeit substance."[49] As currently written, however, counterfeit Xanax tablets containing alprazolam imported unlawfully from abroad would expose a trafficker to the same Schedule IV penalty ("not more than 5 years" and a fine) as one would be exposed for distributing, dispensing, or possessing with intent to distribute or dispense, a noncounterfeit version of the same API. Because of the added risks in consuming a counterfeit drug of dubious origin, purity, and dosing strength, we believe the CSA should provide for enhanced penalties when the drug in question is counterfeit.

viii. A study of regulatory and law enforcement sources revealed the average street price for hydrocodone and oxycodone is about one dollar per milligram.[51] This is almost 20 times the price of the drugs at retail pharmacies.

According to the UN's Office of Drugs and Crime, more than 90% of global trade is transported by sea and over 500 million maritime containers that move this trade throughout the world each year, with only 2% of these containers inspected by authorities for contraband.[52] These conditions favor large drug and chemical companies in China and India that are aggressively advertising and distributing bulk supplies of APIs and precursor chemicals despite the fact that this commerce is controlled by international and national laws.[ix] Using second and third countries as transshipment hubs and falsely invoicing the contents of shipments can bring bulk supplies of these drugs to underground counterfeit pill makers anywhere in the world, including—as we showed previously—the United States.

In recent years, several states have considered and at least two (Vermont and Colorado) have adopted regulations permitting the personal importation of pharmaceutical drugs from Canada. The rationale for this is to give patients access to cheaper prices for drugs. The FDA has warned that buying drugs from unregulated foreign sources may result in receiving outdated, counterfeit, and potentially toxic substances. Some foreign-based Internet "pharmacies" offer to sell controlled substances, including BZDs, without requiring a prescription. This, however, remains illegal under federal law. Nonetheless, the expansion of the international market for prescription drugs has provided increased opportunities for criminal organizations to introduce counterfeit drugs, including controlled substances, into the unregulated or loosely regulated international supply chain.

In 2006, the FDA investigated two Canadian companies filling prescriptions for US customers. The companies, Mediplan Prescription Plus Pharmacy and Mediplan Global Health, both of Manitoba, operated 10 Web-based pharmacies purporting to sell Canadian-approved drugs. The FDA's investigation found counterfeits of the following prescription drugs: Lipitor, Crestor, Zetia/Ezetrol, Diovan, Hyzaar, Actonel, Nexium, Celebrex, Arimidex, and Propecia.[53]

Counterfeit controlled substances pose many problems—both for the legitimate patient hoping to save money as well as for public health officials trying to reduce drug-related morbidity and mortality. Until recently, pharmaceutical companies had exclusive control of the patented and/or licensed products they were authorized to make and market. This no longer is the case. As sophisticated drug precursors and finished API become readily available on the Internet (or Dark Web), and the science of pharmaceutics is simplified by information provided in a patent (available online) or via an underground publication or website, the production and distribution of counterfeit drugs likely will increase.

ix. India and China (including Hong Kong, Taiwan, and Macao) are parties to the 1971 UN Convention on Psychotropic Substances and the 1988 Convention Against the Illicit Traffic in Narcotic Drugs and Psychotropic Substances that contains a number of provisions specifically calling for internal controls on the manufacturing and export of Schedule I to IV drugs, including BZDs. Enforcement of these controls, however, are left to the discretion of each party.

CONCLUSION

In this chapter we presented information about BZDs and how they contribute to morbidity and mortality among drug abusers. Rather than focus solely on the prevalence of BZD nonmedical use—something we do in greater detail in another chapter and throughout this volume—we looked at the general environment and societal circumstances surrounding or influencing the misuse of these drugs as well as the riskier and potentially deadly co-ingestion of BZDs with opioids.

A military proverb of uncertain origin warns that generals always prepare to fight the last war. The same might be said for government agencies and officials tasked with reducing drug abuse. As we note in the text, the data systems used to measure drug-related morbidity and mortality were designed almost a half-century ago. They are inadequate to assess today's needs and incapable of assessing the emerging world of extreme substances and high-dose API counterfeit drugs. They are not designed to collect information about drugs obtained from unregulated commercial pharmaceutical and chemical industries that deal exclusively on the Dark Web segment of the Internet. In short, none of these data collection efforts, including the ICD taxonomy we discussed in the text, cannot meet today's needs for protecting the public health and safety. The emerging threat from counterfeit drugs containing authentic API obliterates the line between the licit and illicit drug channels, thus further complicating an already difficult task for regulators and patients alike.

The counterfeit drugs as previously noted in the 2006 FDA investigation of two Canadian pharmacies were popular therapeutic substances for treating conditions and illnesses. They were not controlled substances. We may assume that those who intended to consume these products would not do so unless they considered them necessary to maintain their health. Controlled substances differ from this paradigm in that people choose to use controlled substances for nonmedical purposes—for the psychic effect they provide—as well as for unsupervised medical purposes. This important distinction builds a customer base for controlled substances far larger than what might be expected based on therapeutic needs alone.

The handful of cases we mention in this chapter are indeed commendable for what they represent in global liaison, investigative acumen, and technology, but they also warn that the vulnerabilities that permitted authorities to intervene are not permanent and that in the future traffickers may be able to work around these vulnerabilities to avoid detection. To have a chance against such odds, government authorities, especially those in the United States, must move aggressively to design and implement dynamic systems capable of effectively dealing with the threats identified in this chapter.

In October 2018, Congress enacted the Support for Patients and Communities Act.[54] Among its many provisions, the act instructs the CDC to modernize its system for coding causes of death related to drug overdoses. It also calls for creating a system to collect data on drug and alcohol abuse cases from hospital emergency departments. This, in effect, authorizes and calls for the reinstitution of DAWN that we described in this chapter and which, for more than three decades, monitored hospital emergency department admissions for drug misuse/abuse. As we mentioned in the text, it was abruptly terminated by HHS in 2011 at the very height of the opioid abuse crisis. This act is a good first step in the right direction, but it hardly encourages the type of innovative thinking needed to address the emerging drug threats that we identified in this chapter.

This act followed the recommendations of the 2017 report of the *President's Commission on Combatting Drug Addiction and the Opioid Crisis* to reinstate the DAWN system.[55] We applaud these efforts by the Commission and Congress even though, in truth, like military generals, they are fighting the last war. For example, we question the wisdom of SAMHSA in awarding a contract to the vendor who supplied DAWN services when the system was terminated in 2011. Although it can be said that this vendor is familiar with the program of tracking hospital emergency departments and medical examiners for drug-related morbidity and mortality, its management of the program and the timeliness of its data when it managed the program were criticized.[56,57]

We think it would have been better for SAMHSA to have solicited competitive bidding for this program using a statement of work to describe a system that avoids the limitations in the former DAWN program and ensures a more reliable and timelier data set. Virtually all US hospitals with emergency care facilities depend upon HHS for funding and support. This should facilitate cooperative agreements that expand DAWN's sampling base and enhance its information collection.

In addition, we urge federal authorities tasked with modernizing the CDC's system for coding drug overdose deaths and reinstituting DAWN to go beyond these 1970s-era programs and include a new generation of forensic tools and methodologies to identify specific agents causing or contributing to drug-related morbidity and mortality. As noted in the text, the states are ahead of the CDC in performing these tasks, and many are funded and supported by the CDC in this effort. We believe that the newly reinstituted DAWN program could serve as a vehicle to acquire detailed drug overdose death data from all the states and territories.

When it comes to addressing the nation's persistent and changing drug abuse problem, there is a need for rapid response capability—something that clearly is not present in the capabilities of HHS, the world's largest bureaucracy. A review of internal correspondence between SAMHSA officials and others within the HHS, obtained by this author pursuant to the Freedom of Information Act, reveals a corporate environment in which even the most minuscule decision must be vetted through multiple levels of approval. This may explain why it takes agencies within HHS years to accomplish even simple tasks and why programs like DAWN are allowed to vanish overnight and be forgotten.

REFERENCES

1. Canadian Agency for Drugs and Technologies in Health. *Discontinuation Strategies for Patients with Long-term Benzodiazepine Use: A Review of Clinical Evidence and Guidelines.* Ottawa, ON: Canadian Agency for Drugs and Technologies in Health; 2015.
2. American Psychiatric Association. *Benzodiazepine Dependence, Toxicity, and Abuse: A Task Force Report of the American Psychiatric Association.* Washington, DC: APA; 1990.

3. World Health Organization. WHO model list of essential medicines. http://apps.who.int/iris/bitstream/handle/10665/273826/EML-20-eng.pdf?ua=1. Published 2017. Accessed November 24, 2018.

4. Doweiko HE, Evans AL. *Concepts of Chemical Dependency*. 10th ed. Boston, MA: Cengage; 2018.

5. United Nations, Office on Drugs and Crime. Non-medical use of benzodiazepines: a growing threat to public health? https://www.unodc.org/documents/scientific/Global_SMART_Update_2017_Vol_18.pdf. Published 2017. Accessed October 16, 2019.

6. United Nations, Treaty Collection. Convention on psychotropic substances. https://treaties.un.org/Pages/ViewDetails.aspx?src=TREATY&mtdsg_no=VI-16&chapter=6&lang=en. Published February 1971. Accessed October 16, 2019.

7. Comprehensive Drug Abuse Prevention and Control Act of 1970; Pub. L. 91-51; Controlled Substances Act, Title 21, Food and Drugs, Chapter 13: Drug Abuse Prevention Control, Sec. 801, et seq. (1970). Accessed March 22, 2019.

8. United Nations, Office of Drugs and Crime. Scheduling procedures. https://www.unodc.org/documents/commissions/CND/Scheduling_Resource_Material/Scheduling_procedures_detailed.pdf. Published July 2019. Accessed October 18, 2019.

9. Code of Federal Regulations. Title 21, Section 1308.14, Schedule IV Controlled Substances. 2018. Accessed January 19, 2019.

10. Drug Enforcement Administration. Benzodiazepines: street names: benzos, downers, nerve pills, tranks. https://www.deadiversion.usdoj.gov/drug_chem_info/benzo.pdf#search=benzodiazepine%20. Published 2013. Accessed November 24, 2018.

11. European Monitoring Centre for Drugs and Drug Addiction. Classification of controlled drugs (according to 1961 Single Convention). http://www.emcdda.europa.eu/publications/topic-overviews/classification-of-controlled-drugs/html_en. Accessed October 18, 2019.

12. Code of Federal Regulations. 21 CFR 1301.18 (Research protocols) (2018). https://www.govinfo.gov/content/pkg/CFR-2018-title21-vol9/xml/CFR-2018-title21-vol9-chapII.xml. Accessed May 25, 2019.

13. Hillory J. Farias and Samantha Reid Date-Rape Drug Prohibition Act of 2000; Pub. L. 106–172 (2000). http://www.gpo.gov/fdsys/pkg/PLAW-106publ172/pdf/PLAW-106publ172.pdf. Accessed January 3, 2012.

14. Controlled Substances Act, Title II, 21 USC 812(b)(4)(A), Pub. L. 91-513, 84 Stat. 1242 (1970). http://uscode.house.gov/. Accessed February 25, 2019.

15. Food and Drug Administration. FDA news release: FDA requires strong warnings for opioid analgesics, prescription opioid cough products, and benzodiazepine labeling related to serious risks and death from combined use. https://www.fda.gov/NewsEvents/Newsroom/PressAnnouncements/ucm518697.htm. Published August 31, 2016. Accessed January 12, 2019.

16. Hwang CS, Kang EM, Kornegay CJ, et al. Trends in the concomitant prescribing of opioids and benzodiazepines, 2002–2014. *Am J Prev Med.* 2016;51(2):151–160.

17. Paulozzi LJ, Mack KA, Hockenberry JM. Variation among states in prescribing of opioid pain relievers and benzodiazepines—United States, 2012. *J Safety Res.* 2014;51:125–129.

18. Paulozzi LJ, Strickler GK, Kreiner PW, Koris CM. Controlled substance prescribing patterns: prescription behavior surveillance system, eight states, 2013. *MMWR Surveill Summ.* 2015;64(9):1–14.

19. Seth P, Rudd RA, Noonan RK, Haegerich TM. Quantifying the epidemic of prescription opioid overdose deaths. *Am J Public Health.* 2018;108(4):500–502.

20. Centers for Disease Control and Prevention, NCHS. ICD-10-CM Table of drugs and chemicals. ftp://ftp.cdc.gov/pub/Health_Statistics/NCHS/Publications/ICD10CM/2019/icd10cm_drug_2019.pdf. Published 2019. Accessed January 30, 2019.

21. Hedegaard H, Bastian BA, Trinidad JP, et al. Drugs most frequently involved in drug over-dose deaths: United States, 2011–2016. *Natl Vital Stat Rep.* 2018;67(9):14.

22. Delany PJ, Draft of letter from Director Delany to DAWN-participating hospitals announcing the termination of DAWN. [Obtained by John J. Coleman via Freedom of Information Act, December 27, 2011, from SAMHSA (unpublished document)].

23. Centers for Disease Control and Prevention. Enhanced state opioid overdose surveillance. https://www.cdc.gov/drugoverdose/foa/state-opioid-mm.html. Accessed May 21, 2019.

24. Centers for Disease Control and Prevention, National Center for Health Statistics. A guide to state implementation of ICD-10 for mortality. ftp://ftp.cdc.gov/pub/Health_Statistics/NCHS/Publications/ICD9_10Con/let2.txt. Published July 31, 1998. Accessed January 12, 2017.

25. Florida Department of Law Enforcement. Medical Examiners Commission. https://www.fdle.state.fl.us/MEC/MEC-Home.aspx. Accessed May 25, 2019.

26. State of Florida, Medical Examiners Commission, Department of Law Enforcement. 2017 Annual report: drugs identified in deceased persons by Florida Medical Examiners. http://www.fdle.state.fl.us/MEC/Publications-and-Forms/Documents/Drugs-in-Deceased-Persons/2017-Annual-Drug-Report.aspx. Published November 2018. Accessed January 14, 2019.

27. Dowell D, Haegerich TM, Chou R. CDC guideline for prescribing opioids for chronic pain—United States, 2016. *MMWR Recomm Rep.* 2016;65(No. RR-1):1–49. http://dx.doi.org/10.15585/mmwr.rr6501e1.

28. Controlled Substances Act, Title II, 21 USC 811; Authority and criteria for classification of substances, Pub. L. 91-513, 84 Stat. 1242 (1970). http://uscode.house.gov/. Accessed February 24, 2019.

29. Controlled Substances Act, Title II, 21 USC 812; Schedules of controlled substances, Pub. L. 91-513, 84 Stat. 1242 (1970). http://uscode.house.gov/. Accessed February 24, 2019.

30. Final rule: placement of chlordiazepoxide, diazepam, oxazepam, clorazepate, flurazepam, and clonazepam in Schedule IV. *Fed Regist.* 1975;40(108):40FR23998.

31. Schedules of controlled substances; placement of alprazolam in Schedule IV. *Fed Regist.* 1981;46(18):46FR23998.

32. Schedules of controlled substances; temporary placement of bromazepam, camazepam, clobazam, clotiazepam, cloxazolam, delorazepam, estazolam, ethyl loflazepate, fludiazepam, fiunitrazepam, haloxazolam, ketazolam, loprazolam, lormetazepam, medazepam, nimetazepam, nitrazepam, nordiazepam, oxazoiam, pinazepam, and tetrazepam into Schedule IV. *Fed Regist.* 1984;49(195):49FR39307.

33. Comprehensive Drug Abuse Prevention and Control Act, Title II: Controlled Substances Act. Pub. L. No. 91-513, 84 Stat. 1236, Title 21, USC, Sect 811(d)(1) *International treaties, conventions, and protocols requiring control, etc.* 1970; http://uscode.house.gov/. Accessed May 25, 2019.

34. Controlled Substances Act. Title 21, USC, Sect. 811(b); Evaluation of drugs and other substances. 1970; http://uscode.house.gov/. Accessed August 29, 2016.

35. Controlled Substances Act, Title II, 21, USC 811(a); Authority and criteria for classification of substances, Pub. L. 91-513, 84 Stat. 1242 (1970). http://uscode.house.gov/. Accessed January 15, 2012.

36. Controlled Substances Act. Title 21, USC, Sect. 812(b)(2)(A & C); Schedules of controlled substances, Pub. L. 91-513, 84 Stat. 1236 (1970).

37. Bureau of Narcotics and Dangerous Drugs, Department of Justice. Final rule: amphetamine, methamphetamine, and optical isomers. *Fed Regist.* 1971;36:12734.

38. Anabolic Steroid Control Act. 21 USC 802, as amended (1990). http://uscode.house.gov/.

39. US District Court, District of Vermont. Criminal Complaint and Affidavit, *United States of America v Yazid Al Fayyad Finn*, Case 5:18-cr-00019-gwc, Doc. #1, filed February 1, 2018.

40. Drug Enforcement Administration. 2018 national drug threat assessment. https://www. dea.gov/sites/default/files/2018-11/DIR-032-18%202018%20NDTA%20final%20 low%20resolution.pdf?utm_medium=email&utm_source=govdelivery. Published November 2018. Accessed November 16, 2018.

41. US District Court, District of Utah. *USA v. Arron Michael Shamo, et al.*; Case 2:16-cr-00631-PMW, Doc. #32 (Superseding indictment). Filed May 31, 2017.

42. US District Court, District of Utah. *USA v. Arron Michael Shamo, et al.*; Case 2:16-cr-00631-PMW, Doc. #136 (Second superseding indictment). Filed October 18, 2018.

43. US District Court, District of Utah. *US v Aaron Michael Shamo*; Verdict form, Case No. 2:16-cr-631 DAK, Doc. #280. Filed August 30, 2019.

44. Young Californian dies after accidentally taking counterfeit Xanax. Partnership for Safe Medicines. https://www.safemedicines.org/2017/09/young-californian-dies-after-accidentally-taking-counterfeit-xanax-made-with-fentanyl.html. Published 2019. Accessed January 14, 2019.

45. Mahoney E. Update: man arrested in connection to fake "Xanax" in Santa Cruz KION News Channel 5/46. https://www.kion546.com/news/monterey-county/update-man-arrested-in-connection-to-fake-xanax-in-santa-cruz/66796210. Updated August 30, 2016. Accessed January 23, 2019.

46. Eurojust. Background: history. http://www.eurojust.europa.eu/about/background/Pages/History.aspx. Accessed May 7, 2019.

47. Europol. About Europol. https://www.europol.europa.eu/about-europol. Accessed May 7, 2019.

48. Drug Enforcement Administration. Global investigation of Dark Web drug network leads to arrest of 3 German nationals. https://www.dea.gov/press-releases/2019/05/03/global-investigation-dark-web-drug-network-leads-arrest-3-german. Published May 3, 2019. Accessed May 7, 2019.

49. 21 USC 841, Prohibited Acts, *Section* (a)(2). (1970). http://uscode.house.gov/. Accessed May 16, 2019.

50. Food and Drug Administration. Guidance for industry: incorporation of physical-chemical identifiers into solid oral dosage form drug products for anticounterfeiting. https://www.fda.gov/downloads/drugs/guidances/ucm171575.pdf. Published October 2011. Accessed March 9, 2019.

51. Surratt H, Kurtz S, Cicero T, Dart R, Baker G, Vorsanger G. Street prices of prescription opioids diverted to the illicit market: data from a national surveillance program. *J Pain*. 2013;*14*(4):S40.

52. United Nations Office on Drugs and Crime. UN drugs and crime office, World Customs Organization make a dent in counterfeit goods and drug shipments. https://www.unodc. org/unodc/en/press/releases/2012/June/un-drugs-and-crime-office-world-customs-organization-make-a-dent-on-counterfeit-goods-and-drug-shipments.html. Published June 2012. Accessed May 25, 2019.

53. Hitti, M. FDA: fake Drugs on Canadian Web sites. WebMD.com. https://www.webmd. com/drug-medication/news/20060831/fda-fake-drugs-on-canadian-web-sites. Published August 31, 2006. Accessed May 25, 2019.

54. Support for Patients and Communities Act, H.R. 6, 115th Congr, Pub L. 115-271 (October 24, 2018). https://www.congress.gov/bill/115th-congress/house-bill/6/actions?q=% 7B%22search%22%3A%5B%22HR+6%22%5D%7D&r=1&s=1. Accessed December 24, 2018.

55. Report of the President's Commission on Combating Drug Addiction and the Opioid Crisis. https://www.whitehouse.gov/sites/whitehouse.gov/files/images/Final_Report_Draft_11-1-2017.pdf. Published November 1, 2017. Accessed December 17, 2017.

56. Westat wins Drug Abuse Warning Network (DAWN) contract. *Westat.com.* https://www.westat.com/articles/westat-wins-drug-abuse-warning-network-dawn-contract. Published November 12, 2018. Accessed January 22, 2019.

57. Caulkins JP, Ebener PA, McCaffrey DF. Describing DAWN's dominion. *Contemp Drug Probl.* 1995;22:547–567.

CHAPTER 12

In Search of Benzodiazepine Guidelines

JO ANN LEQUANG

HIGHLIGHTS

- There are currently no definitive focused guidelines for benzodiazepine (BZD) use and cessation (titration, tailoring, and tapering).
- Consistent recommendations are that BZDs should be used at the lowest effective doses for the shortest amount of time.
- BZDs are first-line considerations for alcohol withdrawal, status epilepticus, anesthesia, and crisis anxiety in the absence of features of psychosis.
- BZDs are no longer considered first-line treatment for anxiety disorders, but may be used short-term if the initially-prescribed standard treatment is ineffective or not well-tolerated.
- BZDs are indicated to treat insomnia, but should not be used as first-line therapy, should only be used short term (less than 4 weeks), and should not be used in geriatric patients.

The development of benzodiazepines (BZDs) in the 1950s eclipsed the role of the more addictive barbiturates as the main treatment for insomnia and anxiety, making BZDs among the most frequently prescribed drugs in the world today.[1,2] With widespread use came growing concerns about adverse safety data, tolerance, and their abuse potential, yet BZD prescribing to outpatients in the United States doubled from 2003 to 2015.[3] While much is known today about the risks and benefits of BZD therapy, there is no definitive focused guideline for their use. What can be learned about BZDs comes to us piecemeal, primarily through disorder-specific guidance, package insert indications, and small clinical trials in specific populations. Prescribing practices do not always align even with this paucity of evidence.[4] The objective of this chapter is to list some of the main conditions for which BZDs are prescribed and what is known about their use in that setting. It is not a guideline, but rather a case for why guidelines are urgently needed.

There are four main indications for BZDs: procedural sedation, alcohol withdrawal, insomnia, and anxiety.[5] The anxiety indication was granted for "anxiety states" and "anxiety disorders" before the publication of the third edition of the *Diagnostic and Statistical Manual*, which established specific diagnostic criteria for many mental disorders that had previously come under the broad umbrella of "anxiety disorders." Thus, unless a specific indication was granted by the U.S. Food and Drug Administration (FDA) retrospectively, the use of BZD in many anxiety-related conditions may be technically off-label.[6] For example, posttraumatic stress disorder (PTSD) was originally described as an "anxiety disorder" (for which BZDs might be indicated) but is today recognized as a condition quite distinct from an anxiety disorder (and so BZDs are not indicated). This has created confusion, in particular since not every disorder previously included under "anxiety disorder"—including PTSD—is appropriate for BZD therapy.[6]

There are a few other approved indications; for example, alprazolam is indicated for panic disorder with or without agoraphobia; clonazepam is indicated for panic disorder, restless leg syndrome, and nystagmus; diazepam is indicated for status epilepticus and drug-induced seizures; lorazepam is indicated for status epilepticus and chemotherapy-induced nausea and vomiting (as prophylaxis or adjunctive therapy with an antiemetic); midazolam is indicated for sedation during rapid-sequence intubation.[4,7] These are specific indications and, by and large, not particularly controversial or the subject of misuse. The most frequent uses of BZDs occur in the settings in which they are likely to be inappropriately prescribed, namely, for treating insomnia and mental health disorders.

THE USE OF BZDS FOR INSOMNIA

BZDs relieve insomnia by acting as sedative anxiolytic agents or hypnotic, soporific agents through the actions of the BZD on the gamma-aminobutyric acid (GABA) system. All BZDs may produce both anxiolytic and hypnotic effects, although only certain BZDs are approved to treat insomnia (estazolam, temazepam, lorazepam, triazolam).[6] The so-called Z-drugs are sometimes grouped together with BZDs as sleep aids but fall outside the scope of this chapter.

BZDs are recommended by the European Sleep Research Society guideline for the diagnosis and treatment of insomnia for short-term use (<4 weeks), but this recommendation is based on moderate-quality evidence.[8] BZDs confer what might be called a "modest benefit" for insomnia patients.[9] In fact, the number needed to treat with BZD for any to have improved sleep quality is 13 patients (95% confidence interval, 6.7 to 62.9).[10] Over time, these modest benefits are overcome by risks to the extent that insomnia patients are more likely to have an adverse event associated with BZD use than improved sleep quality.[10] Furthermore, BZDs may exacerbate insomnia by decreasing the relative amount of deep sleep, thus impairing healthy sleep architecture.[11] The American College of Physicians found low-strength evidence in support of BZD for insomnia in adults but added that their use was associated with a slight risk for serious harms.[12] Guidance for treating insomnia asserts that BZDs not be considered first-line therapy for insomnia.[13]

The use of BZD treatment for insomnia becomes more problematic because BZDs should only be used short term and insomnia tends to be a persistent condition. Clinical practice deviates markedly from evidence and labeling, because it has been estimated that 50% to 70% of those who take BZD (or a similar Z-drug) for insomnia take them chronically, sometimes for years.[14,15] Moreover, BZDs are often prescribed to patients in long-term care (55%) and hospital (69%) to help patients sleep.[16,17] Geriatric patients may be at risk, because insomnia is prevalent in this population, but Canadian Insomnia Clinical Practice Guidelines do not recommend BZD use, even short term, in adults ≥65 years.[18] Nonpharmacological interventions, such as sleep hygiene practices and cognitive behavioral therapy may be options considered.[19]

In summary, BZDs are indicated to treat insomnia but should not be used as first-line therapy, should only be used short term (<4 weeks), and should not be used in geriatric patients.

THE USE OF BZDS FOR MENTAL DISORDERS

Acute Disturbances

In some cases, BZDs may be administered to manage an urgent case of acute anxiety, agitation, and/or aggression in the setting of another disorder. Guidelines from the British Association of Psychopharmacology and the National Association of Psychiatric Intensive Care and Low Secure Units define these events as "acute disturbances," a collective term encompassing episodes of intense agitation, aggression, and violence in the setting of an acute mental state associated with a mental and/or physical disorder.[20] While this is not a commonly used medical term in all parts of the world, it is helpful here to define the use of BZDs for urgent treatment of acute episodes of anxiety/aggression, where it is necessary to achieve a rapid tranquilization of the patient to reduce the risk of harm to the patient or others. For optimal therapy, this rapid tranquilization should avoid the patient's loss of consciousness, somnolence, and sedation. An oral or parenteral BZD may be used alone or in combination with an antipsychotic medication. In 90% of cases, lorazepam is the preferred BZD in this setting with a median dose of 1 mg.[20] The use of BZDs for acute disturbances occurs in a clinical setting (emergency department, hospital, etc.) and does not involve prolonged dosing.

Anxiety Disorders

Anxiety disorders are among the most prevalent mental health conditions. The term *anxiety disorder* collectively encompasses numerous conditions: generalized anxiety disorder (GAD), panic disorder, agoraphobia (which may occur with or without panic disorder), social anxiety disorder, specific phobias, and others, some of which are described in more detail later in this chapter.[21] BZDs are indicated for certain anxiety disorders, and it is estimated that between 55% and 94% of U.S. patients diagnosed with anxiety disorders are prescribed BZDs.[21] Despite this widespread use, BZDs are not indicated for all anxiety disorders, they are not recommended as first-line treatment, they are contraindicated in certain patients and certain conditions, and their long-term use is not recommended, even when they are indicated.[21]

The World Federation of Societies of Biological Psychiatry recommends the use of selective serotonin reuptake inhibitors (SSRIs), selective norepinephrine reuptake inhibitors (SNRIs), and pregabalin for first-line treatment of anxiety with BZDs to be used only when other treatments are not effective and then only in patients with no history of substance use disorder.[22] The Canadian Clinical Practice Guidelines recommend cognitive behavioral therapy as the first-line approach and pharmacological therapy only if psychological therapy is not effective. If the patient is to advance to pharmacological therapy, these Canadian guidelines recommend SSRIs and SNRIs as preferred agents for first-line therapy and suggest if they fail that noradrenergic and specific serotonergic antidepressants, tricyclic antidepressants, monoamine oxidase inhibitors, and reversible inhibitors of monoamine oxidase A be considered. The Canadian Guidelines state that BZDs may be appropriate in anxiety patients early in treatment as an adjunctive agent if the patient suffers acute agitation or is in crisis but advises that BZDs should be discontinued once the SSRI or other preferred agent goes into effect. Due to treatment-limiting side effects and concerns about dependency, cognitive impairment, and abuse, BZDs should be used in anxiety patients only short term and dosed regularly rather than as-needed.[23] Further guidance from Bandelow and colleagues supports the view that BZDs not be considered as a first-line treatment for anxiety disorders, but these investigators advise that BZDs may be used short-term if the initially prescribed standard treatment was ineffective or not well tolerated.[21,24]

Bipolar Disorder

Bipolar disorder is a potentially disabling mental illness with significant morbidity and mortality that presents with multiple subtypes.[25] Although BZDs are not indicated for bipolar disorder and may even worsen symptoms, they are often prescribed. The Systematic Treatment Enhancement Program for Bipolar Disorder (STEP-BD) clinical study found 25.6% of the study population of bipolar I and II patients ($N = 1,365$) were prescribed a BZD at the time they remitted from an episode and that the use of a BZD was associated with a greater risk for recurrence of such an episode in these patients.[26] The Canadian Network for Mood and Anxiety Treatments and the International Society for Bipolar Disorders in their joint 2018 guidelines for managing patients with bipolar disorder recommend the use of oral BZDs only for the management of acute episodes of intense agitation common in mania, with intramuscular lorazepam among first-line treatments.[25] Likewise, BZD therapy is not recommended by the Kaiser Permanente healthcare system for patients diagnosed with bipolar disorder except for the urgent management of an acute episode of severe mania.[27]

Borderline Personality Disorder

Despite its name, borderline personality disorder is not a true personality disorder but is rather a psychiatric syndrome of specific symptoms (such as emotional dysregulation) and personality traits (such as impulsivity). It is often comorbid with other mental health conditions as well as chronic pain. There is no specific drug indicated for the treatment of borderline personality disorder, although pharmacological therapy is common.[28] The recommended first-line approach to borderline personality disorder involves nonpharmacological therapies (cognitive behavior therapy, psychotherapy) plus pharmacological care with antipsychotics, mood stabilizers, and SSRIs but not BZDs.[29] The American Psychiatric Association recommends that, overall, BZDs should be used with caution (if at all) in the borderline personality population because of the potential for misuse and issues of tolerance with protracted exposure.[30] Despite this guidance, a retrospective observational study found that 85.2% of patients diagnosed with borderline personality disorder were prescribed BZDs or other non-BZD hypnotics.[31] Of particular concern in this population is the concomitant use of polypharmacy. A survey from 2001 to 2009 in the Netherlands found that 30% of patients were treated with four or more drugs.[28] Furthermore, the comorbidities of borderline personality disorder and chronic pain may result in patients being concurrently prescribed opioids and BZDs, against which the Centers for Disease Control and Prevention (CDC) advise.[32,33] Both BZDs and opioids depress the central nervous system and may increase the risk of potentially life-threatening respiratory depression.

Generalized Anxiety Disorder

GAD is characterized by a persistent, exaggerated, and largely uncontrollable sense of fear, worry, and concern about multiple subjects that can cause diffuse psychological symptoms as well as physical ailments.[34] GAD is often comorbid with substance use disorder, depression, or general health problems (headaches, back pain, insomnia, and so on). Patients with GAD may be restless or edgy and find it nearly impossible to stop worrying. First-line therapy for GAD includes cognitive behavioral therapy with pharmacological support from an SSRI or an SNRI. In the case of treatment-resistant GAD, BZDs may be considered for certain appropriate patients, but their long-term use is not advised.[34] The National Institute for Health and Care Excellence guidelines recommend an SSRI as first-line treatment for GAD, followed by SNRI or pregabalin as second-line treatment, cautioning against the use of BZDs, except for short-term management of an acute crisis.[35]

Major Depressive Disorder

A synthesis of guidelines from Europe and America regarding the treatment of major depressive disorder (MDD) reports first-line recommendations as antidepressant monotherapy and/or psychotherapy. There is only a very limited role for BZDs, namely, for the short-term management of acute episodes of anxiety, agitation, or insomnia.[36] Since MDD may be comorbid with anxiety disorder(s) or acute episodes of agitation, patients may sometimes be prescribed both antidepressants and BZDs. A Cochrane meta-analysis reported that this combination therapy was more effective than antidepressants alone in reducing the severity of depression but only in the early phase, and benefits were not sustained over time. Combined therapy led to fewer patients discontinuing pharmacological therapy in the early phase but was also associated with a higher rate of adverse events.[37] Despite the fact that BZD monotherapy for the treatment of depression is generally discouraged with BZDs recommended at most for short-term adjunctive treatment, 9.3% of adult patients treated for depression in a national cross-sectional analysis from 2012 to 2015 data collected by the United States National Ambulatory Medical Care Survey were treated with BZD monotherapy.[38] Specialists seem less likely to prescribe BZDs for MDD. For example, psychiatrists were less likely to prescribe BZD monotherapy for MDD than other healthcare providers (odds ratio 0.42, 95% confidence interval, 0.29 to 0.61).[38]

Obsessive-Compulsive Disorder

Obsessive-compulsive disorder (OCD) involves recurrent persistent thoughts or urges and responding repetitive behaviors that the patient perceives as unwanted and intrusive but nevertheless performs.[23] In some cases, compulsions may be adaptive mechanisms aimed at reducing anxiety. OCD was at first categorized as an "anxiety disorder," but today is seen as its own category along with conditions such as hoarding or trichotillomania. A combination approach of psychological therapy, such as cognitive behavioral therapy, plus pharmacological treatment is preferred with escitalopram, fluoxetine, fluvoxamine, paroxetine, and sertraline the preferred first-line agents; BZDs are not recommended.[23] An international study of OCD treatments found considerable variations among nations in terms of treatment with SSRIs the most common.[39] Although BZDs are not indicated for OCD patients, a study of 955 OCD patients in Brazil found 38.4% were treated with BZDs, mostly (96.7%) as part of a polypharmacy regimen.[40] An international multicenter survey ($N = 361$) found that 24.9% of OCD patients were taking BZD therapy.[41]

Panic Disorder

A panic attack is described as an intense and sudden surge of fearful emotions and discomfort that peaks in minutes and may include sweating, heart palpitations, chest pain, nausea, a sensation of choking, chest pain, dizziness, chills or sensations of heat, fear of dying, and feelings of detachment or unreality.[23] Recurrent panic attacks can lead to a diagnosis of panic disorder, which is further exacerbated by worry about recurring panic attacks and maladaptive coping behaviors. Panic disorder may be accompanied by agoraphobia, which includes anxiety related to at least two of the following: public transportation, open spaces, being in shops or theaters, being in a crowd or standing in line, and being alone outside the house in other situations. Most people with agoraphobia develop maladaptive avoidance behaviors. The first line of treatment is combination therapy with psychotherapy plus pharmacological treatment using SSRIs and SNRIs as the preferred agents. BZDs, specifically alprazolam, clonazepam, lorazepam, and diazepam, are considered effective but are second-line options although they may be helpful in the management of acute episodes of severe anxiety/agitation.[23] A Cochrane systematic review and meta-analysis found low-quality evidence supported the possible advantage of BZD versus placebo for acute treatment of panic disorders; no longer-term studies were available.[42] In this population, BZDs are recommended for short-term use only.[23] The National Institute for Health and Care Excellence guidelines do not recommend the use of BZD for panic disorder and caution that long-term outcomes with BZDs are inferior to long-term outcomes using antidepressant therapy.[35]

Phobias

A specific phobia involves an intense fear of a certain situation, animal, or object, with 90% of phobic patients having multiple specific phobias (mean number: 3).[43] The object of the phobia produces an immediate and disproportionate fear response, and it can sometimes be clinically challenging to distinguish a phobia from a panic attack. Phobias are typically treated using exposure therapy so that patients can, with support, gradually learn to experience the phobia without fear. Novel therapeutic options are now exploring virtual reality and computer-based simulations for treating phobias. In light of exposure therapy, pharmacological treatment for phobias has been more limited. BZDs may be appropriate to provide acute relief of symptoms when the patient must face an unavoidable but temporally limited situation (e.g., visit to dentist, airline travel, claustrophobia associated with magnetic resonance imaging).[23] Where BZDs have been used as an adjunct to exposure therapy, BZDs conferred no additional benefits to patients.[44]

Posttraumatic Stress Disorder

PTSD occurs when a patient is exposed to a traumatic event, such as a physical or sexual assault, unexpected death of someone close, serious injury, and then has recurrent, intrusive memories of the events, upsetting dreams, dissociative reactions, and persistent distress.[23] PTSD can involve avoidance behaviors, mood dysregulation, sudden episodes of anger and aggression, hypervigilance, disordered sleep, and feelings of detachment from others. Some people with PTSD cannot clearly remember the traumatic event and may be confused by their intense symptoms. PTSD can be comorbid with other mental health disorders, such as MDD and substance use disorders. The appropriate pharmacotherapy for PTSD remains to be elucidated. In the 1990s, BZDs were given prophylactically to people who might experience a trauma that could lead to PTSD, but

BZDs conferred no beneficial effect in this situation. In fact, they may have even elevated the risk that the patient would develop PTSD.[45] Although often prescribed to PTSD patients, BZD therapy is considered ineffective and, as such, is not recommended.[23,46] Although BZDs are indicated for insomnia, they are not recommended for PTSD-related sleep disturbances.[47]

Social Anxiety Disorder

In social anxiety disorder (SAD), an individual has a disproportionate fear of social groups or individuals that are perceived to be highly judgmental or critical.[23] First-line treatment is cognitive behavioral therapy and if pharmacological treatment is needed, SSRIs are the preferred agents. BZDs, specifically clonazepam, may be effective, but the risk of dependency is treatment limiting. BZDs may be used for SAD patients who require initial rapid relief of acute symptoms or as adjunctive therapy in a patient who is not responding well to other drug therapy, but they should not be administered to patients with substance use disorder or concomitant depression.[23] BZDs must be considered a second-line treatments and only for short-term use in SAD patients.[23] Nevertheless, BZDs are often prescribed to SAD patients.[48] A Cochrane database meta-analysis found low-to-moderate quality evidence for the use of SSRIs in SAD patients but did not report on BZD use.[49]

Stage Fright

Stage fright and other forms of performance anxiety are typically temporally limited situations in which a patient becomes distressed and overly fearful when asked to speak in public or perform in a specific situation, such as singing onstage.[50] This form of anxiety disorder differs from SAD and the recommended first-line treatment is beta-blockers (such as propranolol) taken about an hour before the performance. BZDs are sometimes administered for stage fright, but this is not the recommended first-line treatment as BZDs can result in sedation or fatigue.[50] There are no BZD indications for forms of performance anxiety.

THE USE OF BZDS FOR OTHER CONDITIONS
Alcohol Withdrawal

Alcohol withdrawal syndrome (AWS) is a potentially life-threatening condition arising in those with alcohol use disorder who stop drinking; it may require hospitalization.[51] AWS is associated with glutamate overactivity and may be described a hyperexcitation of the central nervous system (CNS). AWS involves initial symptoms, which may progress to severe symptoms, including hallucinations, seizures, and delirium tremens.[52] The use of BZDs is recognized as the first-line of treatment, with rapid BZD dose escalation as needed.[53] Treatment-resistant AWS may require the adjunctive use of propofol and/phenobarbital.[52] The short-term use of BZD therapy for AWS is a means to control agitation, manage anxiety, and prevent other unpleasant symptoms; the use of BZDs for AWS is supported by placebo-controlled trials.[54] The best evidence exists for diazepam, chlordiazepoxide, oxazepam, lorazepam, and alprazolam. A loading dose is recommended.[55] Short-acting BZDs may be better suited than long-acting BZDs for patients with liver dysfunction.[54] Symptom-triggered therapy with BZDs is preferred for AWS[53] because of the agonism of BZDs at the GABA type A $(GABA_A)$ receptors, which mimics the inhibition on neuronal effect caused by alcohol.[52,56] Fixed-schedule administration is recommended once symptoms develop.[55]

During the detoxification process, patients should be made as comfortable as possible, and steps should be taken to limit BZD use to the short-term and avoid their prolonged use.[55]

Epilepsy, Status Epilepticus, Seizures

The American Epilepsy Society published an evidence-based guideline for the treatment of convulsive status epilepticus (prolonged seizure) in children and adults and recommended intramuscular midazolam, intravenous (IV) lorazepam, IV diazepam, and IV phenobarbital as first-line initial treatment.[57] The Working Group guidelines from the Polish Society of Epileptology recommend BZDs as first-line treatment for status epilepticus with phenytoin, valproic acid, ad phenobarbital as second-line agents.[58] A retrospective study of 44 patients treated for generalized convulsive status epilepticus found BZD monotherapy aborted seizures in 50% of patients; in this study, all patients required hospitalization, and BZD doses were lower than recommended.[59] This study further reported that medical services tended to use midazolam while the hospital emergency room utilized lorazepam.[59] The Hong Kong Epilepsy Guideline recommends intramuscular midazolam for early-stage status epilepticus, favored over IV lorazepam.[60] While BZDs are recommended for treating early status epilepticus events, there are no guidelines with respect to how to treat established, refractory status epilepticus.[61] Rectal diazepam is the most frequently used rescue medication for prolonged epileptic seizures in all age groups, along with intranasal midazolam and oral clonazepam.[62]

PRESCRIBING CONSIDERATIONS

Dependence

Dependence is the normal and expected result of prolonged exposure to BZDs, and it is estimated that about half of all patients who take BZDs for over a month will become dependent.[63] The abrupt discontinuation of BZDs or a marked dose decrease may precipitate withdrawal symptoms in dependent patients.

Drug–Drug Interactions

Sedation, respiratory depression, and other potentially severe CNS adverse effects may occur if BZDs are taken together with alcohol, opioids, barbiturates, and tricyclic antidepressants.[7] CDC guidelines advise specifically against the use of BZDs in patients on opioid therapy.[33]

Duration of Use

BZDs are recommended for short-term use, usually defined as <4 to 12 consecutive weeks.[64] Guidelines from insurance providers recommend that patients be advised at the outset of BZD therapy that the duration of treatment will not exceed two weeks.[27] This advice adds that patients should also be informed about risks and benefits of BZD therapy, exit plans (such as tapering), and alternative treatments (e.g., cognitive behavioral therapy, antidepressants, and so on).[27] Guidelines for BZD use published in Ireland do not recommend BZD prescriptions of more than four weeks and advocate phased dispensing if possible (usually no more than a week's supply at once).[65] Moreover, BZDs should be used at the lowest effective doses for the shortest amount of time; the Irish guidance sets the limit at diazepam 5 mg three times daily or equivalent.[65]

THE USE OF BZDS IN SPECIAL POPULATIONS
Benzodiazepine Patients

The healthcare system Kaiser Permanente does not recommend that any patient take any two of the following: a BZD, Z-drug, or muscle relaxant.[27] When BZD use is recommended, only one BZD should be used.

Cancer Patients

Cancer patients may be prescribed BZDs to manage disease-related symptoms of stress, anxiety, and insomnia. Their use should be considered in light of other drugs the cancer patient may be taking, the underlying disease processes, and age. For example, BZDs can cause confusion and delirium in the critically ill. In some cases, BZDs can exacerbate fatigue and weakness.[66] Important in this regard are findings from a meta-analysis that found the use of BZDs increased cancer risk and potential immunosuppressive effects of BZDs.[67]

Cancer treatment may cause distressing symptoms, such as chemotherapy-induced nausea and vomiting (CINV). This condition is typically treated with antiemetics. In the event of breakthrough CINV, the National Comprehensive Cancer Network recommends adding one agent to the regimen from a different class of drugs; BZDs (lorazepam 0.5 to 2 mg) are among the choices.[68] This is for short-term use only to address breakthrough CINV symptoms.

Comorbid Patients

BZDs may exacerbate certain conditions that may be comorbid in a patient who otherwise has an indication for BZD therapy.[27] For example, in patients with fibromyalgia, chronic fatigue syndrome, somatization disorders, depression, attention deficit/hyperactivity disorder, kleptomania, and certain cardiopulmonary conditions, BZDs may worsen those symptoms even if they are otherwise indicated. [27]

Intensive Care Unit Patients

Guidelines for the care of intensive care unit patients suffering pain, agitation, and/or delirium recommend that sedation strategies emphasize light sedation and use propofol or dexmedetomidine rather than BZDs to confer better outcomes on mechanically ventilated adults.[69,70] Further, the guidelines caution that the use of BZDs may be a risk factor for development of delirium in intensive care unit patients. Delirious patients (when the delirium is not related to alcohol or benzodiazepine withdrawal) should not be sedated with a BZD.[69,70] Furthermore, critically ill adults with agitation should be managed using an analgesia-first approach, with the possibility of adding antipsychotics as adjuncts for severe agitation in patients with extensive trauma and/or high levels of pain intensity.[71] The use of propofol or dexmedetomidine instead of BZD therapy in critically ill adults may reduce hospital length of stay and/or duration of mechanical ventilation.[72]

Patients Already on BZD Therapy

A patient may be referred to a new clinic, come to the emergency room, or enter long-term care with a history of chronic and/or high-dose BZD therapy. These are the so-called legacy patients This is a complicated area as the new provider must assess the patient's BZD use and indications and arrive at a decision about BZD therapy.[73] This involves assessment of the patient's history and diagnosis combined with a review of potential harms. When feasible, a shared decision-making model should be used to evaluate the role of BZD treatment and whether it should be maintained, decreased, or discontinued and, in the case of the latter, which alternative treatments are to be trialed. BZD should not be discontinued abruptly; a systematic tapering plan should be utilized, discussed later in this chapter.[73]

Older Patients

In general, the use of BZDs is not appropriate for older patients because of side effects and the comparatively long half-lives of these agents. The 2015 Beers Criteria do not recommend the use of BZDs in older adults.[74] The Kaiser Permanente healthcare system allows for BZD therapy in older patients with a dose reduction. For patients >65 years and for older and/or frail patients, Kaiser Permanente states that BZD dose should be half of the adult dose and administered under close clinical monitoring, as patients may be susceptible to BZD side effects as well as polypharmacy-related drug–drug interactions.[27] Despite the fact that the American Geriatric Society recommends not using BZD at all in geriatric patients, the most common[75] CNS polypharmacy in older adults remains the use of opioids together with BZDs.[33] An evidence-based clinical practice guideline recommended deprescribing (slow-tapering) BZDs to adults ≥65 years taking BZDs for insomnia, regardless of duration of use.[18]

BZDs are associated with specific risks in older patients. For example, BZDs may put geriatric patients at greater risk for falls and fractures.[76,77] There is some evidence that BZDs may increase the risk of Alzheimer's disease.[78] Irish guidelines from 2002 advise that long-acting BZDs with active metabolites, such as diazepam, be avoided in older patients in favor of short-acting BZDs with few active metabolites, such as lorazepam or alprazolam.[65] Late-life depression in geriatric patients should be treated with antidepressant therapy and not BZDs.[65] The prevalence of many anxiety disorders lessens with advanced age,[21] yet the long-term use of BZD is common in geriatric patients in residential care.[79]

Opioid Patients

The CDC state in their opioid prescribing guidelines for primary care physicians that patients taking opioids should not be administered a concomitant BZD.[33] Both drugs depress the CNS, and their combined use poses a safety risk. Yet opioids and BZDs are often prescribed together, even over the long term. In a year-long study of osteoarthritis outpatients (N = 31,123 outpatient encounters), 27% of patients had prescriptions for both BZDs and opioids and of that population, 43% were >65 years of age.[80] The Kaiser Foundation Health Plan provides specific guidance for BZD prescribing and states explicitly that they are not to be prescribed to any patient currently taking any opioid.[27]

Pain Patients

Pain patients taking opioid analgesics are not indicated for BZD use. Furthermore, BZDs may increase the action of GABA at the $GABA_A$ receptors associated with pain modulation and, in that way, may counteract the analgesic benefits of opioids such as morphine.[81]

Patients with Substance Use Disorder

Patients with active substance use disorder or a history of substance use disorder should not be treated with BZDs, particularly those patients with a prior history of BZD misuse.[21] As much as possible, people with substance use disorder (including opioid use disorder and alcoholism) should not be initiated on BZD as it is a drug that can be misused and may cause altered consciousness or euphoric effects in certain situations.[65]

Pediatric Patients

Anxiety, phobias, panic disorder, and other distressing conditions can occur in pediatric patients.[23] In some cases, children may express fear and anxiety by crying, throwing a tantrum, freezing, clinging, or shrinking. In general, psychological therapy is preferred to drug therapy. There is little evidence for the use of BZDs in pediatric patients overall.[23]

Pregnant Patients

Kaiser Permanente guidance contraindicates the use of BZDs in pregnant patients.[27] However, it may be urgently necessary to treat AWS during pregnancy, which could require BZD use. Alcohol exposure during pregnancy may cause irreversible neurodevelopmental problems in the child. For AWS during pregnancy, the World Federation of Societies of Biological Psychiatry recommends the lowest possible effective dose of BZD be used for the shortest possible time to help mitigate symptoms.[82]

Anxiety disorders can be common during pregnancy and postpartum, but the use of BZDs in pregnant and lactating patients is not well studied. BZDs are secreted in breast milk[83] and should not be administered to nursing mothers.[65] Babies born to mothers who used BZD over the long term during their pregnancy (particularly late in the pregnancy) may be born with physical dependence on the drugs and be at risk for withdrawal symptoms after birth.[65] There are no guidelines available for BZD detoxification or tapering during pregnancy or how to manage babies born with BZD dependence.[84,85]

DISCONTINUATION AND WITHDRAWAL

Dependent patients will experience some degree of withdrawal symptoms upon BZD discontinuation/tapering, often including anxiety, insomnia, muscle spasms, and hypersensitivity. Abrupt discontinuation of BZD or even abrupt dose decreases may precipitate withdrawal symptoms. Fits or psychotic episodes are rare but have been observed.[86] Patients on high-dose BZD therapy who have undergone BZD withdrawal perceive it as difficult and distressing; relapse is common.[87] BZD dose should not be substantially decreased or discontinued abruptly, as it likely will lead to withdrawal symptoms in dependent patients. Withdrawal symptoms are not rare; about 90% of those who have taken BZDs for ≥8 months will experience clinically significant withdrawal as they are discontinued.[7] By contrast, patients taking BZDs for two weeks or less may expect few or no withdrawal symptoms. Typical withdrawal symptoms include gastrointestinal symptoms, diaphoresis, increased heart rate, increased blood pressure, tremors, lethargy, dizziness, headaches, restlessness, irritability, insomnia, anxiety, disturbed perception, depression, tinnitus, delirium, panic attacks, hallucinations, and abnormal muscle movements. Seizures, delirium, confusion, and psychosis may occur but are rare.[7] In patients with a concomitant mental health disorder, withdrawal symptoms may exacerbate or trigger symptoms of the underlying disorder, for example, mania or anxiety.[7]

Shared Decision-Making

Safe and effective BZD therapy cessation demands the active participation of the patient as well as close clinical monitoring. Preceding discontinuation, clinicians may discuss the risks and benefits of BZD therapy with patients (and their families, as appropriate) in an effort to educate the patient and obtain informed consent to discontinue BZD therapy. Such discussions may not always be comfortable, and in some cases, several conversations may be required before action is taken.

Once the patient understands the medical need to discontinue BZD therapy, a slow tapering plan should be set up and discussed with the patient. Symptoms of panic and anxiety may in some cases be managed with cognitive behavioral therapy interventions.[7] Just as there is a paucity of guidance about BZD indications and use, there is little in the literature about how to effectively manage withdrawal symptoms that may occur during BZD tapers. It is not clear if pharmacological therapy is of benefit. There is some evidence for the use of propranolol and valproic acid to mitigate withdrawal symptoms, but there is no evidence supporting the use of antipsychotics (exacerbates symptoms) or antidepressants, although the latter may be used in selected cases.[7] One drawback to certain SSRIs, such as fluoxetine or citalopram 40 to 60 mg/day or buspirone, is that while they may ultimately be effective, they can take three to four weeks to show efficacy.[7] Beta-blockade may be an option for certain appropriate patients. For example, propranolol 20 to 40 mg twice a day blocks somatic symptoms of anxiety and offers a rapid onset of action.

Withdrawal may be more severe in patients who took high-potency BZDs (alprazolam, lorazepam, triazolam), those on high-dose therapy, and/or those with prolonged exposure to BZDs. Patients who are unmotivated to discontinue BZDs or those equivocal about their BZD use may have increased difficulties with cessation. Other patient-related factors that can complicate BZD discontinuation include a diagnosis of panic disorder, high levels of depression and/or anxiety before starting the tapering plan, other substance abuse, and certain personality pathologies (neurotic or dependent patients).[7]

Unlike the withdrawal symptoms associated with opioids or alcohol, BZD withdrawal symptoms can take months or years to resolve. About 15% of BZD patients who discontinue BZD therapy will experience protracted withdrawal. Anxiety diminishes gradually but may last a year.[7] Insomnia may persist 6 to 12 months after BZD discontinuation.

Depression may last a few months, and individual decisions must be made in terms of how to treat it. Cognitive impairment improves slowly, but cognitive deficits can persist for a year. BZDs can cause distorted perceptions, such as tinnitus, paresthesia, and pain in the extremities, which may improve gradually. In some cases, symptoms last for years or never entirely resolve. Motor symptoms improve over time, but normal motor function can take months to regain. Gastrointestinal symptoms typically resolve only very slowly, if ever.[7] Clinicians should discuss these symptoms with their patients to encourage realistic expectations. In some cases, supportive care may be used to help with symptoms.

Tapering

BZD is active at the GABA receptors in the brain, which modulate feelings of relaxation; a reduction in BZD reduces this relaxation and increases excitement, which, in turn, can trigger feelings of agitation, restlessness, anxiety, insomnia, and confusion. As the patient gets used to having less and less BZD, the brain starts to regenerate new GABA receptors, which then increase in number and allow for better relaxation. Thus, to manage withdrawal, a systematic tapering plan should be put in place, which is slow enough to allow time for the GABA receptors in the brain to regenerate.[7] In general, rapid tapers can be more distressing and provoke more symptoms than slower plans.

With a shared decision-making model, patients are informed prior to the start of the taper, accept and acknowledge the goals of BZD discontinuation, and understand the specific steps ahead. BZD discontinuation should be based on a systematic tapering plan with specific milestones; patients should be seen regularly throughout the discontinuation process and be made to feel that they can contact the clinic as needed as they navigate the withdrawal.

Tapering Plans

There is limited evidence and no official guidance with regard to BZD tapering, but some general concepts in the literature can help the clinician and patient craft a realistic and workable plan. If necessary and at all possible, the BZD should be rotated to a longer-acting BZD (such as diazepam) rather than a short-acting formulation.[7] Diazepam has a long half-life (20 to 200 hours) and thus reduces gradually in serum concentration.[7] If time and the patient's condition permits, a slow taper is more comfortable for the patient than a more rapid plan. A slow taper means modest dose decreases in each step, allowing the patient to plateau for a week or two (or longer) at each new dose step before it is decreased further. During a taper, it is better to prolong a plateau for a struggling patient than to temporarily increase a dose; in fact, during the taper, doses should only be maintained or decreased, not increased. Supportive care may be required to manage withdrawal symptoms, but as much as possible new medications, such as sleep aids, should be avoided. Nonpharmacological interventions may be helpful to manage symptoms. As a rule, antidepressants are not recommended except in carefully selected cases to treat clinical depression or panic attacks.[7]

Based on 40 mg/day dose of diazepam, a tapering plan might be[7]

- Reduce 2 mg to 4 mg every one or two weeks until the dose is 20 mg/day.
- Reduce 1 mg to 2 mg every one or two weeks until dose is 10 mg/day.
- Reduce 1 mg every one or two weeks until dose is 5 mg/day.
- Reduce 0.5 to 1 mg every 1 to 2 weeks until discontinued.

Using this plan, it would take a patient on 40 mg/day of diazepam a year or more to discontinue (30 to 60 weeks). Even patients taking 20 mg/day diazepam would need 20 to 40 weeks for this type of slow taper. The last step in the taper is often perceived by patients as the most difficult, but the challenge may be more psychological than physical as the final step will achieve the major milestone of complete cessation of BZD therapy.[7] Throughout the taper, the patient may benefit from close clinical supervision with in-clinic visits (ideally prior to each dose decrement) and occasional supportive phone calls. Relapse is common in BZD discontinuation and should not be taken as a reason to abandon the goal of discontinuing BZD treatment.[7]

CONCLUSION

BZDs are familiar and frequently prescribed drugs with not inconsiderable risks, including adverse effects, drug–drug interactions, dependency, and misuse. Despite the fact that they are among the most prescribed drugs in the world, there is a paucity of guidance in terms of how they should be used, their appropriate indications, and how to discontinue therapy, particularly in patients who experience protracted withdrawal symptoms. BZDs are often used off-label in many mental health conditions and sometimes in direct contradiction to evidence that they may exacerbate certain conditions, such as PTSD. Greater guidance is urgently need for BZDs so that these important and versatile drugs are appropriate used in patients who can benefit from them and potential adverse events and drug–drug interactions are avoided.

REFERENCES

1. Ashton H. The diagnosis and management of benzodiazepine dependence. *Curr Opin Psychiatry.* 2005;18(3):249–255.
2. Bushnell GA, Sturmer T, Gaynes BN, Pate V, Miller M. Simultaneous antidepressant and benzodiazepine new use and subsequent long-term benzodiazepine use in adults with depression, United States, 2001–2014. *JAMA Psychiatry.* 2017;74(7):747–755.
3. Agarwal SD, Landon BE. Patterns in outpatient benzodiazepine prescribing in the United States. *JAMA Network Open.* 2019;2(1):e187399.

4. Dell'Osso B, Albert U, Atti AR, et al. Bridging the gap between education and appropriate use of benzodiazepines in psychiatric clinical practice. *Neuropsychiatr Dis Treat.* 2015;*11*:1885–1909.

5. Olfson M, King M, Schoenbaum M. Benzodiazepine use in the United States. *JAMA Psychiatry.* 2015;*72*(2):136–142.

6. Guina J, Merrill B. Benzodiazepines I: upping the care on downers: the evidence of risks, benefits and alternatives. *J Clin Med.* 2018;*7*(2):17.

7. Parks J. Safe and effective use of benzodiazepines in clinical practice. *Substance Abuse and Mental Health Services Administration.* https://www.integration.samhsa.gov/about-us/Benzodiazepines_Presentation.pdf. Published 2017. Accessed July 26, 2019.

8. Riemann D, Baglioni C, Bassetti C, et al. European guideline for the diagnosis and treatment of insomnia. *J Sleep Res.* 2017;*26*(6):675–700.

9. Huedo-Medina TB, Kirsch I, Middlemass J, Klonizakis M, Siriwardena AN. Effectiveness of non-benzodiazepine hypnotics in treatment of adult insomnia: meta-analysis of data submitted to the Food and Drug Administration. *BMJ (Clinical Research Ed).* 2012;*345*:e8343.

10. Glass J, Lanctot KL, Herrmann N, Sproule BA, Busto UE. Sedative hypnotics in older people with insomnia: meta-analysis of risks and benefits. *BMJ (Clinical Research Ed).* 2005;*331*(7526):1169.

11. Parrino L, Terzano MG. Polysomnographic effects of hypnotic drugs. A review. *Psychopharmacology.* 1996;*126*(1):1–16.

12. Wilt TJ, MacDonald R, Brasure M, et al. Pharmacologic treatment of insomnia disorder: an evidence report for a clinical practice guideline by the American College of Physicians. *Ann Intern Med.* 2016;*165*(2):103–112.

13. Tannenbaum C, Farrell B, Shaw J, et al. An ecological approach to reducing potentially inappropriate medication use: Canadian Deprescribing Network. *Can J Aging.* 2017;*36*(1):97–107.

14. Moore TJ, Mattison DR. Assessment of patterns of potentially unsafe use of zolpidem. *JAMA Intern Med.* 2018;*178*(9):1275–1277.

15. Neutel CI. The epidemiology of long-term benzodiazepine use. *Int Rev Psychiatr (Abingdon, Engl).* 2005;*17*(3):189–197.

16. Hogan DB, Maxwell CJ, Fung TS, Ebly EM. Prevalence and potential consequences of benzodiazepine use in senior citizens: results from the Canadian Study of Health and Aging. *Can J Clin Pharmacol.* 2003;*10*(2):72–77.

17. Ng BJ, Le Couteur DG, Hilmer SN. Deprescribing benzodiazepines in older patients: impact of interventions targeting physicians, pharmacists, and patients. *Drugs Aging.* 2018;*35*(6):493–521.

18. Pottie K, Thompson W, Davies S, et al. Deprescribing benzodiazepine receptor agonists: evidence-based clinical practice guideline. *Can Fam Physician.* 2018;*64*(5):339–351.

19. Lam S, Macina LO. Therapy update for insomnia in the elderly. *Consult Pharm.* 2017;*32*(10):610–622.

20. Patel MX, Sethi FN, Barnes TR, et al. Joint BAP NAPICU evidence-based consensus guidelines for the clinical management of acute disturbance: De-escalation and rapid tranquillisation. *J Psychopharmacol (Oxford, Engl).* 2018;*32*(6):601–640.

21. Bandelow B, Michaelis S, Wedekind D. Treatment of anxiety disorders. *Dialogues Clin Neurosci.* 2017;*19*(2):93–107.

22. Bandelow B, Zohar J, Hollander E, et al. World Federation of Societies of Biological Psychiatry (WFSBP) guidelines for the pharmacological treatment of anxiety, obsessive-compulsive and post-traumatic stress disorders: first revision. *World J Biol Psychiatry.* 2008;*9*(4):248–312.

23. Katzman MA, Bleau P, Blier P, et al. Canadian clinical practice guidelines for the management of anxiety, posttraumatic stress and obsessive-compulsive disorders. *BMC Psychiatry.* 2014;*14*(Suppl 1):S1.

24. Stone MH. Borderline personality disorder: clinical guidelines for treatment. *Psychodyn Psychiatry.* 2019;*47*(1):5–26.

25. Yatham LN, Kennedy SH, Parikh SV, et al. Canadian Network for Mood and Anxiety Treatments (CANMAT) and International Society for Bipolar Disorders (ISBD) 2018 guidelines for the management of patients with bipolar disorder. *Bipolar Dis.* 2018;*20*(2):97–170.

26. Perlis RH, Ostacher MJ, Miklowitz DJ, et al. Benzodiazepine use and risk of recurrence in bipolar disorder: a STEP-BD report. *J Clin Psychiatry.* 2010;*71*(2):194–200.

27. Kaiser Permanente. Benzodiazepine and Z-drug safety guideline. https://wa.kaiserpermanente.org/static/pdf/public/guidelines/benzo-zdrug.pdf. Published January 2019. Accessed August 5, 2019.

28. Pascual JC, Martin-Blanco A, Soler J, et al. A naturalistic study of changes in pharmacological prescription for borderline personality disorder in clinical practice: from APA to NICE guidelines. *Int Clin Psychopharmacol.* 2010;*25*(6):349–355.

29. Korkeila J, Kantojarvi L, Koivisto M, et al. [Update on current care guideline: borderline personality disorder]. *Duodecim.* 2015;*131*(16):1484–1485.

30. Oldham J, Gabbard G, Goin M, et al. Practice guideline for the treatment of patients with borderline personality disorder. *American Psychiatric Association.* http://psychiatryonline.org/pb/assets/raw/sitewide/practice_guidelines/guidelines/bpd.pdf. Published 2001. Accessed July 30, 2019.

31. Paolini E, Mezzetti FA, Pierri F, Moretti P. Pharmacological treatment of borderline personality disorder: a retrospective observational study at inpatient unit in Italy. *Int J Psychiatry Clin Pract.* 2017;*21*(1):75–79.

32. Kalira V, Treisman GJ, Clark MR. Borderline personality disorder and chronic pain: a practical approach to evaluation and treatment. *Curr Pain Headache Rep.* 2013;*17*(8):350.

33. Dowell D, Haegerich TM, Chou R. CDC guideline for prescribing opioids for chronic pain—United States, 2016. *JAMA.* 2016;*315*(15):1624–1645.

34. Stein MB, Sareen J. Clinical practice: generalized anxiety disorder. *N Engl J Med.* 2015;*373*(21):2059–2068.

35. National Institute for Health and Care Excellence. Generalised anxiety disorder and panic disorder in adults: management. https://www.nice.org.uk/guidance/cg113/chapter/1-Guidance#principles-of-care-for-people-with-generalised-anxiety-disorder-gad. Published 2011. Updated July 2019. Accessed July 30, 2019.

36. Davidson JR. Major depressive disorder treatment guidelines in America and Europe. *J Clin Psychiatry.* 2010;*71*(Suppl E1):e04.

37. Ogawa Y, Takeshima N, Hayasaka Y, et al. Antidepressants plus benzodiazepines for adults with major depression. *Cochrane Database Syst Rev.* 2019;*6*:Cd001026.

38. Soric MM, Paxos C, Dugan SE, et al. Prevalence and predictors of benzodiazepine monotherapy in patients with depression: a national cross-sectional study. *J Clin Psychiatry.* 2019;*80*(4):18m12588.

39. Brakoulias V, Starcevic V, Albert U, et al. Treatments used for obsessive-compulsive disorder-An international perspective. *Hum Psychopharmacol.* 2019;*34*(1):e2686.

40. Starcevic V, Berle D, do Rosario MC, et al. Use of benzodiazepines in obsessive-compulsive disorder. *Int Clin Psychopharmacol.* 2016;*31*(1):27–33.

41. Van Ameringen M, Simpson W, Patterson B, et al. Pharmacological treatment strategies in obsessive compulsive disorder: a cross-sectional view in nine international OCD centers. *J Psychopharmacol (Oxford, Engl).* 2014;*28*(6):596–602.

42. Breilmann J, Girlanda F, Guaiana G, et al. Benzodiazepines versus placebo for panic disorder in adults. *Cochrane Database Syst Rev.* 2019;3:Cd010677.
43. Stinson FS, Dawson DA, Patricia Chou S, et al. The epidemiology of DSM-IV specific phobia in the USA: results from the National Epidemiologic Survey on Alcohol and Related Conditions. *Psychol Med.* 2007;37(7):1047–1059.
44. Choy Y, Fyer AJ, Lipsitz JD. Treatment of specific phobia in adults. *Clin Psychol Rev.* 2007;27(3):266–286.
45. Gelpin E, Bonne O, Peri T, Brandes D, Shalev AY. Treatment of recent trauma survivors with benzodiazepines: a prospective study. *J Clin Psychiatry.* 1996;57(9):390–394.
46. Guina J, Rossetter SR, De RB, Nahhas RW, Welton RS. Benzodiazepines for PTSD: A systematic review and meta-analysis. *J Psychiatr Pract.* 2015;21(4):281–303.
47. Lipinska G, Baldwin DS, Thomas KG. Pharmacology for sleep disturbance in PTSD. *Hum Psychopharmacol.* 2016;31(2):156–163.
48. Laurito LD, Loureiro CP, Dias RV, et al. Predictors of benzodiazepine use in a transdiagnostic sample of panic disorder, social anxiety disorder, and obsessive-compulsive disorder patients. *Psychiatry Res.* 2018;262:237–245.
49. Williams T, Hattingh CJ, Kariuki CM, et al. Pharmacotherapy for social anxiety disorder (SAnD). *Cochrane Database Syst Rev.* 2017;10:Cd001206.
50. Leichsenring F, Leweke F. Social anxiety disorder. *N Engl J Med.* 2017;376(23):2255–2264.
51. Morrison M, Udeh E, Burak M. Retrospective analysis of a gabapentin high dose taper compared to lorazepam in acute inpatient alcohol withdrawal. *Am J Drug Alcohol Abuse.* 2019;45(4):385–391.
52. Long D, Long B, Koyfman A. The emergency medicine management of severe alcohol withdrawal. *Am J Emerg Med.* 2017;35(7):1005–1011.
53. Mayo-Smith MF. Pharmacological management of alcohol withdrawal: a meta-analysis and evidence-based practice guideline: American Society of Addiction Medicine Working Group on Pharmacological Management of Alcohol Withdrawal. *JAMA.* 1997;278(2):144–151.
54. Soyka M, Kranzler HR, Hesselbrock V, Kasper S, Mutschler J, Moller HJ. Guidelines for biological treatment of substance use and related disorders, Part 1: Alcoholism, first revision. *World J Biol Psychiatry.* 2017;18(2):86–119.
55. Airagnes G, Ducoutumany G, Laffy-Beaufils B, Le Faou AL, Limosin F. Alcohol withdrawal syndrome management: is there anything new? *La Revue de medecine interne.* 2019;40(6):373–379.
56. Perry EC. Inpatient management of acute alcohol withdrawal syndrome. *CNS Drugs.* 2014;28(5):401–410.
57. Glauser T, Shinnar S, Gloss D, et al. Evidence-based guideline: treatment of convulsive status epilepticus in children and adults: report of the Guideline Committee of the American Epilepsy Society. *Epilepsy Curr.* 2016;16(1):48–61.
58. Jedrzejczak J, Mazurkiewicz-Beldzinska M, Szmuda M, et al. Convulsive status epilepticus management in adults and children: report of the Working Group of the Polish Society of Epileptology. *Neurologia i neurochirurgia polska.* 2018;52(4):419–426.
59. Braun J, Gau E, Revelle S, Byrne L, Kumar A. Impact of non-guideline-based treatment of status epilepticus. *J Neurol Sci.* 2017;382:126–130.
60. Fung EL, Fung BB. Review and update of the Hong Kong epilepsy guideline on status epilepticus. *Hong Kong Med J.* 2017;23(1):67–73.
61. Unterberger I. Status epilepticus: do treatment guidelines make sense? *J Clin Neurophysiol.* 2016;33(1):10–13.
62. Wallace A, Wirrell E, Payne E. Seizure rescue medication use among us pediatric epilepsy providers: a survey of the Pediatric Epilepsy Research Consortium. *J Pediatr.* 2019;212:111–116.

63. de las Cuevas C, Sanz E, de la Fuente J. Benzodiazepines: more "behavioural" addiction than dependence. *Psychopharmacology.* 2003;*167*(3):297–303.

64. Panes A, Pariente A, Benard-Laribiere A, et al. Use of benzodiazepines and Z-drugs not compliant with guidelines and associated factors: a population-based study. *Eur Arch Psychiatry Clin Neurosci.* 2020;*270*(1):3–10.

65. Department of Health and Children. Benzodiazepines: good practice guidelines for clinicians. https://health.gov.ie/wp-content/uploads/2014/04/Benzodiazepines-Good-Practice-Guidelines.pdf. Published July 25, 2002. Accessed August 5, 2019.

66. Caruso R, Grassi L, Nanni MG, Riba M. Psychopharmacology in psycho-oncology. *Curr Psychiatry Rep.* 2013;*15*(9):393.

67. Kim HB, Myung SK, Park YC, Park B. Use of benzodiazepine and risk of cancer: a meta-analysis of observational studies. *Int J Cancer.* 2017;*140*(3):513–525.

68. Berger MJ, Ettinger DS, Aston J, et al. NCCN guidelines insights: antiemesis, version 2.2017. *JNCCN.* 2017;*15*(7):883–893.

69. Barr J, Fraser GL, Puntillo K, et al. Clinical practice guidelines for the management of pain, agitation, and delirium in adult patients in the intensive care unit: executive summary. *Am J Health-System Pharm.* 2013;*70*(1):53–58.

70. Barr J, Fraser GL, Puntillo K, et al. Clinical practice guidelines for the management of pain, agitation, and delirium in adult patients in the intensive care unit. *Crit Care Med.* 2013;*41*(1):263–306.

71. McGinn K, Davis SN, Terrry E, Simmons J, Brevard S. Elimination of routine benzodiazepine administration for nonprocedural sedation in a trauma intensive care unit is feasible. *Am Surgeon.* 2018;*84*(6):947–951.

72. Fraser GL, Devlin JW, Worby CP, et al. Benzodiazepine versus nonbenzodiazepine-based sedation for mechanically ventilated, critically ill adults: a systematic review and meta-analysis of randomized trials. *Crit Care Med.* 2013;*41*(9 Suppl 1):S30–S38.

73. Guina J, Merrill B. Benzodiazepines II: waking up on sedatives: providing optimal care when inheriting benzodiazepine prescriptions in transfer patients. *J Clin Med.* 2018;*7*(2):20.

74. American Geriatrics Society 2015 updated Beers Criteria for potentially inappropriate medication use in older adults. *J Am Geriatr Soc.* 2015;*63*(11):2227–2246.

75. Gerlach LB, Olfson M, Kales HC, Maust DT. Opioids and other central nervous system-active polypharmacy in older adults in the United States. *J Am Geriatr Soc.* 2017;*65*(9):2052–2056.

76. Petrovic M, Mariman A, Warie H, Afschrift M, Pevernagie D. Is there a rationale for prescription of benzodiazepines in the elderly? Review of the literature. *Acta Clinica Belgica.* 2003;*58*(1):27–36.

77. Allain H, Bentue-Ferrer D, Polard E, Akwa Y, Patat A. Postural instability and consequent falls and hip fractures associated with use of hypnotics in the elderly: a comparative review. *Drugs Aging.* 2005;*22*(9):749–765.

78. Billioti de Gage S, Moride Y, Ducruet T, et al. Benzodiazepine use and risk of Alzheimer's disease: case-control study. *BMJ (Clin Res Ed).* 2014;*349*:g5205.

79. Kalisch Ellett LM, Kassie GM, Pratt NL, Kerr M, Roughead EE. Prevalence and duration of use of medicines recommended for short-term use in aged care facility residents. *Pharmacy (Basel, Switzerland).* 2019;*7*(2):E55.

80. Alamanda VK, Wally MK, Seymour RB, Springer BD, Hsu JR. Opioid and benzodiazepine prescriptions for osteoarthritis remain prevalent. *Arthritis Care research.* 2019. [Epub ahead of print] https://doi.org/10.1002/acr.23933

81. Nielsen S, Lintzeris N, Bruno R, et al. Benzodiazepine use among chronic pain patients prescribed opioids: associations with pain, physical and mental health, and health service utilization. *Pain Med. (Malden, Mass).* 2015;*16*(2):356–366.

82. Thibaut F, Chagraoui A, Buckley L, et al. WFSBP (*) and IAWMH (**) guidelines for the treatment of alcohol use disorders in pregnant women. *World J Biol Psychiatry.* 2019;20(1):17–50.

83. Kelly LE, Poon S, Madadi P, Koren G. Neonatal benzodiazepines exposure during breastfeeding. *J Pediatr.* 2012;161(3):448–451.

84. Gopalan P, Glance JB, Azzam PN. Managing benzodiazepine withdrawal during pregnancy: case-based guidelines. *Arch Womens Ment Health.* 2014;17(2):167–170.

85. Fenn NE 3rd, Plake KS. Opioid and benzodiazepine weaning in pediatric patients: review of current literature. *Pharmacotherapy.* 2017;37(11):1458–1468.

86. Lader M. Benzodiazepine harm: how can it be reduced? *Br J Clin Pharmacol.* 2014;77(2):295–301.

87. Liebrenz M, Gehring MT, Buadze A, Caflisch C. High-dose benzodiazepine dependence: a qualitative study of patients' perception on cessation and withdrawal. *BMC Psychiatry.* 2015;15:116.

Conclusion

JOHN F. PEPPIN, JOSEPH V. PERGOLIZZI JR.,
ROBERT B. RAFFA, AND STEVEN L. WRIGHT

This volume has set out an academic and scientific discussion of the harmful and understudied aspects of an overused class of drugs, benzodiazepines. Benzodiazepines can be useful in a number of settings, for example, acute seizure management and as a bridge for anxiety disorders. However, over the last few decades, increased and longer-term benzodiazepine use has been observed to be associated with anticipated and unanticipated side effects. Benzodiazepines can have significant adverse effects even when used for more than a few weeks. Unfortunately, many healthcare practitioners are not aware of these relatively recent findings. Patients with anxiety disorders, depression, sleep disturbances, and even pain are still prescribed benzodiazepines for long periods of time. The concomitant use of benzodiazepines and opioids is especially troubling, as data show a correlation between these two drugs and overdose deaths, *vida supra*. However, this combination has only recently been given more attention at professional meetings and is still common in the treatment regimens of chronic pain patients. Benzodiazepines have been on the Beers list for some time, yet prescriptions are still issued to the elderly at an alarming rate.[1,2] The use of benzodiazepines in the elderly should be re-evaluated and their use in this patient population significantly reduced. Benzodiazepines are not indicated for long-term use to treat anxiety, and the literature has been clear that their chronic use in this population is not effective.[3] There is no indication for their use in chronic pain, muscle spasms, or chronic sleep disorders, nor is there much evidence to support such off-label prescribing.[4] There is no indication for their use in chronic pain, chronic muscle spasms (not associated with neurologic abnormalities) nor is there much evidence to support such off-label prescribing.[5] Additionally, there have been suggestions that the long term use of benzodiazepines may increase all-cause mortality.[6,7] Despite these concerns, the use of benzodiazepines continues to increase.

Certainly, side effects such as sedation, cognitive issues, abuse, and dependence are all well known. However, many other side effects have been reported by patients that did not seem to fit the known mechanism of action of benzodiazepines in the central nervous system. The recent discovery of an abundant network of peripheral benzodiazepine receptors offers a plausible explanation for these side effects.

Clinicians have observed some of these adverse effects of benzodiazepine use and many have struggled with finding their appropriate role in patient care. It is time for clinicians, patients, the healthcare system, and the regulatory bodies to get a renewed and updated perspective on benzodiazepines. We hope that in some small way this volume has been a contribution in furtherance of this goal.

It was the goal of this book to offer insights into the historical development of benzodiazepines, their mechanisms of action, and our evolving understanding of how they work and when their use is appropriate. Regulatory agencies are addressing benzodiazepine use, and some states in the United States include benzodiazepines in their prescription drug monitoring programs.[8]

Benzodiazepines are indicated in certain situations for specific patients and must be used with close clinical monitoring and for short-term rather than long-term use. Starting benzodiazepine therapy in a patient without discussing treatment goals and an exit plan is not helpful and can result is poor outcomes as well as morbidity. The public health issue of opioid overdose mortality has caused us to re-examine opioid therapy, and it is time that the same discussion be advanced for benzodiazepine treatment. This volume is a clarion call to change the way Benzodiazepines are used and prescribed. It is a further call to increase the research both at the bench and clinically, on the action and side effects of this class of medications.

REFERENCES

1 https://consultgeri.org/try-this/general-assessment/issue-16;   and   https://www.guidelinecentral.com/summaries/american-geriatrics-society-2015-updated-beers-criteria-for-potentially-inappropriate-medication-use-in-older-adults/#section-society. Accessed October 18, 2019.

2 Olfson, Mark, Marissa King, and Michael Schoenbaum. "Benzodiazepine use in the United States." *JAMA Psychiatry* 72, no. 2 (2015): 136–142.

3 Johnson, Brian, and Jon Streltzer. "Risks associated with long-term benzodiazepine use." *Am Fam Physician* 88, no. 4 (2013): 224–226.

4 Nielsen, Suzanne, Nicholas Lintzeris, Raimondo Bruno, Gabrielle Campbell, Briony Larance, Wayne Hall, Bianca Hoban, Milton L. Cohen, and Louisa Degenhardt. "Benzodiazepine use among chronic pain patients prescribed opioids: associations with pain, physical and mental health, and health service utilization." *Pain Med* 16, no. 2 (2015): 356–366.

5 Béland, Sarah-Gabrielle, Michel Préville, Marie-France Dubois, Dominique Lorrain, Sébastien Grenier, Philippe Voyer, Guilhème Pérodeau, and Yola Moride. "Benzodiazepine use and quality of sleep in the community-dwelling elderly population." *Aging Mental Health* 14, no. 7 (2010): 843–850.

6 Kalum Amarasuriya, Umesh, Puja R Myles, and Robert David Sanders. "Long-term benzodiazepine use and mortality: are we doing the right studies?" *Curr Drug Safety* 7, no. 5 (2012): 367–371.

7 Coleman, J Chapter 10.

8 Coleman, J Chapter 11.

DISCLOSURE AGREEMENTS

Michael M. Miller—Expert Witness consultations, consultations to federal and state agencies, consultations to health systems and other provider organizations, et al.

Jamie L. Hansen—Jamie L. Hansen has no relevant disclosures.

Timothy J. Atkinson—Relevant disclosure:

- Axial Healthcare (Consultant)
- Daiichi Sankyo (Advisory Board)
- Purdue Pharma (Epidemiology Advisory Board)
- ACCP (Honoraria)
- PAINWeek (Honoraria)
- Auburn (Speaker)
- Rockpointe (Speaker)
- Vanguard Pain Management Consulting (Owner)

Brian Merrill—Brian Merrill has no relevant disclosures.

Jeffrey Guina—Chief Medical Officer, Easterseals Michigan

Psychiatry Residency Program Director, Beaumont Health

Clinical Associate Professor, Wright State University and Michigan State University

Jan M. Kitzen—The author is a former employee of Wyeth Pharmaceuticals (currently Pfizer, Inc), manufacturer of Effexor® brand of venlafaxine.

Michael H. Ossipov—Michael H. Ossipov reports no conflicts of interests in the writing of this chapter.

Robert B. Raffa—Dr. Raffa was a previous employee of Johnson & Johnson (1986–1996) prior to a teaching career in academia and has received research support or honoraria from pharmaceutical companies involved in analgesics research and related areas (*e.g.*, recently BDSI, CerSci, Grünenthal, Insys, NEMA, Salix, and US WorldMeds, *etc.*)—but he receives no remuneration based on sales of any product. He is a cofounder of CaRafe Drug Innovation and Enalare, and is the consultant CSO of Neumentum, companies involved in drug discovery and development. He declares that he has no financial interest or conflict of interest in the subject matter of this book.

George F. Koob—George F. Koob has no relevant disclosures

Steven L. Wright—Relevant disclosure:

• Alliance for Benzodiazepine Best Practices—medical consultant

Other current (1year) disclosures

• Cordant Health Solutions—consultant, contracted speaker—drug testing
• Indivior—contracted speaker—Suboxone, Sublocade, Opioid addiction (resigned in April)
• BioDelivery Sciences, Inc—consultant—Belbuca
• Daiichi Sankyo—contracted speaker—Movantik, Morphabone ER, Oxybond
• US World Meds—contracted speaker—Lucemyra
• NEMA research—consultant, contracted speaker—BZ, OIC

John F. Peppin—Relevant disclosures:

• YourEncore: Consulting
• Janssen Pharmaceuticals: Consulting
• Neurana Pharmaceuticals: Consulting
• USWorldMeds: Consulting

John J. Coleman—John J. Coleman has no relevant disclosures.

Jo Ann LeQuang—Jo Ann LeQuang has no relevant disclosures.

INDEX

For the benefit of digital users, indexed terms that span two pages (e.g., 52–53) may, on occasion, appear on only one of those pages.

References to tables and figures are denoted by an italic *t* or *f* following the page number.

inappropriate benzodiazepine
use, 22–24

anxiolytics. *See* benzodiazepine receptor
agonists; benzodiazepines; *specific medications*; Z-drugs

API (active pharmaceutical ingredient), 174,
175, 207–8

apparent tolerance, 103–4

a-process, opponent process theory, 103–4

Ashton, H., xx–xxi, 122, 126, 128–29

Ashton Manual (Ashton), xx–xxi, 126

Ativan. *See* lorazepam

attorney general, role in drug scheduling, 166–67

AUD. *See* alcohol use disorder

AWS. *See* alcohol withdrawal syndrome;
withdrawal

Bakken, M.S., 60, 61–62

balance, effects of aging on, 52–53

Bandelow, B., 219

barbiturates, 83*f*
adverse effects of, 6–7, 18, 42–43
benzodiazepine agonism, 73
benzodiazepine antagonism, 74
BzRAs as improvement over, 82–83
overview, 1

Bartels, John R., Jr., 164

Beers Criteria (AGS), 53–55, 227

behavioral adverse effects, 25*t*

Benzo Buddies online community, 134

benzodiazepine 1 (BZ1) receptor, 13–15

benzodiazepine 2 (BZ2) receptor, 13–15

benzodiazepine adverse effects. *See* adverse
effects

benzodiazepine adverse reactions. *See*
adverse effects

benzodiazepine dependence. *See*
dependence

benzodiazepine discontinuation syndrome.
See benzodiazepine withdrawal
syndrome; discontinuation of
benzodiazepines

benzodiazepine-induced
hyperanxiogenesis, 122

benzodiazepine-induced neurocognitive
disorder, 28–29

benzodiazepine-induced persisting amnestic
disorder, 28–29

benzodiazepine injury syndrome, 137.
See also benzodiazepine withdrawal
syndrome

benzodiazepine pharmacodynamics, 9*f*,
9–10, 51–52

benzodiazepine pharmacokinetics,
10–11, 11*t*
lipid solubility, 10
metabolism, 10–11
protein binding, 10

benzodiazepine physiologic dependence. *See*
dependence

benzodiazepine receptor agonists (BzRAs).
See also γ-aminobutyric acid type A
receptor complex; *specific drugs*; *specific
related topics*; Z-drugs
classification, 81–82, 83*f*
contributions made by, 17–20, 82–83
mechanism of action, 7, 83–84, 85–86
medicinal chemistry, 9*f*, 9
origin, 6–7
overview, 6
and pain management, 149–54
pharmacokinetics, 10–11, 11*t*
teratogenicity, 12–13
therapeutic use, 12
urine toxicology, 13, 14*f*

benzodiazepine receptors, ix, 82, 83–84,
85–86. *See also* γ-aminobutyric acid
receptors; γ-aminobutyric acid type
A receptor complex; peripheral
benzodiazepine receptors

benzodiazepines (BZDs), 17–18. *See also*
benzodiazepine receptor agonists;
specific drugs; *specific related topics*
adverse effects (*see* adverse effects)
approved indications for, 3, 19–20, 19*t*
background, 1–2, 42–43
benefits of use, 18–20, 19*t*
best practices for therapy, 34–35
chronology of use, xxvii–xxix
classification, 81–82, 83*f*
contraindications for use, 20–24,
28–29, 30–31
contributions made by, 17–20, 82–83
counterfeit, 174–78, 187, 197, 205–9, 210
dependence (*see* dependence)
long-term use and effects (*see* long-term
benzodiazepine use)
mechanism of action, 83–84, 85–86
overview, ix, 1–4
and pain management, 149–54
patient example, xvii
physiologic dependence (*see* dependence)

control efforts for benzodiazepines. *See* regulatory history of benzodiazepines

controlled substances, 210

Controlled Substances Act (CSA), 2–3, 167–68
  counterfeit drugs, 207–8n.7
  history of BZD control, 162–63, 164–67, 169–70
  purposes of, 194
  rescheduling BZDs, 183, 203–5
  scheduling schema, 161, 194–95

Convention on Psychotropic Substances (UN), 194

convulsive status epilepticus, 224

corticotropin-releasing factor (CRF), 109

counteradaptation hypothesis of withdrawal, 102–3

counterfeit drugs, 187, 210
  counterfeit-real drugs, 175
  counterfeit-toxic drugs, 176–78
  counterfeit-unreal drugs, 175–76
  current problem of, 205–9
  and detection of drug abuse trends, 184–86
  ICD limitations in regards to, 197
  overview, 174–75

cross tapering, 127–28, 127*t*, 131

CSA. *See* Controlled Substances Act

cut-and-hold method, 129

Dalmane. *See* flurazepam

Dark Web, 177–78, 207

data collection on drug abuse. *See* abuse; Centers for Disease Control and Prevention; Project DAWN

date rape drugs, xv. *See also* flunitrazepam

DAWN. *See* Project DAWN

DBI (diazepam binding inhibitor). *See* peripheral benzodiazepine receptors

DEA. *See* Drug Enforcement Administration

delirium, 226

dementia, benzodiazepines and risk for, 62–63

Department of Health, Education, and Welfare (HEW), 163–64, 166–67

Department of Health and Human Services (HHS), 170, 186, 205, 211

dependence (physiologic dependence), 2, 20–21, 81. *See also* benzodiazepine withdrawal syndrome; tolerance; withdrawal

versus BUD, 25*t*, 31, 119–20
  defined, 30, 119
  motivational aspects, 102
  as normal physiological adaptation, 84–85
  in opponent process theory, 105
  overview, 119–20
  patient example, xx–xxi
  prescribing considerations, 224

deprescribing. *See also* discontinuation of benzodiazepines; tapering
  legacy patients, 132–33
  managing withdrawal, 125–31, 127*t*, 128*t*
  multiple barriers to, 152
  rationality of, 153

depression, 29, 220–21

de Vries, O.J., 61–62

dexmedetomidine, 226

Diagnostic and Statistical Manual of Mental Disorders (DSM), 19, 99–100, 119

diazepam (Valium), 68–69, 162, 183–84, 193–94
  approved indications, 217
  benzodiazepine agonism, 73
  DAWN data for, 170–71, 173, 174*t*, 179, 180*t*
  development, 1–2, 42–43
  dose conversions, 127*t*
  for epilepsy, status epilepticus, and seizures, 224
  FDA-approved indications, 19*t*
  half-life and risk for falls, 61–62
  as inappropriate for geriatric patients, 27
  overdose deaths related to, 184, 197, 199*t*, 201*f*, 202*f*, 203*f*
  for pain, 151
  peripheral benzodiazepine receptor discovery, 88
  pharmacodynamics, 9*f*
  pharmacokinetics, 10–11, 11*t*
  prescribing rates, 196*f*, 196, 198*t*
  regulatory history, 164–65, 169
  rise in prescriptions for, 173–74
  safety of, 68–69
  in tapering plans, 230–31
  teratogenicity, 12–13
  urine toxicology, 13, 14*f*
  in withdrawal or discontinuation management, 127–28

diazepam binding inhibitor (DBI). *See* peripheral benzodiazepine receptors

half-life
  benzodiazepine, 9f, 9, 10
  and risk for falls, 59, 60, 61–62
  and risk of dementia, 62–63
hallucinogenics, 202f
Harrison Narcotic Tax Act, 166
hedonic opponent process, 102–7, 104f, 105f
hematologic adverse effects of BZDs, 25t
hepatic function, effects of aging on, 49–50
hepatic metabolism, 10–11, 11t, 49–50
HEW (Department of Health, Education, and Welfare), 163–64, 166–67
HHS (Department of Health and Human Services), 170, 186, 205, 211
hip fractures, risk factors for, 60, 61t
Historic Estimates from the Drug Abuse Warning Network (SAMHSA), 170–71
Hoffman-La Roche, 6–7, 162
Holy Trinity, 125, 171
Hong Kong Epilepsy Guideline, 224
hydrocodone, 182
hydroxyzine, 130
hyperanxiogenesis, BZD-induced, 122
hyperkatifeia, 97, 99–100, 102, 103–4, 110–11. *See also* motivational component of withdrawal
hypothalamic-pituitary-adrenal axis, 119

ICD (*International Classification of Diseases*), 186, 197
illicit traffic in pharmaceutical drugs, 34, 163. *See also* counterfeit drugs
imipramine, 128t, 129
impulsivity, as risk factor for benzodiazepine use disorder, 33t
IMS America, Ltd., 168–69
IMS Health, 196
incentive salience, role in addiction, 97–98, 106, 131
insomnia. *See also* legacy patients
  approved benzodiazepine indications, 19, 19t
  first-line therapy for, 20
  in geriatric population, 55–58, 57t
  guidelines for benzodiazepine use, 22, 23, 24, 217–18
  in pain patients, 151
  rebound, 3
  as risk factor for benzodiazepine use disorder, 33t
intensive care unit patients, 226

interdose withdrawal symptoms, 123
intermediate-acting benzodiazepines, 9f, 9, 10
International Benzodiazepine Symposium, xvii
International Classification of Diseases (ICD), 186, 197
International Society for Bipolar Disorders, 219
Internet pharmacies, 208–9
Interpol, 177
intoxication, 32t, 34, 97–100, 100f
inverse agonists, benzodiazepine, 68, 72–73, 73f, 75–76, 77f, 86

Kafka, F., 132–33
Kaiser Permanente healthcare system, 219, 225, 227, 228
kidney function, effects of aging on, 47t, 49
kindling, 119
Klonopin. *See* clonazepam
κ-opioid receptors, 109–10

LaCorte, S., 134
Lader, M.H., 130
Langeland, William E., 164
latency to persistent sleep (LPS), 56–57
lavender, 130–31
law enforcement, penetration of Dark Web by, 177–78, 207
League of Nations, 161
lean muscle mass, effects of aging on, 48, 50–51
legacy patients
  clinical aspects, 132–33
  defined, 21, 132
  guidelines for benzodiazepine use, 226
legislative route for rescheduling BZDs, 182–83
Lembke, A., 174
levofloxacin, 76
Librium. *See* chlordiazepoxide
lipophilicity, 10
liquid titration, 128, 134
liver, effects of aging on, 47t, 49–50
L-methyl folate, 130
long-acting benzodiazepines
  pharmacodynamics, 9f, 9
  pharmacokinetics, 10
  risk for falls and fractures, 59, 60, 61–62
  risk of dementia, 62–63

National Association of Psychiatric Intensive Care and Low Secure Units, 218
National Comprehensive Cancer Network, 225–26
National Institute for Health and Care Excellence, 220, 221–22
National Institute on Drug Abuse (NIDA), 168, 169, 170
National Prescription Audit database, 196
National Vital Statistics System (CDC), 201n.4
negative affect stage of substance use disorders. See withdrawal
negative emotionality, role in addiction, 97–98, 106
negative reinforcement, relation to withdrawal, 104f, 104
neural circuitry associated with withdrawal, 105f, 105–10
neuroadaptations, within- and between-system, 105f, 107–10
neuroanatomical changes, age-related, 51
neurochemical changes, age-related, 51
neurocognitive disorder, BZD-induced, 28–29
neuropathic adverse effects of BZDs, 25t
neuropeptide Y (NPY), 110
neurophysiologic withdrawal symptoms, 122–23, 122t
neurotransmitter systems, effects of aging on, 51–52
New DAWN program, 172–74, 174t
niacin, 130–31
nicotinamide adenine dinucleotide, 130–31
nicotine addiction, 98
NIDA (National Institute on Drug Abuse), 168, 169, 170
nociceptin, 110
nonbarbiturate sedative-hypnotics, 1–2
nonmedical use. See abuse
nordiazepam, 202f, 203f
norepinephrine, 109
norfloxacin, 76
NO TEARS tool, 133
NPY (neuropeptide Y), 110
nursing mothers, 27–28, 228
nutritional approaches to withdrawal management, 130–31

obsessive-compulsive disorder (OCD), 133, 221

ofloxacin, 76
older adult patients. See geriatric patients
Olfson, M., 43–44, 46
ondansetron, 130
online communities, 134
opioids. See also polypharmacy
    for acute and chronic pain, 150
    current drug problems, 181
    emergency visits involving BZDs and, 173, 185f
    guidelines for benzodiazepine use, 227
    interactions with benzodiazepines, xiv
opioid use disorder
    between-system neuroadaptations, 109
    physical symptoms of withdrawal, 101t, 102
    stages in, 98, 99–100
    within-system neuroadaptations, 107, 108
opponent process theory, 102–7, 104f, 105f, 119
overdose deaths, 149, 150, 185f
    limitations in DAWN program, 171
    overview, 150
    shortcomings in tracking system, 184–86
    tracking, 181–82, 196, 197–201, 199t, 201f, 202f
overdose management, 125, 152–53
oxaloacetate, 130–31
oxazepam (Serax)
    DAWN data for, 180t
    dose conversions, 127t
    FDA-approved indications, 19t
    for geriatric patients, 27
    half-life and risk for falls, 61–62
    overdose deaths related to, 202f, 203f
    pharmacodynamics, 9f
    pharmacokinetics, 10–11, 11t
    prescribing rates, 198t
    regulatory history, 164–66
oxycodone (OxyContin), 172, 176, 178, 181, 206

pain, 33t, 149–54, 227
Pangea X operation (Interpol), 177
panic disorder, 20, 22, 221–22
Parola, A.L., 88
patient advocacy, xvii–xviii
Paxipam (halazepam), 169–70
PCIDs (physical-chemical identifiers), 178, 187, 207–8
pediatric patients, 228